Metabolomics as a Tool in Nutrition Research

Related titles

Foods, nutrients and food ingredients with authorised EU health claims Volume 2
(ISBN 978-1-78242-382-9)

Dietary supplements
(ISBN 978-1-78242-076-7)

Managing and preventing obesity
(ISBN 978-1-78242-091-0)

Woodhead Publishing Series in Food Science, Technology and Nutrition: Number 266

Metabolomics as a Tool in Nutrition Research

Edited by

J.-L. Sébédio and L. Brennan

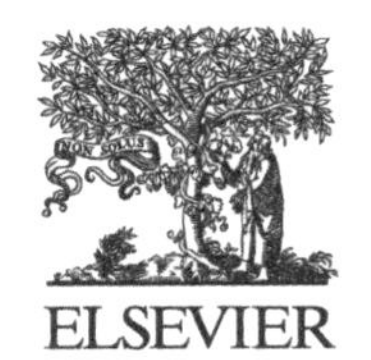

AMSTERDAM • BOSTON • CAMBRIDGE • HEIDELBERG
LONDON • NEW YORK • OXFORD • PARIS • SAN DIEGO
SAN FRANCISCO • SINGAPORE • SYDNEY • TOKYO
Woodhead Publishing is an imprint of Elsevier

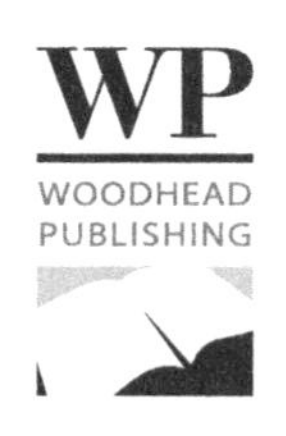

Woodhead Publishing is an imprint of Elsevier
80 High Street, Sawston, Cambridge, CB22 3HJ, UK
225 Wyman Street, Waltham, MA 02451, USA
Langford Lane, Kidlington, OX5 1GB, UK

British Library Cataloguing-in-Publication Data
A catalogue record for this book is available from the British Library.

Library of Congress Control Number: 2014946553

ISBN 978-1-78242-084-2 (print)
ISBN 978-1-78242-092-7 (online)

For information on all Woodhead Publishing publications
visit our website at http://store.elsevier.com

Typeset by SPi Global
www.spi-global.com

Printed and bound in the United Kingdom

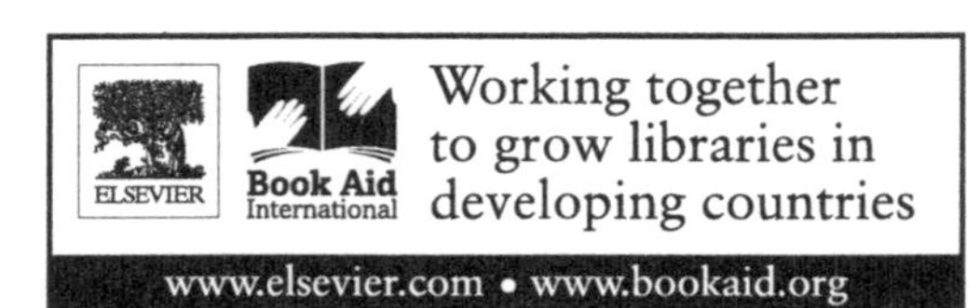

Contents

List of contributors **ix**
Woodhead Publishing Series in Food Science, Technology and Nutrition **xi**
Preface **xxv**

Part One Principles 1

1 Challenges in nutritional metabolomics: from experimental design to interpretation of data sets **3**
M. Ferrara, J.-L. Sébédio
1.1 Introduction **3**
1.2 The experimental design **5**
1.3 The analytical platform **6**
1.4 Extraction of data sets and statistical analyses **7**
1.5 Metabolite identification **8**
1.6 Biological interpretations **10**
1.7 Conclusion: do we need standardisation procedures and repositories? **11**
References **12**

2 Metabolic profiling as a tool in nutritional research: key methodological issues **17**
S.E. Richards, E. Holmes
2.1 Introduction **17**
2.2 Key issues in nutritional research **17**
2.3 The role of genomics, proteomics, metabolomics, and metagenomics in nutritional research **19**
2.4 Applications of metabolomics in nutrition-related research **20**
2.5 The use of metabolomics to assess the effects of diet on health **21**
2.6 Methods for mapping dietary patterns **23**
2.7 Observational and interventional studies into the effects of diet and nutrition on health **25**
2.8 Analytical methods **26**
2.9 Issues in analysing samples **27**
References **29**

3 Chemometrics methods for the analysis of genomics, transcriptomics, proteomics, metabolomics and metagenomics datasets **37**
S.E. Richards, E. Holmes
3.1 Introduction **37**

3.2 Unsupervised and supervised pattern recognition methods **38**
3.3 Multivariate calibration methods for developing predictive models **39**
3.4 Statistical data integration methods **40**
3.5 Data integration: multiblock strategies **41**
3.6 Data integration: calibration transfer methods **43**
3.7 Data integration: multiway/multimodal analysis methods **44**
3.8 Data integration: correlation-based approaches **46**
3.9 Data integration: techniques for analysing different types of genomics datasets **47**
3.10 Statistical data integration of different sample types **48**
3.11 Statistical data integration of different molecular components in samples **49**
3.12 Modelling relationships between molecular components **51**
3.13 Conclusion and future trends **52**
References **52**

Part Two Applications in nutrition research **61**

4 Application of lipidomics in nutrition research **63**
X. Han, Y. Zhou
4.1 Introduction **63**
4.2 Lipids **63**
4.3 Lipidomics **66**
4.4 Lipidomics in nutrition research **73**
4.5 Conclusion and future trends **77**
Acknowledgement **78**
References **78**

5 Analysing human metabolic networks using metabolomics: understanding the impact of diet on health **85**
N. Poupin, F. Jourdan
5.1 Introduction **85**
5.2 Metabolic network reconstruction **86**
5.3 Human metabolic networks **88**
5.4 Linking metabolomics data and metabolic network elements **94**
5.5 Metabolism modelling, from pathways to network **97**
5.6 Subnetwork extraction between identified metabolites **105**
5.7 Conclusion and future directions **109**
Acknowledgements **109**
References **110**

6 Using metabolomics to analyse the role of gut microbiota in nutrition and disease **115**
G. Xie, W. Jia
6.1 Introduction: gut microbiota and human health **115**
6.2 Metagenomics of gut microbiota **117**
6.3 Metabolomics: uncovering complex host–microbe interactions **124**
6.4 The marriage of metagenomics and metabolomics: microbiome–metabolome interactions **127**
6.5 Future trends: personalised nutrition **128**
References **130**

7 Metabotyping: moving towards personalised nutrition **137**
L. Brennan
7.1 Introduction **137**
7.2 The concept of the metabotype **138**
7.3 Examples of metabotyping with a focus on nutrition **138**
7.4 Extension of metabotypes to include markers of dietary origin **141**
7.5 Conclusion and future trends **142**
7.6 Sources of further information and advice **142**
References **142**

8 Using metabolomics to identify biomarkers for metabolic diseases: analytical methods and applications **145**
J.-L. Sébédio, S. Polakof
8.1 Introduction **145**
8.2 Using metabolomics to understand the relationship between nutrition and chronic metabolic diseases **146**
8.3 Cohort studies and biomarker identification **153**
8.4 Isolating *in situ* biomarkers **159**
8.5 Conclusions and future trends **160**
References **161**

9 Using metabolomics to evaluate food intake: applications in nutritional epidemiology **167**
C. Manach, L. Brennan, L.O. Dragsted
9.1 Introduction **167**
9.2 Biomarkers as a complementary approach to questionnaires **170**
9.3 Definition of the food metabolome **172**
9.4 Metabolomics as a tool for dietary biomarker discovery **172**
9.5 Dietary patterns and metabolomic profiles: potential use of nutritypes **184**
9.6 Validation of putative biomarkers **185**
9.7 The future of metabolomics in dietary assessment **186**
9.8 Conclusion **190**
References **190**

10 Metabolomics and nutritional challenge tests: what can we learn? **197**
L. Brennan
10.1 Introduction **197**
10.2 Application of metabolomics to challenge tests **197**
10.3 Conclusion and future trends **201**
References **202**

11 Using metabolomics to describe food in detail **203**
F. Capozzi, A. Trimigno
11.1 Introduction **203**
11.2 Using metabolomics to assess the effects of genetic selection and modification **205**
11.3 Using metabolomics to assess the effects of organic versus conventional farming **208**
11.4 Using metabolomics to identify the geographical origin of food products **211**
11.5 Using metabolomics to assess the effects of rearing conditions on the quality of meat, eggs, and fish **213**
11.6 Using metabolomics to assess the effects of processing on food quality **217**
11.7 Using metabolomics to assess the effects of digestion on nutrient intake from particular foods **219**
11.8 Conclusion **221**
References **225**
Appendix: abbreviations **228**

12 Future perspectives for metabolomics in nutrition research: a nutritionist's view **231**
M. Ferrara
12.1 Introduction **231**
12.2 Metabolites identification and biological relevance **232**
12.3 *In vivo* metabolomics **232**
12.4 Conclusion **233**
References **234**

Index **237**

List of contributors

L. Brennan University College Dublin, Dublin, Ireland, and Newcastle University, Newcastle upon Tyne, United Kingdom

F. Capozzi University of Bologna, Bologna, Italy

L.O. Dragsted University of Copenhagen, Copenhagen, Denmark

M. Ferrara Institut National de la Recherche Agronomique (INRA), Clermont-Ferrand, France

X. Han Sanford-Burnham Medical Research Institute, Orlando, FL, USA

E. Holmes Imperial College, London, United Kingdom

W. Jia University of Hawaii Cancer Center, Honolulu, HI, USA

F. Jourdan Institut National de la Recherche Agronomique (INRA), Paris, France

C. Manach Institut National de la Recherche Agronomique (INRA), Clermont-Ferrand, France

S. Polakof Institut National de la Recherche Agronomique (INRA), and Clermont Université, Clermont-Ferrand, France

N. Poupin Institut National de la Recherche Agronomique (INRA), Paris, France

S.E. Richards Nottingham Trent University, Nottingham, United Kingdom

J.-L. Sébédio Institut National de la Recherche Agronomique (INRA), and Clermont Université, Clermont-Ferrand, France

A. Trimigno University of Bologna, Bologna, Italy

G. Xie University of Hawaii Cancer Center, Honolulu, HI, USA

Y. Zhou Institute for Nutritional Sciences, Shanghai Institutes for Biological Sciences, P.R. China

Woodhead Publishing Series in Food Science, Technology and Nutrition

1 **Chilled foods: A comprehensive guide**
Edited by C. Dennis and M. Stringer
2 **Yoghurt: Science and technology**
A. Y. Tamime and R. K. Robinson
3 **Food processing technology: Principles and practice**
P. J. Fellows
4 **Bender's dictionary of nutrition and food technology Sixth edition**
D. A. Bender
5 **Determination of veterinary residues in food**
Edited by N. T. Crosby
6 **Food contaminants: Sources and surveillance**
Edited by C. Creaser and R. Purchase
7 **Nitrates and nitrites in food and water**
Edited by M. J. Hill
8 **Pesticide chemistry and bioscience: The food-environment challenge**
Edited by G. T. Brooks and T. Roberts
9 **Pesticides: Developments, impacts and controls**
Edited by G. A. Best and A. D. Ruthven
10 **Dietary fibre: Chemical and biological aspects**
Edited by D. A. T. Southgate, K. W. Waldron, I. T. Johnson and G. R. Fenwick
11 **Vitamins and minerals in health and nutrition**
M. Tolonen
12 **Technology of biscuits, crackers and cookies Second edition**
D. Manley
13 **Instrumentation and sensors for the food industry**
Edited by E. Kress-Rogers
14 **Food and cancer prevention: Chemical and biological aspects**
Edited by K. W. Waldron, I. T. Johnson and G. R. Fenwick
15 **Food colloids: Proteins, lipids and polysaccharides**
Edited by E. Dickinson and B. Bergenstahl
16 **Food emulsions and foams**
Edited by E. Dickinson
17 **Maillard reactions in chemistry, food and health**
Edited by T. P. Labuza, V. Monnier, J. Baynes and J. O'Brien
18 **The Maillard reaction in foods and medicine**
Edited by J. O'Brien, H. E. Nursten, M. J. Crabbe and J. M. Ames

19 **Encapsulation and controlled release**
Edited by D. R. Karsa and R. A. Stephenson
20 **Flavours and fragrances**
Edited by A. D. Swift
21 **Feta and related cheeses**
Edited by A. Y. Tamime and R. K. Robinson
22 **Biochemistry of milk products**
Edited by A. T. Andrews and J. R. Varley
23 **Physical properties of foods and food processing systems**
M. J. Lewis
24 **Food irradiation: A reference guide**
V. M. Wilkinson and G. Gould
25 **Kent's technology of cereals: An introduction for students of food science and agriculture Fourth edition**
N. L. Kent and A. D. Evers
26 **Biosensors for food analysis**
Edited by A. O. Scott
27 **Separation processes in the food and biotechnology industries: Principles and applications**
Edited by A. S. Grandison and M. J. Lewis
28 **Handbook of indices of food quality and authenticity**
R. S. Singhal, P. K. Kulkarni and D. V. Rege
29 **Principles and practices for the safe processing of foods**
D. A. Shapton and N. F. Shapton
30 **Biscuit, cookie and cracker manufacturing manuals Volume 1: Ingredients**
D. Manley
31 **Biscuit, cookie and cracker manufacturing manuals Volume 2: Biscuit doughs**
D. Manley
32 **Biscuit, cookie and cracker manufacturing manuals Volume 3: Biscuit dough piece forming**
D. Manley
33 **Biscuit, cookie and cracker manufacturing manuals Volume 4: Baking and cooling of biscuits**
D. Manley
34 **Biscuit, cookie and cracker manufacturing manuals Volume 5: Secondary processing in biscuit manufacturing**
D. Manley
35 **Biscuit, cookie and cracker manufacturing manuals Volume 6: Biscuit packaging and storage**
D. Manley
36 **Practical dehydration Second edition**
M. Greensmith
37 **Lawrie's meat science Sixth edition**
R. A. Lawrie
38 **Yoghurt: Science and technology Second edition**
A. Y. Tamime and R. K. Robinson
39 **New ingredients in food processing: Biochemistry and agriculture**
G. Linden and D. Lorient

40 **Benders' dictionary of nutrition and food technology Seventh edition**
D. A. Bender and A. E. Bender
41 **Technology of biscuits, crackers and cookies Third edition**
D. Manley
42 **Food processing technology: Principles and practice Second edition**
P. J. Fellows
43 **Managing frozen foods**
Edited by C. J. Kennedy
44 **Handbook of hydrocolloids**
Edited by G. O. Phillips and P. A. Williams
45 **Food labelling**
Edited by J. R. Blanchfield
46 **Cereal biotechnology**
Edited by P. C. Morris and J. H. Bryce
47 **Food intolerance and the food industry**
Edited by T. Dean
48 **The stability and shelf-life of food**
Edited by D. Kilcast and P. Subramaniam
49 **Functional foods: Concept to product**
Edited by G. R. Gibson and C. M. Williams
50 **Chilled foods: A comprehensive guide Second edition**
Edited by M. Stringer and C. Dennis
51 **HACCP in the meat industry**
Edited by M. Brown
52 **Biscuit, cracker and cookie recipes for the food industry**
D. Manley
53 **Cereals processing technology**
Edited by G. Owens
54 **Baking problems solved**
S. P. Cauvain and L. S. Young
55 **Thermal technologies in food processing**
Edited by P. Richardson
56 **Frying: Improving quality**
Edited by J. B. Rossell
57 **Food chemical safety Volume 1: Contaminants**
Edited by D. Watson
58 **Making the most of HACCP: Learning from others' experience**
Edited by T. Mayes and S. Mortimore
59 **Food process modelling**
Edited by L. M. M. Tijskens, M. L. A. T. M. Hertog and B. M. Nicolaï
60 **EU food law: A practical guide**
Edited by K. Goodburn
61 **Extrusion cooking: Technologies and applications**
Edited by R. Guy
62 **Auditing in the food industry: From safety and quality to environmental and other audits**
Edited by M. Dillon and C. Griffith
63 **Handbook of herbs and spices Volume 1**
Edited by K. V. Peter

64 **Food product development: Maximising success**
M. Earle, R. Earle and A. Anderson
65 **Instrumentation and sensors for the food industry Second edition**
Edited by E. Kress-Rogers and C. J. B. Brimelow
66 **Food chemical safety Volume 2: Additives**
Edited by D. Watson
67 **Fruit and vegetable biotechnology**
Edited by V. Valpuesta
68 **Foodborne pathogens: Hazards, risk analysis and control**
Edited by C. de W. Blackburn and P. J. McClure
69 **Meat refrigeration**
S. J. James and C. James
70 **Lockhart and Wiseman's crop husbandry Eighth edition**
H. J. S. Finch, A. M. Samuel and G. P. F. Lane
71 **Safety and quality issues in fish processing**
Edited by H. A. Bremner
72 **Minimal processing technologies in the food industries**
Edited by T. Ohlsson and N. Bengtsson
73 **Fruit and vegetable processing: Improving quality**
Edited by W. Jongen
74 **The nutrition handbook for food processors**
Edited by C. J. K. Henry and C. Chapman
75 **Colour in food: Improving quality**
Edited by D. MacDougall
76 **Meat processing: Improving quality**
Edited by J. P. Kerry, J. F. Kerry and D. A. Ledward
77 **Microbiological risk assessment in food processing**
Edited by M. Brown and M. Stringer
78 **Performance functional foods**
Edited by D. Watson
79 **Functional dairy products Volume 1**
Edited by T. Mattila-Sandholm and M. Saarela
80 **Taints and off-flavours in foods**
Edited by B. Baigrie
81 **Yeasts in food**
Edited by T. Boekhout and V. Robert
82 **Phytochemical functional foods**
Edited by I. T. Johnson and G. Williamson
83 **Novel food packaging techniques**
Edited by R. Ahvenainen
84 **Detecting pathogens in food**
Edited by T. A. McMeekin
85 **Natural antimicrobials for the minimal processing of foods**
Edited by S. Roller
86 **Texture in food Volume 1: Semi-solid foods**
Edited by B. M. McKenna
87 **Dairy processing: Improving quality**
Edited by G. Smit

88 **Hygiene in food processing: Principles and practice**
Edited by H. L. M. Lelieveld, M. A. Mostert, B. White and J. Holah
89 **Rapid and on-line instrumentation for food quality assurance**
Edited by I. Tothill
90 **Sausage manufacture: Principles and practice**
E. Essien
91 **Environmentally-friendly food processing**
Edited by B. Mattsson and U. Sonesson
92 **Bread making: Improving quality**
Edited by S. P. Cauvain
93 **Food preservation techniques**
Edited by P. Zeuthen and L. Bøgh-Sørensen
94 **Food authenticity and traceability**
Edited by M. Lees
95 **Analytical methods for food additives**
R. Wood, L. Foster, A. Damant and P. Key
96 **Handbook of herbs and spices Volume 2**
Edited by K. V. Peter
97 **Texture in food Volume 2: Solid foods**
Edited by D. Kilcast
98 **Proteins in food processing**
Edited by R. Yada
99 **Detecting foreign bodies in food**
Edited by M. Edwards
100 **Understanding and measuring the shelf-life of food**
Edited by R. Steele
101 **Poultry meat processing and quality**
Edited by G. Mead
102 **Functional foods, ageing and degenerative disease**
Edited by C. Remacle and B. Reusens
103 **Mycotoxins in food: Detection and control**
Edited by N. Magan and M. Olsen
104 **Improving the thermal processing of foods**
Edited by P. Richardson
105 **Pesticide, veterinary and other residues in food**
Edited by D. Watson
106 **Starch in food: Structure, functions and applications**
Edited by A.-C. Eliasson
107 **Functional foods, cardiovascular disease and diabetes**
Edited by A. Arnoldi
108 **Brewing: Science and practice**
D. E. Briggs, P. A. Brookes, R. Stevens and C. A. Boulton
109 **Using cereal science and technology for the benefit of consumers: Proceedings of the 12th International ICC Cereal and Bread Congress, 24 – 26th May, 2004, Harrogate, UK**
Edited by S. P. Cauvain, L. S. Young and S. Salmon
110 **Improving the safety of fresh meat**
Edited by J. Sofos

111 **Understanding pathogen behaviour: Virulence, stress response and resistance**
Edited by M. Griffiths
112 **The microwave processing of foods**
Edited by H. Schubert and M. Regier
113 **Food safety control in the poultry industry**
Edited by G. Mead
114 **Improving the safety of fresh fruit and vegetables**
Edited by W. Jongen
115 **Food, diet and obesity**
Edited by D. Mela
116 **Handbook of hygiene control in the food industry**
Edited by H. L. M. Lelieveld, M. A. Mostert and J. Holah
117 **Detecting allergens in food**
Edited by S. Koppelman and S. Hefle
118 **Improving the fat content of foods**
Edited by C. Williams and J. Buttriss
119 **Improving traceability in food processing and distribution**
Edited by I. Smith and A. Furness
120 **Flavour in food**
Edited by A. Voilley and P. Etievant
121 **The Chorleywood bread process**
S. P. Cauvain and L. S. Young
122 **Food spoilage microorganisms**
Edited by C. de W. Blackburn
123 **Emerging foodborne pathogens**
Edited by Y. Motarjemi and M. Adams
124 **Benders' dictionary of nutrition and food technology Eighth edition**
D. A. Bender
125 **Optimising sweet taste in foods**
Edited by W. J. Spillane
126 **Brewing: New technologies**
Edited by C. Bamforth
127 **Handbook of herbs and spices Volume 3**
Edited by K. V. Peter
128 **Lawrie's meat science Seventh edition**
R. A. Lawrie in collaboration with D. A. Ledward
129 **Modifying lipids for use in food**
Edited by F. Gunstone
130 **Meat products handbook: Practical science and technology**
G. Feiner
131 **Food consumption and disease risk: Consumer–pathogen interactions**
Edited by M. Potter
132 **Acrylamide and other hazardous compounds in heat-treated foods**
Edited by K. Skog and J. Alexander
133 **Managing allergens in food**
Edited by C. Mills, H. Wichers and K. Hoffman-Sommergruber
134 **Microbiological analysis of red meat, poultry and eggs**
Edited by G. Mead

135 **Maximising the value of marine by-products**
Edited by F. Shahidi
136 **Chemical migration and food contact materials**
Edited by K. Barnes, R. Sinclair and D. Watson
137 **Understanding consumers of food products**
Edited by L. Frewer and H. van Trijp
138 **Reducing salt in foods: Practical strategies**
Edited by D. Kilcast and F. Angus
139 **Modelling microorganisms in food**
Edited by S. Brul, S. Van Gerwen and M. Zwietering
140 **Tamime and Robinson's Yoghurt: Science and technology Third edition**
A. Y. Tamime and R. K. Robinson
141 **Handbook of waste management and co-product recovery in food processing Volume 1**
Edited by K. W. Waldron
142 **Improving the flavour of cheese**
Edited by B. Weimer
143 **Novel food ingredients for weight control**
Edited by C. J. K. Henry
144 **Consumer-led food product development**
Edited by H. MacFie
145 **Functional dairy products Volume 2**
Edited by M. Saarela
146 **Modifying flavour in food**
Edited by A. J. Taylor and J. Hort
147 **Cheese problems solved**
Edited by P. L. H. McSweeney
148 **Handbook of organic food safety and quality**
Edited by J. Cooper, C. Leifert and U. Niggli
149 **Understanding and controlling the microstructure of complex foods**
Edited by D. J. McClements
150 **Novel enzyme technology for food applications**
Edited by R. Rastall
151 **Food preservation by pulsed electric fields: From research to application**
Edited by H. L. M. Lelieveld and S. W. H. de Haan
152 **Technology of functional cereal products**
Edited by B. R. Hamaker
153 **Case studies in food product development**
Edited by M. Earle and R. Earle
154 **Delivery and controlled release of bioactives in foods and nutraceuticals**
Edited by N. Garti
155 **Fruit and vegetable flavour: Recent advances and future prospects**
Edited by B. Brückner and S. G. Wyllie
156 **Food fortification and supplementation: Technological, safety and regulatory aspects**
Edited by P. Berry Ottaway
157 **Improving the health-promoting properties of fruit and vegetable products**
Edited by F. A. Tomás-Barberán and M. I. Gil
158 **Improving seafood products for the consumer**
Edited by T. Børresen

159 **In-pack processed foods: Improving quality**
Edited by P. Richardson
160 **Handbook of water and energy management in food processing**
Edited by J. Klemeš, R. Smith and J.-K. Kim
161 **Environmentally compatible food packaging**
Edited by E. Chiellini
162 **Improving farmed fish quality and safety**
Edited by Ø. Lie
163 **Carbohydrate-active enzymes**
Edited by K.-H. Park
164 **Chilled foods: A comprehensive guide Third edition**
Edited by M. Brown
165 **Food for the ageing population**
Edited by M. M. Raats, C. P. G. M. de Groot and W. A Van Staveren
166 **Improving the sensory and nutritional quality of fresh meat**
Edited by J. P. Kerry and D. A. Ledward
167 **Shellfish safety and quality**
Edited by S. E. Shumway and G. E. Rodrick
168 **Functional and speciality beverage technology**
Edited by P. Paquin
169 **Functional foods: Principles and technology**
M. Guo
170 **Endocrine-disrupting chemicals in food**
Edited by I. Shaw
171 **Meals in science and practice: Interdisciplinary research and business applications**
Edited by H. L. Meiselman
172 **Food constituents and oral health: Current status and future prospects**
Edited by M. Wilson
173 **Handbook of hydrocolloids Second edition**
Edited by G. O. Phillips and P. A. Williams
174 **Food processing technology: Principles and practice Third edition**
P. J. Fellows
175 **Science and technology of enrobed and filled chocolate, confectionery and bakery products**
Edited by G. Talbot
176 **Foodborne pathogens: Hazards, risk analysis and control Second edition**
Edited by C. de W. Blackburn and P. J. McClure
177 **Designing functional foods: Measuring and controlling food structure breakdown and absorption**
Edited by D. J. McClements and E. A. Decker
178 **New technologies in aquaculture: Improving production efficiency, quality and environmental management**
Edited by G. Burnell and G. Allan
179 **More baking problems solved**
S. P. Cauvain and L. S. Young
180 **Soft drink and fruit juice problems solved**
P. Ashurst and R. Hargitt
181 **Biofilms in the food and beverage industries**
Edited by P. M. Fratamico, B. A. Annous and N. W. Gunther

182 **Dairy-derived ingredients: Food and neutraceutical uses**
Edited by M. Corredig
183 **Handbook of waste management and co-product recovery in food processing Volume 2**
Edited by K. W. Waldron
184 **Innovations in food labelling**
Edited by J. Albert
185 **Delivering performance in food supply chains**
Edited by C. Mena and G. Stevens
186 **Chemical deterioration and physical instability of food and beverages**
Edited by L. H. Skibsted, J. Risbo and M. L. Andersen
187 **Managing wine quality Volume 1: Viticulture and wine quality**
Edited by A. G. Reynolds
188 **Improving the safety and quality of milk Volume 1: Milk production and processing**
Edited by M. Griffiths
189 **Improving the safety and quality of milk Volume 2: Improving quality in milk products**
Edited by M. Griffiths
190 **Cereal grains: Assessing and managing quality**
Edited by C. Wrigley and I. Batey
191 **Sensory analysis for food and beverage quality control: A practical guide**
Edited by D. Kilcast
192 **Managing wine quality Volume 2: Oenology and wine quality**
Edited by A. G. Reynolds
193 **Winemaking problems solved**
Edited by C. E. Butzke
194 **Environmental assessment and management in the food industry**
Edited by U. Sonesson, J. Berlin and F. Ziegler
195 **Consumer-driven innovation in food and personal care products**
Edited by S. R. Jaeger and H. MacFie
196 **Tracing pathogens in the food chain**
Edited by S. Brul, P. M. Fratamico and T. A. McMeekin
197 **Case studies in novel food processing technologies: Innovations in processing, packaging, and predictive modelling**
Edited by C. J. Doona, K. Kustin and F. E. Feeherry
198 **Freeze-drying of pharmaceutical and food products**
T.-C. Hua, B.-L. Liu and H. Zhang
199 **Oxidation in foods and beverages and antioxidant applications Volume 1: Understanding mechanisms of oxidation and antioxidant activity**
Edited by E. A. Decker, R. J. Elias and D. J. McClements
200 **Oxidation in foods and beverages and antioxidant applications Volume 2: Management in different industry sectors**
Edited by E. A. Decker, R. J. Elias and D. J. McClements
201 **Protective cultures, antimicrobial metabolites and bacteriophages for food and beverage biopreservation**
Edited by C. Lacroix
202 **Separation, extraction and concentration processes in the food, beverage and nutraceutical industries**
Edited by S. S. H. Rizvi

203 **Determining mycotoxins and mycotoxigenic fungi in food and feed**
Edited by S. De Saeger
204 **Developing children's food products**
Edited by D. Kilcast and F. Angus
205 **Functional foods: Concept to product Second edition**
Edited by M. Saarela
206 **Postharvest biology and technology of tropical and subtropical fruits Volume 1: Fundamental issues**
Edited by E. M. Yahia
207 **Postharvest biology and technology of tropical and subtropical fruits Volume 2: Açai to citrus**
Edited by E. M. Yahia
208 **Postharvest biology and technology of tropical and subtropical fruits Volume 3: Cocona to mango**
Edited by E. M. Yahia
209 **Postharvest biology and technology of tropical and subtropical fruits Volume 4: Mangosteen to white sapote**
Edited by E. M. Yahia
210 **Food and beverage stability and shelf life**
Edited by D. Kilcast and P. Subramaniam
211 **Processed Meats: Improving safety, nutrition and quality**
Edited by J. P. Kerry and J. F. Kerry
212 **Food chain integrity: A holistic approach to food traceability, safety, quality and authenticity**
Edited by J. Hoorfar, K. Jordan, F. Butler and R. Prugger
213 **Improving the safety and quality of eggs and egg products Volume 1**
Edited by Y. Nys, M. Bain and F. Van Immerseel
214 **Improving the safety and quality of eggs and egg products Volume 2**
Edited by F. Van Immerseel, Y. Nys and M. Bain
215 **Animal feed contamination: Effects on livestock and food safety**
Edited by J. Fink-Gremmels
216 **Hygienic design of food factories**
Edited by J. Holah and H. L. M. Lelieveld
217 **Manley's technology of biscuits, crackers and cookies Fourth edition**
Edited by D. Manley
218 **Nanotechnology in the food, beverage and nutraceutical industries**
Edited by Q. Huang
219 **Rice quality: A guide to rice properties and analysis**
K. R. Bhattacharya
220 **Advances in meat, poultry and seafood packaging**
Edited by J. P. Kerry
221 **Reducing saturated fats in foods**
Edited by G. Talbot
222 **Handbook of food proteins**
Edited by G. O. Phillips and P. A. Williams
223 **Lifetime nutritional influences on cognition, behaviour and psychiatric illness**
Edited by D. Benton
224 **Food machinery for the production of cereal foods, snack foods and confectionery**
L.-M. Cheng

225 **Alcoholic beverages: Sensory evaluation and consumer research**
Edited by J. Piggott
226 **Extrusion problems solved: Food, pet food and feed**
M. N. Riaz and G. J. Rokey
227 **Handbook of herbs and spices Second edition Volume 1**
Edited by K. V. Peter
228 **Handbook of herbs and spices Second edition Volume 2**
Edited by K. V. Peter
229 **Breadmaking: Improving quality Second edition**
Edited by S. P. Cauvain
230 **Emerging food packaging technologies: Principles and practice**
Edited by K. L. Yam and D. S. Lee
231 **Infectious disease in aquaculture: Prevention and control**
Edited by B. Austin
232 **Diet, immunity and inflammation**
Edited by P. C. Calder and P. Yaqoob
233 **Natural food additives, ingredients and flavourings**
Edited by D. Baines and R. Seal
234 **Microbial decontamination in the food industry: Novel methods and applications**
Edited by A. Demirci and M.O. Ngadi
235 **Chemical contaminants and residues in foods**
Edited by D. Schrenk
236 **Robotics and automation in the food industry: Current and future technologies**
Edited by D. G. Caldwell
237 **Fibre-rich and wholegrain foods: Improving quality**
Edited by J. A. Delcour and K. Poutanen
238 **Computer vision technology in the food and beverage industries**
Edited by D.-W. Sun
239 **Encapsulation technologies and delivery systems for food ingredients and nutraceuticals**
Edited by N. Garti and D. J. McClements
240 **Case studies in food safety and authenticity**
Edited by J. Hoorfar
241 **Heat treatment for insect control: Developments and applications**
D. Hammond
242 **Advances in aquaculture hatchery technology**
Edited by G. Allan and G. Burnell
243 **Open innovation in the food and beverage industry**
Edited by M. Garcia Martinez
244 **Trends in packaging of food, beverages and other fast-moving consumer goods (FMCG)**
Edited by N. Farmer
245 **New analytical approaches for verifying the origin of food**
Edited by P. Brereton
246 **Microbial production of food ingredients, enzymes and nutraceuticals**
Edited by B. McNeil, D. Archer, I. Giavasis and L. Harvey
247 **Persistent organic pollutants and toxic metals in foods**
Edited by M. Rose and A. Fernandes
248 **Cereal grains for the food and beverage industries**
E. Arendt and E. Zannini

249 **Viruses in food and water: Risks, surveillance and control**
Edited by N. Cook
250 **Improving the safety and quality of nuts**
Edited by L. J. Harris
251 **Metabolomics in food and nutrition**
Edited by B. C. Weimer and C. Slupsky
252 **Food enrichment with omega-3 fatty acids**
Edited by C. Jacobsen, N. S. Nielsen, A. F. Horn and A.-D. M. Sørensen
253 **Instrumental assessment of food sensory quality: A practical guide**
Edited by D. Kilcast
254 **Food microstructures: Microscopy, measurement and modelling**
Edited by V. J. Morris and K. Groves
255 **Handbook of food powders: Processes and properties**
Edited by B. R. Bhandari, N. Bansal, M. Zhang and P. Schuck
256 **Functional ingredients from algae for foods and nutraceuticals**
Edited by H. Domínguez
257 **Satiation, satiety and the control of food intake: Theory and practice**
Edited by J. E. Blundell and F. Bellisle
258 **Hygiene in food processing: Principles and practice Second edition**
Edited by H. L. M. Lelieveld, J. Holah and D. Napper
259 **Advances in microbial food safety Volume 1**
Edited by J. Sofos
260 **Global safety of fresh produce: A handbook of best practice, innovative commercial solutions and case studies**
Edited by J. Hoorfar
261 **Human milk biochemistry and infant formula manufacturing technology**
Edited by M. Guo
262 **High throughput screening for food safety assessment: Biosensor technologies, hyperspectral imaging and practical applications**
Edited by A. K. Bhunia, M. S. Kim and C. R. Taitt
263 **Foods, nutrients and food ingredients with authorised EU health claims: Volume 1**
Edited by M. J. Sadler
264 **Handbook of food allergen detection and control**
Edited by S. Flanagan
265 **Advances in fermented foods and beverages: Improving quality, technologies and health benefits**
Edited by W. Holzapfel
266 **Metabolomics as a tool in nutrition research**
Edited by J.-L. Sébédio and L. Brennan
267 **Dietary supplements: Safety, efficacy and quality**
Edited by K. Berginc and S. Kreft
268 **Grapevine breeding programs for the wine industry: Traditional and molecular technologies**
Edited by A. G. Reynolds
269 **Handbook of natural antimicrobials for food safety and quality**
Edited by M. Taylor
270 **Managing and preventing obesity: Behavioural factors and dietary interventions**
Edited by T. P. Gill

271 **Electron beam pasteurization and complementary food processing technologies**
Edited by S. D. Pillai and S. Shayanfar
272 **Advances in food and beverage labelling: Information and regulations**
Edited by P. Berryman
273 **Flavour development, analysis and perception in food and beverages**
Edited by J. K. Parker, S. Elmore and L. Methven
274 **Rapid sensory profiling techniques and related methods: Applications in new product development and consumer research**
Edited by J. Delarue, J. B. Lawlor and M. Rogeaux
275 **Advances in microbial food safety: Volume 2**
Edited by J. Sofos
276 **Handbook of antioxidants in food preservation**
Edited by F. Shahidi
277 **Lockhart and Wiseman's crop husbandry including grassland: Ninth edition**
H. J. S. Finch, A. M. Samuel and G. P. F. Lane
278 **Global legislation for food contact materials: Processing, storage and packaging**
Edited by J. S. Baughan
279 **Colour additives for food and beverages: Development, safety and applications**
Edited by M. Scotter
280 **A complete course in canning and related processes 14th Edition: Volume 1**
Revised by S. Featherstone
281 **A complete course in canning and related processes 14th Edition: Volume 2**
Revised by S. Featherstone
282 **A complete course in canning and related processes 14th Edition: Volume 3**
Revised by S. Featherstone

Preface

Many studies carried out on animals and humans using nutritional interventions and/or epidemiological observations have shown that many diseases are linked to poor nutrition. In the past two decades, we have witnessed nutrition research moving from disease treatment to promotion of health and disease prevention. With this, there has been an increased emphasis placed on nutritional recommendations. However, considering the interindividual variability in response to food components, optimum levels of physiological functions of individuals have to be determined to optimize recommendations, the purpose being to reach personalized nutrition. The recent development of high-throughput technologies (transcriptomics, proteomics, and metabolomics) that enable the generation of large-scale molecular-level measurements has increased attention of scientists in medical, biological, and nutritional sciences as these tools offer the possibility of characterizing global alterations associated with disease conditions or nutritional exposure and subtle changes in metabolism due to a stimuli.

Among the "omics" technologies, the metabolomics field has been mainly developed in pharmaceutical and plant sciences. However, its application to nutrition is still relatively new although this topic constitutes a growing domain of interest with potential large impacts in nutrition research. The main objectives of this book are on one hand to show the recent progress made in the utilization of metabolomics as a tool in nutrition research and its major applications and on another hand to discuss the major challenges that scientists still have to face and solve in order to allow metabolomics to reach its real potential and to move nutrition from a rather reductionist approach to a global one.

To achieve the aims of the book, we have divided this book in two major parts. The first one deals with principles and methodology issues of metabolomics. The focus of this section is on major challenges for using metabolomics in nutrition research, starting from the experimental design to data integration using bioinformatics tools. Details on the principle of the analytic techniques are well covered in other books, so instead, we chose to focus on challenges with respect to nutrition research.

Part 2 of the book has been divided into nine chapters dealing with application of metabolomics in nutrition research. Chapter 4 summarizes the applications of lipidomic platforms for identifying biomarkers of diseases and metabolic processes associated with diet and for controlling food quality and detecting fraud in food products. Chapter 5 presents how human metabolism can be modelled using metabolic network and how this model can be used to analyse metabolomics data, to interpret the metabolic relationships connecting a set of biomarkers for assessing the metabolic impact of different diets. The role of gut microbiota in nutrition and disease using a metagenomic approach is discussed in Chapter 6, while Chapter 7 focuses on the role of metabolomics and in particular metabotyping in moving towards personalized nutrition.

Chapter 8 describes the application of metabolomics in biomarker discovery for early disease detection and biomarkers for the prediction of the evolution of the health status towards metabolic pathologies. In Chapter 9, the potential of metabolomics for the identification of new biomarkers of intake is discussed. It also describes the challenges that lie ahead, including the validation of identified biomarkers and the development of sharing tools for data and resources. Chapter 10 describes how analysing dynamic metabolomics data (obtained during challenge tests) has been successful in identifying metabolic phenotypes in the predisease state and identifying subtle metabolic changes following dietary interventions. Chapter 11 ("Foodomics") highlights how metabolomics offers the possibility to analyse the effects of cultivation, processing, and digestion on the nutritional value of food. The last chapter (Chapter 12) not only summarizes the perspectives outlined in the different chapters but also discusses a long-term view of the future direction.

We hope that you will enjoy this book and that it encourages you to employ metabolomics techniques in your research. We look forward to seeing this field grow and follow the developments in nutrition research as a result of the use of metabolomics as a tool.

Part One

Principles

Challenges in nutritional metabolomics: from experimental design to interpretation of data sets

1

M. Ferrara, J.-L. Sébédio
Institut National de la Recherche Agronomique (INRA), Clermont-Ferrand, France

1.1 Introduction

Many studies have shown that diseases are often linked to poor nutrition (Aburto et al., 2013; Micha et al., 2013; Simopoulos, 2013; Wang et al., 2013). Nutrition research has identified the functions of essential nutrients, and researchers have established nutrition recommendations that allow the public to meet the needs of their bodies by optimising metabolic pathways. As an example, nutrition research led to the discovery of linoleic (18:2n−6) and linolenic acids (18:3n−3), which are fatty acids involved in essential functions that must be provided by food components because they cannot be synthesised by the body (Holman, 1996). However, considering interindividual variability in response to food components, an individual's optimum physiological function must first be determined in order to optimise recommendations and achieve personalised nutrition (Zivkovic and German, 2009). Food science and nutrition not only focus on the relationship between diseases and macro- and micronutrient consumption, but these disciplines also attempt to identify bioactive molecules that may be present in the diet in low quantities for the purpose of understanding the protective effects that these molecules may have and their mechanisms of action. These non-essential bioactive compounds interact with a number of metabolic pathways and may modulate health status, either directly or indirectly, after being metabolised by the gut microbiota. Dietary polyphenols are a typical example of the importance that gut microbiota may play (Moco et al., 2012).

Consequently, identifying specific early-responding molecules in biofluids, such as blood and urine, is crucial for diagnosis and intervention, or process reversal (Reezi et al., 2008), because these substances may be connected to underlying metabolic dysfunctions. For this purpose, researchers must obtain accurate data on dietary intake in natural populations, which is a great challenge for epidemiological studies (Ismail et al., 2013). The recent development of high-throughput technologies (transcriptomics, proteomics, and metabolomics), which permit large-scale molecular measurements, has drawn the attention of scientists in the medical, biological, and nutritional fields because these tools offer the possibility of characterising global alterations associated with disease conditions, exposing overall nutritional activities and moving nutrition from a rather reductionist approach to a global one. The

Metabolomics as a Tool in Nutrition Research. http://dx.doi.org/10.1016/B978-1-78242-084-2.00001-0

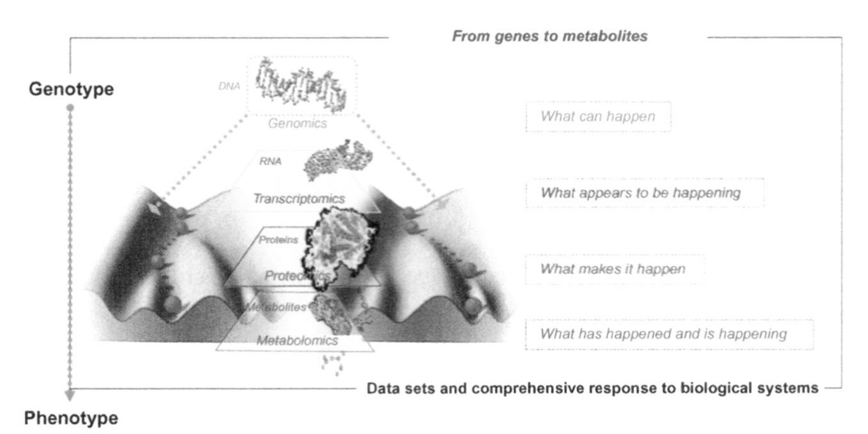

Figure 1.1 Metabolomics: bridging the genotype–phenotype gap. The "omic" technologies are used to obtain a more holistic view of how biological systems work and underpin the fields of functional genomics and systems biology. Genes encode mRNAs that encode proteins that, with environmental factors (e.g., diet), lead to the metabolite.

production and utilisation of metabolites is more directly connected to the phenotype exhibited by an organism than the presence of mRNAs or proteins (Figure 1.1).

Among the "omic" technologies, the metabolomics has mainly grown out of the pharmaceutical and plant sciences. Yet, despite its relatively recent application to nutrition, this topic constitutes a growing domain of interest, considering the shift observed in dietary habits (German et al., 2002; Gibney et al., 2005). The rapidly expanding field of metabolomics has been driven by major advances in analytical tools, such as Nuclear Magnetic Resonance (NMR) (Eisenreich and Bacher, 2007) and mass spectrometry, and the corresponding hyphenated methods, such as high-performance liquid chromatography coupled with mass spectrometry (LC-MS) and gas–liquid chromatography coupled with mass spectrometry (GC-MS) (Dettmer et al., 2007; Pan and Raftery, 2007; Wilson et al., 2005). Advances in chemometric and bioinformatic technologies (Idle and Gonzalez, 2007; Moco et al., 2007; Wishart, 2007) also play an important role. Metabolomics (Fienh et al., 2000; Nicholson et al., 1999) can be described as a global analysis of small molecules of a biofluid (blood, urine, culture broth, cell extract, etc.), which are produced or modified as the result of a stimulus (nutritional intervention, environmental stressors, drug, etc.). At the moment the study of lipid molecules (lipidomics) is a major area in the metabolomics field (Morris and Watkins, 2005; see Chapter 3 for detailed discussion). Some chapters of this book will also discuss the use of metabolomics for discovering biomarkers in nutritional interventions (Brennan, 2013; Lodge, 2010), for predicting the risk of a health state involving into a disease state, and for monitoring food/nutrient biomarker consumption (Hedrick et al., 2012; Pujos-Guillot et al., 2013).

A typical metabolomic experiment (Figure 1.2) includes six elements: (1) design of the experiment and preparation of the sample; (2) analysis of biofluids or tissues via LC-MS, NMR, GC-MS, or a multiplatform approach to maximise metabolite

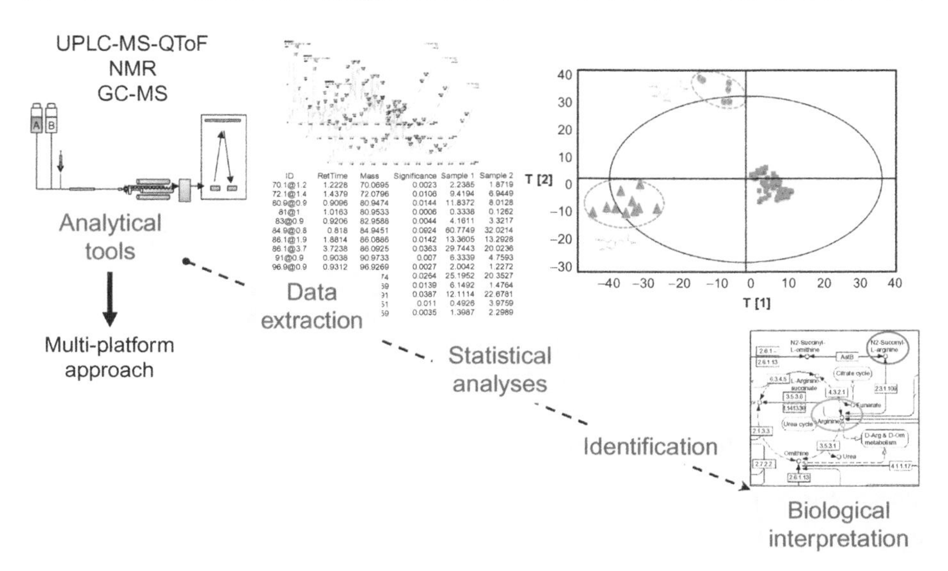

Figure 1.2 Workflow of a metabolomic analysis.

coverage; (3) extraction and treatment of the data set; (4) statistical analyses; (5) identification of key or discriminatory metabolites; and (6) biological interpretation of the data. Data acquisition and retrieval may be achieved by a targeted analysis during which specific pathways are analysed or an untargeted analysis where no prior selection of pathways is performed, which is a hypothesis-driven approach. Both have advantages and disadvantages, and the approach taken ultimately depends on the study in question. In this introductory chapter, we outline the major challenges involved with such an approach. Subsequent chapters provide detailed discussions of the crucial points.

1.2 The experimental design

So far, metabolomic studies have mainly used animal nutritional interventions and human clinical trials. More recently, cohorts with 7–12 year follow-up have largely been utilised for discovering predictive biomarkers for the evolution of a health state towards a disease state. These studies are described in Chapter 6. As previously reported, metabolomics was first developed and applied to toxicology and pharmacology, which usually induce major changes in the blood or urine metabolome after the administration of a drug (Nicholson et al., 2002; Pujos-Guillot et al., 2012). This is not the case when applying metabolomics to nutrition research because dietary interventions most often generate subtle changes in metabolic profiles, which may sometimes be difficult to detect (Solanky et al., 2003). Considering interindividual response to diet (Walsh et al., 2006), the effects of many factors, such as age, sex, and various genetic and environmental stimuli on the metabolic profiles of the biofluids (Johnson and Gonzalez, 2011), researchers must take great care when designing the experimental protocol of a metabolomics approach, especially when using humans, as subtle variations between subjects may induce large variations in metabolite concentrations in the plasma and/or urine. Therefore, the protocol should be designed to reduce confounders as much as possible, allowing retrieval of optimised information from the analytical data (Smilowitz et al., 2013).

For metabolomic studies of predictive biomarkers, the use of cohorts and epidemiological approaches benefit from very comprehensive data sets that have been acquired during the follow-up years. These data include clinical measurements (blood and urine biochemistry, anthropometric and body-composition measurements), number of events (cardiovascular diseases, type 2 diabetes, etc.), food frequency questionnaires, socioeconomic data, and blood and urine samples for further metabolomic analyses. One of the major challenges of this type of study is to correctly evaluate the dietary intake of the individuals. At the moment, 24-h recalls, weighed food diaries, and food frequency questionnaires are being used, but the issues surrounding their use are well documented (Fave et al., 2009). Consequently, researchers are trying to use metabolomics to identify the food metabolome (Llorach et al., 2012; Pujos-Guillot et al., 2013), in order to evaluate dietary exposure based on markers of specific food intake (Fave et al., 2009). Chapter 9 discusses this important topic.

1.3 The analytical platform

Human biofluids are a complex mixture of thousands of metabolites that include endogenous and exogenous molecules, as reported for serum (Psychogios et al., 2011) and urine (Bouatra et al., 2013). A combination of literature mining and a multiplatform approach allowed David Wishart and colleagues to report 445 urine metabolites, while quantifying 378 species (Bouatra et al., 2013). For serum and urine, an examination of the published literature using a similar approach identified reports of 4229 and 2600 confirmed compounds. Importantly, both biofluids are complex mixtures of molecule classes that have a wide range of polarity and of concentrations. Furthermore, blood samples also contain proteins that may interfere with the analytical technique and thus need to be removed before analysis in most cases. Removal must be done in such a way that metabolites of interest are not lost during this pre-fractionation step.

Considering the complexity of the human metabolome, choosing the analytical method is often a critical step. NMR does not require extensive sample preparation time, has high reproducibility, and little inter-laboratory variability, but it is limited by its sensitivity, compared to mass spectrometry, which needs extensive sample treatments or pre-fractionation steps (Scalbert et al., 2009; Yang et al., 2013). On the other hand, NMR is a good method when large-sample sets have to be analysed, as is generally the case for clinical trials, and thus, NMR could be a tool "at the patients' bed" (Johnson and Gonzalez, 2011) even if the number of detected metabolites is smaller compared to those detected by MS. NMR was widely used when metabolomics started

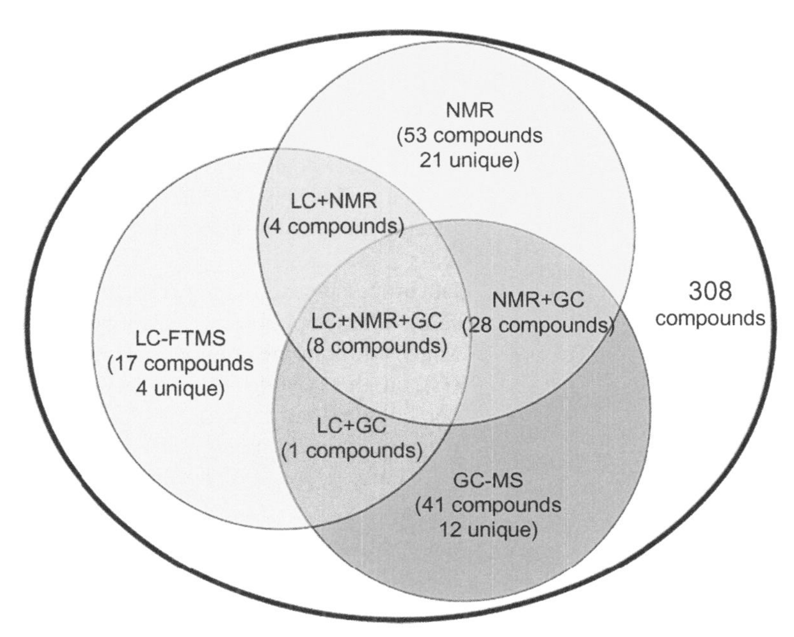

Figure 1.3 Venn diagram showing the overlap of cerebrospinal fluid (CSF) metabolites detected by NMR, GC-MS, and LC-FTMS methods, as compared to the detectable CSF metabolome. GC-MS, gas chromatography-mass spectrometry; LC-FTMS, liquid chromatography-Fourier transform mass spectrometry.
Reproduced by permission from Wishart et al. (2008).

to be applied to nutrition research, but now many studies use LC-MS (see Chapter 2 for a detailed discussion).

Analysing one special chemical class of molecules, such as lipids, by UPLC-MS or other appropriate analytical tools (targeted analysis) is probably the easiest task to accomplish, and metabolites may then be quantified if appropriate standards are available or if those can be synthesised. The most difficult task is to carry out an untargeted approach when no hypothesis is available. Due to the complexity of the biofluid composition, one technique is likely not able to cover the wide range of polarity and structural features of the metabolites. A typical example is illustrated in Figure 1.3, which deals with the analysis of the human cerebrospinal fluid metabolome (Wishart et al., 2008), in which the three above-mentioned analytical techniques were used in order to obtain a comprehensive metabolite data set.

1.4 Extraction of data sets and statistical analyses

Metabolomics in nutrition is primarily interested in the responses of biological systems that result in metabolite-level regulation related to diet changes. It is therefore important to separate pertinent biological variations from noisy sources of variability introduced into studies of metabolites. The determining quality of data processing is thus an essential step in properly analysing and interpreting metabolomic data. The data treatment is generally divided into two steps: data processing and data analysis. The data-processing step consists to transform the raw data into format that is easy to use in the subsequent data analysis steps. The data analysis stage includes tasks for the analysis and interpretation of processed data. This stage typically includes multivariate analyses, such as the clustering of metabolic profiles or the discovery of important differences between groups of samples.

In order to improve metabolomic data processing, software packages are constantly being developed. New tools are still being released, and some existing tools are being further developed (Lommen, 2009). Many solutions are commercial and freely available tools (Katajamaa and Oresic, 2007), but the existing software tools are often difficult to combine with one another or not flexible enough to allow for the rapid prototyping of a new analysis workflow. As a result, many novel algorithms fitting with automatic processing have been recently developed (Kenar et al., 2014; Kuhl et al., 2012)

Regardless of the analytical technique(s) selected, metabolic analyses create a great amount of data, and analysis of these data by multivariate statistics represents an important and time-consuming part of the metabolomics workflow. Current methods of statistical analysis include principal component analysis (PCA), which is an unsupervised technique; partial least square discriminant analysis (PLS-DA); and orthogonal PLS-DA (O-PLSDA), with the two latter being supervised techniques. PCA allows identification and grouping of samples due to similarity in metabolic profile, and supervised techniques require a priori knowledge of sample classification, thus permitting identification of the metabolites that are discriminating the groups. Supervised techniques also allow the construction of models that have to be further validated using, for example, a cross-validation procedure in which samples are left out and their classification is predicted. These different methods are often used in combination. Nevertheless, researchers need more effective and robust bioinformatics tools for metabolomic data analysis, especially when dealing with clinical samples with large individual variability. More recently, a machine learning method, random forest (RF), which has been reported to be an excellent classifier, was used in clinical metabolomics for phenotypic discrimination and biomarker selection (Chen et al., 2013).

1.5 Metabolite identification

Metabolite identification remains one of the biggest challenges in metabolomics, despite major published advances in this area during the past decade. When metabolomics started to be applied in nutrition research, many papers in the literature did not contain much structural information about the discriminant metabolites, although data obtained by NMR, which existed spectral databases, were of great help (Nicholson and Wilson, 1989). Nowadays, mass spectrometry-based approaches are increasingly used in nutrition research. Even if databases have been constructed (Johnson and

Gonzalez, 2011), such as the Human Metabolome database (Wishart et al., 2013), identifying metabolites still represents the limiting step of a metabolomics workflow

Lipid extracts from biofluids or tissues have been revealed as mixtures of lipid species of varying complexity, and, at the moment, the lipidomics field (Smilowitz et al., 2013) is the more advanced metabolomics area for metabolite identification, because a generation of researchers has focused on techniques for fractionating and identifying lipid species (Christie and Han, 2010). Furthermore, the international lipid classification and nomenclature committee, along with the Lipid Maps consortium (see Section 1.7 for further details), developed a classification system for lipids that is compatible with existing databases and that has been accepted by the lipid community around the world (Fahy et al., 2009). As a result, researchers have begun to use a uniform language available online at the LIPID MAPS website (http://www.lipidmaps.org). Data exchange, communication, and sharing experimental protocols and data interpretations are thus assets for this community.

In comparison, when dealing with unknown complex mixtures of different families of molecules, identifying metabolites using untargeted metabolic approaches represents an important challenge, especially when using a combination of liquid chromatography and mass spectrometry. Even if no full agreement on how to solve this problem has been published, guidelines and pipelines have been reported for identifying metabolites. For example, in Figure 1.4, we have reported the metabolite identification procedure recently published by (Peironcely et al., 2013) using LC-MS^n data exploration. Usually, the identification of metabolites involves the determination of the exact mass, database searches, and MS^n fragmentation studies. There are different levels of confidence for the identifications. The highest level of confidence is achieved

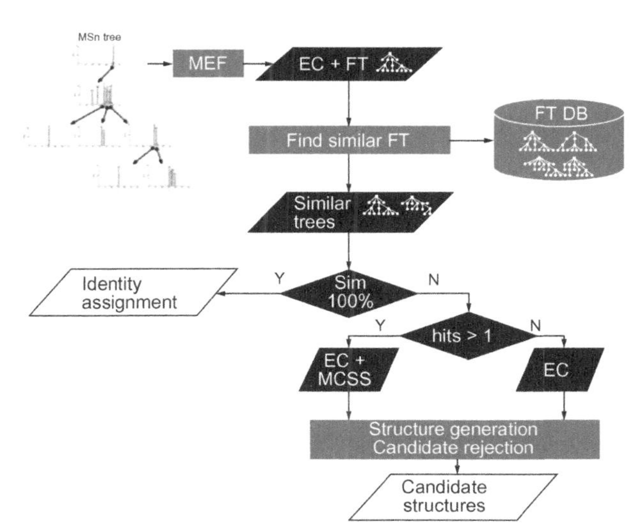

Figure 1.4 Metabolite identification pipeline. Abbreviations: MEF, multistage elemental formula; EC, elemental composition; FT, fragmentation tree; MCSS, maximum common substructure; Sim, similarity.
Reproduced by permission from Peironcely et al. (2013).

when the identity of the molecule is validated using an authentic standard and a subsequent MS analysis. The second highest level involves a putative identification, when a structure is proposed based on MS/MS, MS^n spectral similarities, or fragmentation trees, or it is based on a compound spectrum present in a database. At this level, the putative identification is not validated using a standard molecule, however. Lastly, for the identification with the lowest level of confidence, only the exact molecular mass may be available, and only the raw chemical formula can be obtained. Collaborations between biologists and chemists specialising in metabolite synthesis are sometimes the only way to answer the question, but this technique should only be used in large collaborative projects dealing with major societal outcomes, considering the cost of chemical synthesis. Detailed descriptions of the existing identification techniques and automated pipelines, using LC-MS, are debated in Chapter 2.

1.6 Biological interpretations

After the identification of metabolites, the results of the analysis are, at best, one list of metabolites with relative contents differing between the studied conditions. The task is then to define the relevance and biological significance of these observations, even when the changes in the relative content of metabolites are low, as is generally the case in nutrition research.

Interpretation of these data essentially relies on computational approaches used in large-scale data analysis and data visualisation, which are most often built upon interdependencies between metabolites. The correlations found do not necessarily relate to metabolites that are neighbours on the metabolic level, but they may involve more distant pathways (Steuer et al., 2003). Indeed, most biological processes are regulated by mechanisms that overlap, and ideally metabolomics data should describe the physiological processes in different situations and identify which pathways are altered in specific diseases.

In order to interpret metabolomics data, the first step is commonly the construction of a network structure (see Chapter 4), which helps to highlight the most relevant biological molecules. The published work of Zhang et al. (2013) illustrates network method analysis, showing the key aspects of mapping altered metabolites onto KEGG pathways.

However, some theoretical considerations limit the direct interpretation of metabolic networks generated from metabolic snapshots. First, any subcellular compartmentalisation is lost in the process of sample preparation, and most biofluids used in human studies are either transit compartment (blood, plasma) or collection and elimination metabolic pools (urine, faecal water). Second, most current metabolite profiling approaches rely on the measurement of steady-state levels, therefore, they do not necessarily reflect the flux of metabolites through a network pathway.

Different tissue-specific metabolic networks can be built to overcome these limitations and exclude some non-physiological metabolites associations (see Chapter 4 for detailed information). An outline of dynamic network description reveals interactions between primary and secondary metabolism by the direct link of statistical analysis (Granger causality) and mathematical processes such as those developed by Doerfler et al. (2013). Such approaches provide clues to pathway regulation, but the flux is important for bringing to light alterations in metabolism. Flux profiling is possible in artificial biological systems such as cell cultures, microorganism cultures, or tissue samples. But in humans and other animals, metabolomics approaches the question of whether steady-state measurements can be exploited to reveal flux alterations. Early work by Arkin and Ross (Arkin et al., 1997) demonstrated the need to introduce stochastic models for the interpretation of metabolic networks. In fact, the development of various model systems that interpret the metabolite correlations observed in metabolomics datasets allows the investigation of the whole metabolite network dynamics base on correlation network topologies (Weckwerth, 2003).

The combination of multiple data sources provides the metabolomics data integration in a global evaluation of biological systems. The modules of the omics field, transcriptome, proteome, and metabolome, are not disjoint. The combination of these forms of information can provide a more comprehensive understanding of biological entities. In the human nutrition field, various studies have jointly analysed different metabolomics or proteomics data in order to improve the overall understanding of the system (Oberbach et al., 2011; Pellis et al., 2012).

Thus, metabolomics can be considered as the most functional part among the omics technologies, and it has been promoted as a potent tool for assessing biochemical process related to complex phenotypes.

1.7 Conclusion: do we need standardisation procedures and repositories?

The application of metabolomics in the field of nutrition research has been growing rapidly during the past 10 years. Yet, some challenges discussed in this book must still be solved if we want this approach to reach its real potential. Considering the recent technical progress in analytical techniques, bioinformatics, and statistical tools, as well as advances in potential applications for this approach, more researchers are going to use this tool. Consequently, the need to compare and share datasets will increase, emphasising the need to minimise inter-laboratory variability. Furthermore, scientists working with the "omics approaches" will have to share standard operating procedures (Holmes et al., 2010). The standardisation of protocols, to guide data production, quality, and robustness, is central to coordinating efforts between scientists working in different places.

Some efforts have been made in this direction, and some recommendations were published to standardise metabolic exploration and reporting (Sansone et al., 2007). A recent publication (Griffin and Steinbeck, 2010), again stressed the need to make real efforts towards standardising data in metabolomics in order to build central repositories so that data can be shared by the metabolomics community and very large projects can be distributed across multiple sites, as was done for transcriptomics and proteomics approaches. The metabolomics community has not yet achieved this level of sharing and site distribution even if some databases, including NMR and MS data, are available as described in Section 1.5 (Human Metabolome database, the Madison Metabolomics database, the INTERNET database, etc.). Individual initiatives have also been published. For example, Kanani et al. (2008) proposed a typical workflow for GC-MS metabolomics analyses, using optimised derivatisation procedures, data acquisition, peak identification, and quantification. However, even if GC-MS has been used for a long time and even if extensive databases and experimental protocols are available for this technique, it is not an easy task if one considers the complexity of biological samples, the number of chemical families that have to be quantified and the number of derivatisation reactions that have to be fully controlled for optimising reaction yield in order to obtain reliable data. A comprehensive procedure has also recently been described for faecal water metabolomics analysis (Gao et al., 2009), using a GC-MS approach.

Created in 2003, the LIPID Metabolites and Pathways Strategy (LIPID MAPS) consortium was initiated by a large collaborative project funded by the NIH, and it is a good example of a coordinated multicenter effort for standardisation (Schmelzer et al., 2007) (Dennis, 2009). The objectives of the LIPID MAPS were to identify and quantify all the major and minor lipid species in mammalian species and to identify changes due to perturbations, in order to understand the role that lipids play in major diseases such as diabetes and cardiovascular events. Protocols were defined and carried out in the laboratories of the different participants, and extraction protocols were optimised for each lipid class, analysed by LC-MS in order to facilitate the sharing and comparison of the data sets, further leading to the development of biochemical pathways and interaction networks. Three hundred and forty-two lipid species in the yeast lipidome were quantified, and their changes related to specific gene deletions or growing temperatures were determined (Dennis, 2009).

By providing global biochemical information, metabolomics represents a promising way to monitor changes in compounds from the metabolism, endogenous and food metabolites. Yet, metabolomics is not limited to the physicochemical analysis of tissues and biofluids, and its development includes all upstream and downstream stages from experimental design to data analysis for a biological interpretation. Each of these steps must be developed to optimise the use of metabolomics in nutrition science.

References

Aburto, N.J., Ziolkovska, A., Hooper, L., Elliott, P., Cappuccio, F.P., Meerpohl, J.J., 2013. Effect of lower sodium intake on health: systematic review and meta-analyses. BMJ 346, f1326.

Arkin, A., Shen, P., Ross, J., 1997. A test case of correlation metric construction of a reaction pathway from measurements. Science 277, 1275–1279.

Bouatra, S., Aziat, F., Mandal, R., Guo, A.C., Wilson, M.R., Knox, C., Bjorndahl, T.C., Krishnamurthy, R., Saleem, F., Liu, P., Dame, Z.T., Poelzer, J., Huynh, J., Yallou, F.S., Psychogios, N., Dong, E., Bogumil, R., Roehring, C., Wishart, D.S., 2013. The human urine metabolome. PLoS One 8, e73076.

Brennan, L., 2013. Metabolomics in nutrition research: current status and perspectives. Biochem. Soc. Trans. 41, 670–673.

Chen, T., Cao, Y., Zhang, Y., Liu, J., Bao, Y., Wang, C., Jia, W., Zhao, A., 2013. Random forest in clinical metabolomics for phenotypic discrimination and biomarker selection. Evid. Based Complement. Alternat. Med. 2013, 298183.

Christie, W.W., Han, X., 2010. Lipid analysis: Isolation, Separation, Identification and Lipidomic Analysis. Bridgwater, England.

Dennis, E.A., 2009. Lipidomics joins the omics evolution. Proc. Natl. Acad. Sci. U. S. A. 106, 2089–2090.

Dettmer, K., Aronov, P.A., Hammock, B.D., 2007. Mass spectrometry-based metabolomics. Mass Spectrom. Rev. 26, 51–78.

Doerfler, H., Lyon, D., Nagele, T., Sun, X., Fragner, L., Hadacek, F., Egelhofer, V., Weckwerth, W., 2013. Granger causality in integrated GC-MS and LC-MS metabolomics data reveals the interface of primary and secondary metabolism. Metabolomics 9, 564–574.

Eisenreich, W., Bacher, A., 2007. Advances of high-resolution NMR techniques in the structural and metabolic analysis of plant biochemistry. Phytochemistry 68, 2799–2815.

Fahy, E., Subramaniam, S., Murphy, R.C., Nishijima, M., Raetz, C.R., Shimizu, T., Spener, F., van Meer, G., Wakelam, M.J., Dennis, E.A., 2009. Update of the LIPID MAPS comprehensive classification system for lipids. J. Lipid Res. 50 (Suppl), S9–S14.

Fave, G., Beckmann, M.E., Draper, J.H., Mathers, J.C., 2009. Measurement of dietary exposure: a challenging problem which may be overcome thanks to metabolomics? Genes Nutr. 4, 135–141.

Fienh, O., Kopka, J., Dormann, P., Altmann, T., Trethewey, R.N., Willmitzer, L., 2000. Metabolite profiling for plant functional genomics. Nat. Biotechnol. 18, 1157–1161.

Gao, X., Pujos-Guillot, E., Martin, J.F., Galan, P., Juste, C., Jia, W., Sebedio, J.L., 2009. Metabolite analysis of human fecal water by gas chromatography/mass spectrometry with ethyl chloroformate derivatization. Anal. Biochem. 393, 163–175.

German, J.B., Roberts, M.A., Fay, L., Watkins, S.M., 2002. Metabolomics and individual metabolic assessment: the next great challenge for nutrition. J. Nutr. 132, 2486–2487.

Gibney, M.J., Walsh, M., Brennan, L., Roche, H.M., German, B., van Ommen, B., 2005. Metabolomics in human nutrition: opportunities and challenges. Am. J. Clin. Nutr. 82, 497–503.

Griffin, J., Steinbeck, C., 2010. So what have data standards ever done for us? The view from metabolomics. Genome Med. 2, 38.

Hedrick, V.E., Dietrich, A.M., Estabrooks, P.A., Savla, J., Serrano, E., Davy, B.M., 2012. Dietary biomarkers: advances, limitations and future directions. Nutr. J. 11, 109.

Holman, R.T., 1996. How I got my start in lipids, and where it led me. FASEB J. 10, 931–934.

Holmes, C., McDonald, F., Jones, M., Ozdemir, V., Graham, J.E., 2010. Standardization and omics science: technical and social dimensions are inseparable and demand symmetrical study. OMICS 14, 327–332.

Idle, J.R., Gonzalez, F.J., 2007. Metabolomics. Cell Metab. 6, 348–351.

Ismail, N.A., Posma, J.M., Frost, G., Holmes, E., Garcia-Perez, I., 2013. The role of metabonomics as a tool for augmenting nutritional information in epidemiological studies. Electrophoresis 34 (19), 2776–2786, 10.1002/elps.201300066.

Johnson, C.H., Gonzalez, F.J., 2011. Challenges and opportunities of metabolomics. J. Cell. Physiol. 227 (8), 2975–2981, 10.1002/jcp.24002.

Kanani, H., Chrysanthopoulos, P.K., Klapa, M.I., 2008. Standardizing GC-MS metabolomics. J. Chromatogr. B Anal. Technol. Biomed. Life Sci. 871, 191–201.

Katajamaa, M., Oresic, M., 2007. Data processing for mass spectrometry-based metabolomics. J. Chromatogr. A 1158, 318–328.

Kenar, E., Franken, H., Forcisi, S., Wormann, K., Haring, H.U., Lehmann, R., Schmitt-Kopplin, P., Zell, A., Kohlbacher, O., 2014. Automated label-free quantification of metabolites from liquid chromatography-mass spectrometry data. Mol. Cell. Proteomics 13, 348–359.

Kuhl, C., Tautenhahn, R., Bottcher, C., Larson, T.R., Neuman, S., 2012. CAMERA: an integrated strategy for coumpound spectra extraction and annotation of liquid chromatography/mass spectrometry data sets. Anal. Chem. 84, 283–289.

Llorach, R., Garcia-Aloy, M., Tulipani, S., Vazquez-Fresno, R., Andres-Lacueva, C., 2012. Nutrimetabolomic strategies to develop new biomarkers of intake and health effects. J. Agric. Food Chem. 60 (36), 8797–8808, 10.1021/jf301142b.

Lodge, J.K., 2010. Symposium 2: modern approaches to nutritional research challenges: targeted and non-targeted approaches for metabolite profiling in nutritional research. Proc. Nutr. Soc. 69, 95–102.

Lommen, A., 2009. MetAlign: interface-driven, versatile metabolomics tool for hyphenated full-scan mass spectrometry data preprocessing. Anal. Chem. 81, 3079–3086.

Micha, R., Michas, G., Lajous, M., Mozaffarian, D., 2013. Processing of meats and cardiovascular risk: time to focus on preservatives. BMC Med. 11, 136.

Moco, S., Vervoort, J., Moco, S., Bino, R.J., De Vos, R.C.H., Bino, R., 2007. Metabolomics technologies and metabolite identification. TrAC Trends Anal. Chem. 26, 855–866.

Moco, S., Martin, F.P., Rezzi, S., 2012. A metabolomics view on gut microbiome modulation by polyphenol-rich foods. J. Proteome Res. 11 (10), 4781–4790, 10.1021/pr300581s.

Morris, M., Watkins, S.M., 2005. Focused metabolomic profiling in the drug development process: advances from lipid profiling. Curr. Opin. Chem. Biol. 9, 407–412.

Nicholson, J.K., Wilson, I.D., 1989. High resolution proton magnetic resonance spectroscopy of biological fluids. Prog. Nucl. Magn. Reson. Spectrosc. 21, 449–501.

Nicholson, J.K., Lindon, J.C., Holmes, E., 1999. 'Metabonomics': understanding the metabolic responses of living systems to pathophysiological stimuli via multivariate statistical analysis of biological NMR spectroscopic data. Xenobiotica 29, 1181–1189.

Nicholson, J.K., Connelly, J., Lindon, J.C., Holmes, E., 2002. Metabonomics: a platform for studying drug toxicity and gene function. Nat. Rev. 1, 153–161.

Oberbach, A., Bluher, M., Wirth, H., Till, H., Kovacs, P., Kullnick, Y., Schlichting, N., Tomm, J.M., Rolle-Kampczyk, U., Murugaiyan, J., Binder, H., Dietrich, A., von Bergen, M., 2011. Combined proteomic and metabolomic profiling of serum reveals association of the complement system with obesity and identifies novel markers of body fat mass changes. J. Proteome Res. 10, 4769–4788.

Pan, Z., Raftery, D., 2007. Comparing and combining NMR spectroscopy and mass spectrometry in metabolomics. Anal. Bioanal. Chem. 387, 525–527.

Peironcely, J., Rojas-Chertó, M., Tas, A., Vreeken, R., Reijmers, T., Coulier, L., Hankemeier, T., 2013. An automated pipeline for de novo metabolite identification using mass spectrometry-based metabolomics. Anal. Chem. 85, 3576–3583. http://dx.doi.org/10.1021/ac303218u.

Pellis, L., van Erk, M.J., van Ommen, B., Bakker, G.C., Hendriks, H.F., Cnubben, N.H., Kleemann, R., van Someren, E.P., Bobeldijk, I., Rubingh, C.M., Wopereis, S., 2012. Plasma metabolomics and proteomics profiling after a postprandial challenge reveal subtle diet effects on human metabolic status. Metabolomics 8, 347–359.

Psychogios, N., Hau, D.D., Peng, J., Guo, A.C., Mandal, R., Bouatra, S., Sinelnikov, I., Krishnamurthy, R., Eisner, R., Gautam, B., Young, N., Xia, J., Knox, C., Dong, E.,

Huang, P., Hollander, Z., Pedersen, T.L., Smith, S.R., Bamforth, F., Greiner, R., McManus, B., Newman, J.W., Goodfriend, T., Wishart, D.S., 2011. The human serum metabolome. PLoS One 6, e16957.
Pujos-Guillot, E., Pickering, G., Lyan, B., Ducheix, G., Brandolini-Bunlon, M., Glomot, F., Dardevet, D., Dubray, C., Papet, I., 2012. Therapeutic paracetamol treatment in older persons induces dietary and metabolic modifications related to sulfur amino acids. Age (Dordr) 34, 181–193.
Pujos-Guillot, E., Hubert, J., Martin, J.F., Lyan, B., Quintana, M., Claude, S., Chabanas, B., Rothwell, J.A., Bennetau-Pelissero, C., Scalbert, A., Comte, B., Hercberg, S., Morand, C., Galan, P., Manach, C., 2013. Mass spectrometry-based metabolomics for the discovery of biomarkers of fruit and vegetable intake: citrus fruit as a case study. J. Proteome Res. 12 (4), 1645–1659, 10.1021/pr300997c.
Reezi, S., Martin, F.-P.J., Kochhar, S., 2008. Defining personal nutrition and metabolic through metabonomics. Ernst Schering Found. Symp. Proc. 4, 251–264.
Sansone, S.A., Fan, T., Goodacre, R., Griffin, J.L., Hardy, N.W., Kaddurah-Daouk, R., Kristal, B.S., Lindon, J., Mendes, P., Morrison, N., Nikolau, B., Robertson, D., Sumner, L.W., Taylor, C., van der Werf, M., van Ommen, B., Fiehn, O., 2007. The metabolomics standards initiative. Nat. Biotechnol. 25, 846–848.
Scalbert, A., Brennan, L., Fiehn, O., Hankemeier, T., Kristal, B.S., van Ommen, B., Pujos-Guillot, E., Verheij, E., Wishart, D., Wopereis, S., 2009. Mass-spectrometry-based metabolomics: limitations and recommendations for future progress with particular focus on nutrition research. Metabolomics 5, 435–458.
Schmelzer, K., Fahy, E., Subramaniam, S., Dennis, E.A., 2007. The lipid maps initiative in lipidomics. Methods Enzymol. 432, 171–183.
Simopoulos, A.P., 2013. Dietary omega-3 fatty acid deficiency and high fructose intake in the development of metabolic syndrome, brain metabolic abnormalities, and non-alcoholic fatty liver disease. Nutrients 5, 2901–2923.
Smilowitz, J.T., Zivkovic, A.M., Wan, Y.J., Watkins, S.M., Nording, M.L., Hammock, B.D., German, J.B., 2013. Nutritional lipidomics: molecular metabolism, analytics, and diagnostics. Mol. Nutr. Food Res. 57, 1319–1335.
Solanky, K.S., Bailey, N.J., Beckwith-Hall, B.M., Davis, A., Bingham, S., Holmes, E., Nicholson, J.K., Cassidy, A., 2003. Application of biofluid 1H nuclear magnetic resonance-based metabonomic techniques for the analysis of the biochemical effects of dietary isoflavones on human plasma profile. Anal. Biochem. 323, 197–204.
Steuer, R., Kurths, J., Fiehn, O., Weckwerth, W., 2003. Interpreting correlations in metabolomic networks. Biochem. Soc. Trans. 31, 1476–1478.
Walsh, M.C., Brennan, L., Malthouse, J.P., Roche, H.M., Gibney, M.J., 2006. Effect of acute dietary standardization on the urinary, plasma, and salivary metabolomic profiles of healthy humans. Am. J. Clin. Nutr. 84, 531–539.
Wang, Y., Ma, L., Sun, Y., Yang, L., Yue, H., Liu, S., 2013. Metabonomics study on the hot syndrome of traditional Chinese medicine by rapid resolution liquid chromatography combined with quadrupole time-of-flight tandem mass spectrometry. Arch. Pharm. Res. 37 (7), 899–906, 10.1007/s12272-013-0250-z.
Weckwerth, W., 2003. Metabolomics in systems biology. Annu. Rev. Plant Biol. 54, 669–689.
Wilson, I.D., Plumb, R., Granger, J., Major, H., Williams, R., Lenz, E.M., 2005. HPLC-MS-based methods for the study of metabonomics. J. Chromatogr. B Anal. Technol. Biomed. Life Sci. 817, 67–76.
Wishart, D.S., 2007. Current progress in computational metabolomics. Brief. Bioinform. 8, 279–293.

Wishart, D.S., Lewis, M.J., Morrissey, J.A., Flegel, M.D., Jeroncic, K., Xiong, Y., Cheng, D., Eisner, R., Gautam, B., Tzur, D., Sawhney, S., Bamforth, F., Greiner, R., Li, L., 2008. The human cerebrospinal fluid metabolome. J. Chromatogr. B 871, 164–173.

Wishart, D.S., Jewison, T., Guo, A.C., Wilson, M., Knox, C., Liu, Y., Djoumbou, Y., Mandal, R., Aziat, F., Dong, E., Bouatra, S., Sinelnikov, I., Arndt, D., Xia, J., Liu, P., Yallou, F., Bjorndahl, T., Perez-Pineiro, R., Eisner, R., Allen, F., Neveu, V., Greiner, R., Scalbert, A., 2013. HMDB 3.0—the human metabolome database in 2013. Nucleic Acids Res. 41, D801–D807.

Yang, Y., Cruickshank, C., Armstrong, M., Mahaffey, S., Reisdorph, R., Reisdorph, N., 2013. New sample preparation approach for mass spectrometry-based profiling of plasma results in improved coverage of metabolome. J. Chromatogr. 1300, 217–226.

Zhang, A.H., Sun, H., Han, Y., Yan, G.L., Yuan, Y., Song, G.C., Yuan, X.X., Xie, N., Wang, X. J., 2013. Ultraperformance liquid chromatography-mass spectrometry based comprehensive metabolomics combined with pattern recognition and network analysis methods for characterization of metabolites and metabolic pathways from biological data sets. Anal. Chem. 85, 7606–7612.

Zivkovic, A.M., German, J.B., 2009. Metabolomics for assessment of nutritional status. Curr. Opin. Clin. Nutr. Metab. Care 12 (5), 501–507.

Metabolic profiling as a tool in nutritional research: key methodological issues

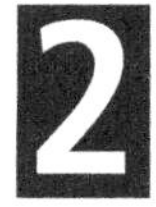

S.E. Richards[1], E. Holmes[2]
[1]Nottingham Trent University, Nottingham, United Kingdom; [2]Imperial College, London, United Kingdom

2.1 Introduction

Understanding the contribution of gene–environment interactions, and in particular the contribution of nutritional factors as drivers for adverse or protective effects in the maintenance of health and in the aetiology of disease, is of prime importance if we are to reduce the global burden of disease in both Western and developing world populations. An array of postgenomic technologies (transcriptomics, proteomics, metabonomics, etc.) have been applied to characterise pathological conditions such as obesity, diabetes, intestinal disorders, and neurodegeneration in animal models and in man, with a view to improving our understanding of the aetiology of disease. These same technologies have also been applied to monitoring therapeutic interventions, including surgical, pharmaceutical, and nutritional, with a view to discovering and implementing new means of therapeutic management.

Of the "omics" technologies, metabonomics provides the most accessible window in investigating the impact of nutritional interventions on human health since metabolic profiles of readily obtainable biofluids such as blood, plasma, and urine carry information relating to both genetic and environmental influences, including contributions from the diet and microbial modulation of dietary components (Stella et al., 2006). Metabolic profiling relies upon the use of high-resolution spectroscopic techniques, typically either nuclear magnetic resonance (NMR) spectroscopy or mass spectrometry (MS)-based platforms, to generate comprehensive low-molecular-weight profiles of biofluids, tissues, or cells that subsequently can be modelled and interpreted using multivariate statistics.

In this chapter, we explore the potential of metabolic profiling as a tool in nutritional research, taking examples from a range of nutritional applications and highlighting the potential of emerging technology.

2.2 Key issues in nutritional research

It is universally acknowledged that nutrition plays a central role in the maintenance of good health. Without good nutrition, the body is prone to a myriad of diseases

Metabolomics as a Tool in Nutrition Research. http://dx.doi.org/10.1016/B978-1-78242-084-2.00002-2

stemming from nutrient deficiency or imbalance. Both over- and undernutrition represent major problems in today's world with profound consequences on health, social, and economic impact. Many developed and developing countries acknowledge an alarming increase in obesity and its comorbidities, with expectation that this trend will increase for the foreseeable future. The prevalence of overweight/obesity and adverse (prehypertensive/hypertensive) blood pressure (BP) levels are at epidemic proportions worldwide. Adverse BP is a major risk factor for stroke and coronary heart disease, the leading cause of death worldwide. Obesity is a major risk factor for type 2 diabetes, insulin resistance, related metabolic disorders, and cardiovascular diseases (CVDs) (Basu and Millett, 2013).

Recently discovered genetic determinants of body weight and obesity, most notably common variants in the *FTO* and *MC4R* genes (Cauchi et al., 2009), explain only a small proportion of the body mass index (BMI) population variance. Environmental factors are overwhelmingly important in explaining the trends and differences in the levels of these risk factors and related disease rates across populations. High sodium intake, inadequate potassium, high BMI, low levels of physical activity, and high alcohol consumption are established risk factors for high BP (Farinaro et al., 1991; Shay et al., 2012).

An enormous body of research has been conducted on "healthy" diets such as the Mediterranean and DASH (Dietary Approaches to Stop Hypertension) diets and has shown that adherence to such diets can reduce the risk of CVD and cancers (Asemi et al., 2014; Schwingshackl and Hoffmann, 2014). Other areas of nutritional research have focused on the effect of antioxidants on health, and many studies have explored the effects of antioxidant-rich foods such as berries, seeds, and other phytochemicals on various diseases. Several studies highlight the positive effect of phytochemicals on neurodegenerative conditions including Parkinson's disease and Alzheimer's disease (Kita et al., 2014; Strathearn et al., 2014; Vepsäläinen et al., 2013).

The role of the gut microbiota in nutritional modification, either in respect to the aetiology and development of disease or as factors to be considered in calculating disease risk, is currently under scrutiny. In addition to their primary function in host immunity, the microbiota are known to be associated with harvesting of energy and metabolism of xenobiotics, including nutrients, and have been implicated in metabolic signalling (Fearnside et al., 2008; Ley et al., 2005; Turnbaugh et al., 2009). The administration of pre- and probiotics has been shown to alter plasma lipids favourably, in addition to inducing changes in a range of urinary gut microbial metabolites (Martin et al., 2009).

The inseparable relationship between the mammalian host, its microbiome, and the diet begins at birth. Infants acquire their microbiota from their mothers. Subsequent introduction of breast milk or bottle milk further diversifies the microbiome. The effects of early nutrition extend well beyond childhood and a growing body of evidence suggests that breast-feeding plays a protective role for several noncommunicable diseases and conditions such as obesity, type 2 diabetes, and heart disease (Kelishadi and Farajian, 2014). As the human grows, nutrition continues to be of prime importance in the maintenance of health and becomes critical in times where the body is challenged such as in severely ill patients and the elderly. It is widely accepted that the importance of correct nutrition is paramount in critically ill patients. The elderly also represent a vulnerable population in which good nutrition can contribute to overall health and quality of life (Brüssow, 2013).

Nutritional research, therefore, has a wide scope and involves multiple layers of analyses targeted at different aspects such as food composition; investigation of the effects of nutrients or foods at the genomic, proteomic, epigenomic, metabonomic, or even metagenomic levels; and more recently the interaction of nutrients with the gut microbiota. Other obvious links between the triad of nutrition, human health, and the gut microbiota are found in the connection between specific foods and adverse responses (Faria et al., 2013).

2.3 The role of genomics, proteomics, metabolomics, and metagenomics in nutritional research

For many decades, medicine and science have been studied in academic silos with researchers specialising in disciplines such as immunology or cell biology. However, increasingly, it is becoming apparent that the human being functions as a system, and in order to understand the cause and effect of diseases or interventions, we must develop a more holistic approach and learn how the different bio-organisational levels communicate with each other.

A prime example is the generation of neuroactive chemicals from dietary components in the intestine by the gut microbiota, which are subsequently absorbed into the circulation and reach the brain to produce an effect. Thus, an event in the gut is translated to an effect in the brain. For example, certain tyramine-containing foods, including cheese and chocolate, have been associated with migraine and with causing nightmares. Since these biological events do not occur in isolation, we need to sample the whole system at multiple levels, ideally in multiple locations.

A major barrier to translating nutritional interventions into clinical settings is the lack of validated biomarkers of intake and efficacy. Beyond the relatively crude tools of dietary recall, food diaries, and traditional epidemiological approaches, the postgenomic technologies also offer new avenues and opportunities for nutritional research in explaining individual differences in response to foods and nutrients and paving the way for personalised nutrition. The nutriomics fields combine traditional nutritional practices and data collection with high-throughput genotyping and phenotyping, molecular epidemiology, and bioinformatics.

Nutrigenomics was the first of the nutriomics fields to emerge and assesses the effect of nutrients on gene expression profiles, exploring how an individual's genotype can influence absorption, distribution, excretion, or activity of specific nutrients. Although genetics is an important determinant of CVD, it is clear that environment also plays a strong role. Here, some progress has been made in studying the interaction between diet and disease risk, and it is known that omega-3 polyunsaturated fatty acids interact with the genetic landscape to influence the development of CVD (Merched and Chan, 2013). It is well established that nutritional factors can alter the epigenome and that they can be used to modulate cancer risk (Hardy and Tollefsbol, 2011; Papoutsis et al., 2010).

Nutriproteomics is an emerging field that characterises molecular and cellular changes in protein expression in response to nutrients and investigates the interaction of proteins with food nutrients (Ganesh and Hettiarachchy, 2012). Sweet cherries are known to have beneficial effects on inflammatory conditions such as gout. In a study by Kelley et al., sweet cherries were found to reduce several markers associated with inflammation including C-reactive protein, ferritin, and some of the cytokines (Kelley et al., 2013).

Metabonomics/metabolomics involves the dynamic and multivariate characterisation of biofluids or tissues in response to a biological stimulus (Nicholson et al., 1999). It involves the measurement of biofluids and tissues using spectroscopic methods such as NMR spectroscopy and MS to generate information-rich metabolic profiles. Due to the complexity of these metabolic profiles, computational modelling is used to analyse and interpret the data and to extract candidate biomarkers of disease or to monitor how a patient responds to a therapeutic intervention, including the modulation of nutritional intake. The term nutrimetabolomics refers to the direct or indirect effect of the diet on metabolism. The role of metabolic profiling in nutritional studies is explored further in the following section.

Metagenomics or *microbiomics* relate to the genetic composition and functional capacity of microbial communities. In the context of nutrition, it is the gut microbiome and its capacity for modification of foods and nutrients that are the most relevant. As mentioned previously, the gut microbiota play an important role as intermediaries between nutrition and host metabolic response. The measurement of faecal bacteria is generally via either 16S rRNA or metagenomic profiling, although fluorescent *in situ* hybridisation is used occasionally to profile the ecology of bacterial communities. The faecal bacterial profiles have limitations in that they do not accurately reflect the community structure or activity of the bacterial communities residing in the intestinal mucosa. However, despite these limitations, many studies have been able to show a relationship between the faecal microbiome and nutritional status (see Chapter 8 for detailed discussion).

2.4 Applications of metabolomics in nutrition-related research

As stated previously, metabolic profiling (metabonomics/metabolomics) has an advantage over other omics in that it can profile chemicals deriving from the food components themselves and map the metabolic effect that a food or nutrient has on the individual. The metabolic profile acts like a mirror that reflects an image of the total system, a looking glass that can capture and display the whole ecosystem of the human body.

The downside of capturing this extra information is that the profiles are a complex mixture of signals deriving from the individual, their diet, other xenobiotic intake, and the gut microbiome and hence sophisticated mathematical modelling is required to handle the data complexity and to assign specific metabolites to their source of origin. Because of this inherent complexity, much of the research in nutrimetabolomics has been carried out in animal models where genetic and environmental background can be better controlled than in human populations.

Metabolic profiling has been used in a wide range of nutritional studies. Examples include: authentication of food composition (Caligiani et al., 2014), identification of adulteration of foods (Alonso-Salces et al., 2010), characterisation of response to nutrients or foods (Stella et al., 2006), validation of nutrient/food intake (Heinzmann et al., 2010), evaluation of the use of functional foods in various diseases (Saulnier et al., 2009), prediction of response to nutritional interventions (Clayton et al., 2009; Wiseman, 2000), and mapping the interaction between food-derived chemicals and the gut microbiota (Claus and Swann, 2013; Heinzmann et al., 2012). It has also been used to assess food quality, safety, and adulteration (Alonso-Salces et al., 2010; Cagliani et al., 2013; Cajka et al., 2014; Caligiani et al., 2014; Wang et al., 2004).

A tantalising proposition for metabolic profiling is the ability to verify the intake of certain foods, in order to validate 24 h recall data or food diaries. For some food components, for example, ascorbic acid (vitamin C) and proline betaine, both found in relatively high concentrations in citrus fruits, metabolism is limited, and it is excreted largely unmetabolised, except for micrometabolites. These compounds can serve as good indicators of recent consumption of these foods and may even be sensitive enough to give an indication of the quantity of food consumed (Heinzmann et al., 2010). Other chemicals are more broadly distributed among the groups of foods. *S*-methyl-L-cysteine sulphoxide (Edmands et al., 2011) is, for example, found in high concentrations in the cruciferous vegetables and, in lower levels, in the alliums and is thought to contribute to the anticarcinogenic properties attributed to cruciferous vegetables (Alvarez-Jubete et al., 2014).

2.5 The use of metabolomics to assess the effects of diet on health

Characterising the metabolic consequences of dietary interventions is perhaps the most widely developed application of metabolic profiling in nutrition. There are plenty of examples in the literature of studies evaluating the effect of single foods or nutrients both in human models and in animal models. The main groups of food studies using this technology are fruits and polyphenols (see Chapter 9 for a detailed discussion), natural products, wheat and fibre, meat and fish, milk products, and functional foods such as pre- and probiotics.

2.5.1 *Natural products*

Both green tea and black tea are purported to have a beneficial effect on health. Compounds such as epicatechins and gallates can be captured in urine spectra. Rodent studies not only have been used to demonstrate the bioavailability of epicatechins from green tea but also showed metabolic changes post consumption including a decrease in the excretion of tricarboxylic acid cycle intermediates and taurine (Solanky et al., 2003). Another NMR-based study measured the direct effects of green tea and green tea extracts on body weight, lipids, and lipid peroxidation in individuals with metabolic syndrome. In addition to a correlation between green tea consumption and weight loss, the NMR profiles revealed a decreasing trend in low-density lipoprotein (LDL) cholesterol and LDL/HDL (high-density lipoprotein) versus controls (Basu et al., 2010).

2.5.2 Wheat and fibre

Other examples of nutritional metabolic profiling studies include a comparison of postprandial differences in metabolism after consumption of white bread versus rye bread, which has a better effect on insulin demand (Bondia-Pons et al., 2011). Several differences in the plasma profile were observed including increased plasma citrate, phenylalanine, and ribitol following rye bread consumption with lower levels of norleucine and picolinic acid. Another study investigating the effect of high-fibre rye bread on the metabolic profiles of postmenopausal women showed modulation of plasma concentrations of ribitol, ribonic acid, and indoleacetic acid (Lankinen et al., 2011). The ribonic acid was correlated to tryptophan, implicating the serotonin pathway in triggering a satiety response.

2.5.3 Meat and fish

Moderate to high consumption of red meat has been associated with adverse health effects with particular association with colon cancer (Pericleous et al., 2013). Various metabolic profiling studies have evaluated the effects of meat versus vegetarian diets and have found increased urinary excretion of creatine, carnosine, acylcarnitine, methylhistidine, and trimethylamine-*N*-oxide in meat eaters, whereas 4-hydroxyphenylacetate and other gut microbial metabolites are associated with urine metabolites of vegetarian (Adlercreutz et al., 1993; Dragsted, 2010; Stella et al., 2006; Yap et al., 2010).

2.5.4 Milk products

Metabolic profiling studies have shown systematic changes in the urinary and plasma metabolic profiles after consumption of milk and dairy products. In a comparison of children supplemented with either milk or meat protein, milk supplementation was found to alter short-chain fatty acid profiles in the plasma and to reduce urinary excretion of hippurate, suggestive of a dietary effect on the gut microbiota (Bertram et al., 2007). Breast milk contains oligosaccharides that serve to feed the gut bacteria rather than the human host and the initial colonisation of the host sets the template for downstream metabolism. Supplementation of human baby microflora-colonised mice with galactosyl-oligosaccharides showed that these milk-derived prebiotics induced a reduction of plasma triglycerides and modulated bile acids (Martin et al., 2009). Metabolic profiling can also be applied directly to the basic characterisation of milk composition (Praticò et al., 2014), similarities in human versus primate milk composition (O'Sullivan et al., 2013), and differences in preterm versus formula milk (Marincola et al., 2012).

2.5.5 *Functional foods*

The role of functional foods in promoting health and improving disease has gained attention from the scientific community and the media. Various claims concerning the efficacy or pre- and probiotics have been made and much of the literature is contradictory. Products such as yoghourts containing live bacteria, raw wheat bran, and inulin have become popular yet limited research has been carried out to substantiate the claims. Animal models that have characterised pre- and probiotics have shown structured metabolic effects reflecting gut bacterial activity, particularly when administered to germ-free animals (Merrifield et al., 2013). Prebiotics such as inulin have also been shown to have an effect on the chemical composition of tissues and biofluids (Duan et al., 2013).

Various hospitals promote the administration of pro- and prebiotics to patients postoperatively. The exact effect of these functional foods is debatable, but since most patients receive a prophylactic dose of antibiotic prior to undergoing surgery, the pre-/probiotics is thought to aid the restoration of a healthy gut microbiome. For some conditions, for example, irritable bowel syndrome, there is an association with low relative concentrations of bifidobacteria, which when supplemented as either a probiotics or prebiotics that stimulates bifidobacteria ameliorates the symptoms (Kerckhoffs et al., 2009).

A multitude of studies have also reported on whole diet modulation, such as caloric restriction or weight-loss diets (Bales and Kraus, 2013). Caloric restriction has been shown to prolong life and reduce inflammatory conditions in many organisms ranging from worms and fruit flies to primates (De Guzman et al., 2013; Wang et al., 2007; Zhang et al., 2012).

2.6 Methods for mapping dietary patterns

In reality, the human diet is complicated and holistic approaches to mapping the effect of dietary patterns rather than single nutrients or food components will give a more realistic picture of the influence of the diet on health. Diets such as the Atkins and South Beach have become popular. One of the newer popular diets is the New Nordic Diet. This is essentially a "healthy" diet advocating the use of fresh and seasonal ingredients, more fruits, grains, and whole foods with a reduction in meat content. LC-MS analysis of 181 individuals randomised to either an average Danish diet (ADD) or a New Nordic Diet (NND) generated predictive models for dietary pattern based on a panel of 52 metabolites. The classification of the ADD was more accurate than NND due to the variation introduced by seasonal food included in the NND, and the fact that due to the dietary constraints of the NND, dietary compliance was lower (Andersen et al., 2014). A study of a murine model of neonatal malnourishment proposed plasma 2-hydroxyisobutyrate (threefold-elevated) and urobilinogen (11-fold increase) as markers in undernourished mice. Differential faecal excretion of deoxycholate also implicated an altered gut microbiome in the malnourished animals (Preidis et al., 2014).

An alternative approach to mapping the diet onto metabolism is to investigate the effect of diet in a free-living population where dietary information has been obtained, usually by either 24 h dietary recall or food diaries. In the INTERMAP (International Study of Macronutrients and Micronutrients and Blood Pressure) study, ~4800 across the United States, the United Kingdom, China, and Japan were interviewed by trained nutritionists to provide 24 h recall information and urine samples were obtained on two separate visits. The premise of the study was to establish the association between diet and hypertension and to explore population differences.

NMR spectroscopic analysis of the urine samples showed population differences with clear differentiation of the Chinese, Japanese, and American populations, reflecting differences in diet and lifestyle (Holmes et al., 2008). Alanine and pentanoic acid were, for example, characteristic of the Chinese urine samples, high trimethylamine-*N*-oxide, reflecting high fish intake, and low hippurate levels were characteristic of the urine of the Japanese population.

Metabolome-wide association studies (MWAS) offer a powerful new means of discovering novel molecular biomarkers and metabolic pathways underlying disease risk. This approach is analogous and complementary to high-throughput genomic screening in genome-wide association studies (GWAS), which have led to deeper understanding of genetic variation underlying common disease. The development of the concept of MWAS, involving the broad, nonselective analysis and statistical characterisation of metabolic phenotypes in relation to epidemiological end points and risk factors, takes its place alongside GWAS and provides a framework for generating novel testable metabolic and physiological hypotheses that relate to disease aetiology. The utility of the MWAS approach has been demonstrated for discovery of novel biomarkers associated with BP variation (Holmes et al., 2008) where formate and alanine were found to correlate directly, while hippurate was inversely correlated.

An important strength of the MWAS approach lies in its scalability and capacity to accomplish comprehensive mapping of population phenotypes and the linkage of phenotypic variation to many types of disease risk factors. In order to assign candidate biomarkers generated from MWAS studies with confidence, the metabolome-wide significance level was developed, which is a combination of permutation and assignment rules (Chadeau-Hyam et al., 2010). The examples of metabolic profiling applications described here represent a snapshot of the nutritional studies performed to date and open a window onto systems biology approaches to understanding the role of nutrition in health.

An obvious route to gaining information at a broader systems level is to correlate GWAS and MWAS data matrices harnessing the power of large-scale epidemiological studies. Some smaller-scale nutritional studies have begun to approach this systems-level analysis. As an example, a GWAS study on 265 individuals, building on the fact that trimethylamine (associated with fish intake) is associated with a microbial gene PYROXD2, confirmed the association and further proposed an association between *N*-acetylated compounds and the ALMS1/NAT8 locus, driven by SNPs in the ALMS1 gene (Montoliu et al., 2013).

2.7 Observational and interventional studies into the effects of diet and nutrition on health

Investigations into the effects of nutrition tend to fall into

- observational (epidemiological) studies
- interventional studies.

Both types of approaches present significant analytic challenges associated with metabolic profiling.

Epidemiological studies typically sample from many hundreds of individuals and are more often cross-sectional than longitudinal. The variation attributed to genetic and environmental factors in humans is vast, and since rarely do we have the luxury of using an individual as their own control, the variation attributed to specific nutrient intakes is difficult to deconvolve from other sources of variation. Here, we are relying on the fact that over the whole population sampled, this extraneous variation should be largely random. The lack of accurate dietary intake assessment in free-living populations makes accurate estimation of how diet is associated with specific disease risk difficult. Typically, studies employ methods such as food diaries or 24 h recall data, both of which are prone to underreporting and inaccuracies.

One approach to improving dietary accuracy is to calculate, and correct for, the total energy expenditure but this is often impractical, as it requires knowledge of resting and physical energy expenditure and the total thermal energy consumption. Given that the measurement of total energy consumption requires calorimetry to be carried out in a defined apparatus, this approach is rarely used. Thus, among the biggest roadblocks to associating food intake with metabolic profiles are as follows: How accurate is the dietary data and what is the effect of the time lag between food intake and its signature as captured in the serum or urine? There are acute markers of dietary intake: proline betaine for citrus fruit, ethyl glucuronide for alcohol, carnitines and carnosines for meat, etc. However, these markers are of little value if chronic dietary exposure is the objective of a study.

Nutritional intervention studies offer more control over food intake versus metabolic output where participants remain in a controlled environment for the duration of the study and the nutrient content of food consumed is carefully monitored, particularly when such studies are carried out in metabolism suites. On a practical level, such studies are limited to a small number of participants and are costly to run. More often, nutritional intervention studies are carried out in free-living populations and rely on the compliance of the participants to achieve accurate results. Given the inherent variation in human metabolite profiles, it is therefore essential to carry out a careful study design before embarking on any analysis.

2.8 Analytical methods

Metabolomic analysis involves the qualitative and quantitative analysis of a diverse range of low-molecular mass compounds over a wide range of concentrations. Metabolic profiling therefore requires very high levels of robustness and accuracy from analytic methods. No one analytic platform can meet all these requirements. The most common techniques used are:

- MS combined with gas chromatography (GC) or liquid chromatography (LC)
- nuclear magnetic resonance (NMR).

These are discussed below.

MS allows the sensitive quantitative determination of metabolites (Wachsmuth et al., 2013). However, MS has a number of disadvantages. The matrix coextracted with the analyte can alter the signal response, resulting in poor accuracy and reproducibility. MS also cannot distinguish between isobaric and isomeric species that yield similar profiles. As a result, MS has been coupled with high-performance separation techniques such as LC and GC using a variety of methods to ionise analytes.

LC is preferred for semi- or nonvolative analytes that can be dissolved in a suitable solvent. An LC assembly consists of a pumping system for one or more solvents that carries the analyte mixture through the LC column. Following separation, analytes are detected and a chromatogram produced. Detection methods include full UV/visible spectra data acquisition using a diode-array detector for fluorescence detection and electrochemical detection. Selective detection is provided by these methods or tandem MS in multiple reaction monitoring mode. Selectivity and sensitivity can be further increased by analyte enrichment methods such as solid-phase extraction or combining different separation mechanisms with different stationary and mobile phases. Coupling of columns of different selectivity further increases the chances of identifying compounds of similar physiochemical properties.

GC is preferred for volatile analytes. A typical extraction step used is headspace solid-phase microextraction (HS-SPME). SPME uses a fibre coated with a stationary phase (either a liquid polymer or a solid sorbent) that extracts the analytes. A technique such as comprehensive two-dimensional GC uses two capillary columns for separation. Separation in the first column is driven by differences in vapour pressure. Separation in the second column arises from the different strengths and types of polar interactions with the stationary phase. Time-of-flight mass analysers are used to record the narrow peaks (which give high detection sensitivity) created by the separation processes. Electron ionisation is used to generate fragment mass spectra for analysis.

NMR is a robust, high-throughput analytic platform characterised by speed, reproducibility and less need for sample preparation (Sotelo and Slupsky, 2013). NMR involves bombarding the targeted nuclei with radio frequency pulses produced by a strong electromagnetic coil. The most common type is ^{1}H-NMR given the abundance of this proton in most molecules. The configuration of electrons around the target nuclei will either augment (deshield) or oppose (shield) the external field around the nuclei, resulting in frequency changes known as chemical shift. In addition, the arrangement of nuclei within a molecule creates distinctive patterns known as scalar coupling. The combination of chemical shift and scalar coupling means that each molecule in an NMR spectrum produces a unique magnetic signature that enables it to be identified within a complex compound. Advances in NMR technology include advanced pulse sequences (which can help to amplify NMR signals), cyroprobes (which lower the temperature of the probe, thereby reducing electronic and thermal interference), microprobes (for smaller volume samples), and stronger magnets that increase the sensitivity of NMR.

These techniques have allowed metabolomic analysis to reach a high level of robustness and automation. Interlaboratory comparisons of metabolomic analysis for both NMR and MS techniques have shown good levels of consistency. Fully automated NMR and MS systems have now been developed. To ensure the robustness of high-throughput methods, statistical techniques such as multivariate analysis are used to assess the reproducibility of analytic methods and identify discriminating variables corresponding to metabolites in metabolomic data sets. Effective sample preparation is also essential.

2.9 Issues in analysing samples

Biological samples are typically composed of thousands of chemicals that derive from multiple sources. Furthermore, each type of biofluid sample carries different information sets (Figure 2.1) on different ranges of molecules and pathways representing

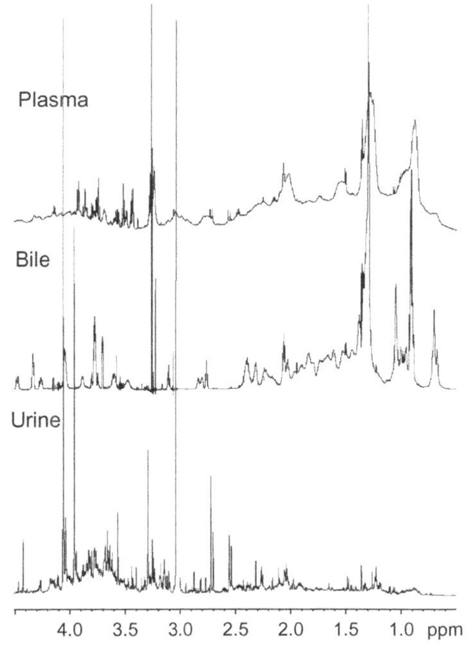

Figure 2.1 ^{1}H-NMR spectra of urine, plasma and bile showing different metabolic profiles.

different systemic timescales (plasma provides a snapshot of metabolism), whereas chemicals in urine are concentrated by the renal tubules and are time-averaged because of collection and storage in the bladder. There are also multiple complex physicochemical interactions and differences in analytic matrix properties that not only determine how samples need to be prepared and analysed but also carry other types of dynamic diagnostic information that is not revealed by simple (molecular identity and concentration) compositional analysis.

NMR spectroscopic approaches do not disturb these complex perturbations in dynamic physicochemical interactions between molecules in biofluids, whereas this occurs of necessity in MS. However, dynamic chemical features have received relatively little attention from the point of view of diagnostics in comparison with purely compositional biomarker analysis despite the fact that some biofluids are highly reactive postcollection. For instance, saliva contains high concentrations of enzymes, which can continue to biochemically degrade samples after collection. Spectroscopic analysis of biofluid samples reflects their complexity and the resulting profiles contain a myriad of overlapping signals. Each chemical entity produces a specific, and in the best case scenario, unique signature in the spectral profile but annotation can be difficult due to the fact that each chemical will typically generate more than one signal.

In the case of ^{1}H-NMR spectroscopy, each proton environment on a molecule will generate a unique signal, and it is possible that two independent compounds will generate signals at the same chemical shift. For example, betaine (associated with choline metabolism) and trimethylamine-*N*-oxide both produce a singlet at 3.27 ppm at pH 7.0 and the CH_3 signal from creatine and creatinine often partially overlap. The expert user will be able to distinguish whether the sample contains betaine, trimethylamine-*N*-oxide, or both by using the additional information that betaine has a second signal at 3.90 ppm and that the signals at 3.27 and 3.9 ppm should reflect the number of contributing protons to each group in a ratio of 9:2.

Some software packages such as Chenomics and BATMAN (Hao et al., 2012) have attempted to use curve-fitting algorithms to achieve automated annotation, but these programmes do not fully accommodate the complexity of biofluid spectra and still rely on human intervention.

With MS, particularly when coupled with a chromatographic separation phase, the problem of signal overlap is not as great. However, MS data have their own problems and chemicals tend to fragment or form adducts resulting in multiple signals reporting on the same metabolite, which can make quantification difficult, without addition of labelled standards. Similarly, ion suppression is common in samples that have a complex chemical matrix, which can also be partially resolved by the addition of labelled samples in targeted assays in which the metabolites of interest are preidentified. Another issue is that after intake of a food or nutrient, it tends to get metabolised, either by endogenous metabolism or by cometabolism with the gut microbiota. Thus, a single starting chemical may translate into many different metabolites and signals in the biofluid.

In order to identify food-derived components, structural elucidation techniques, including multidimensional NMR spectroscopy, MS/MS or MS^n, and hyphenation of LC/NMR/MS, have proven useful (Dear et al., 2000). An example of two-dimensional NMR, for structure elucidation, is given in Figure 2.2. More recently,

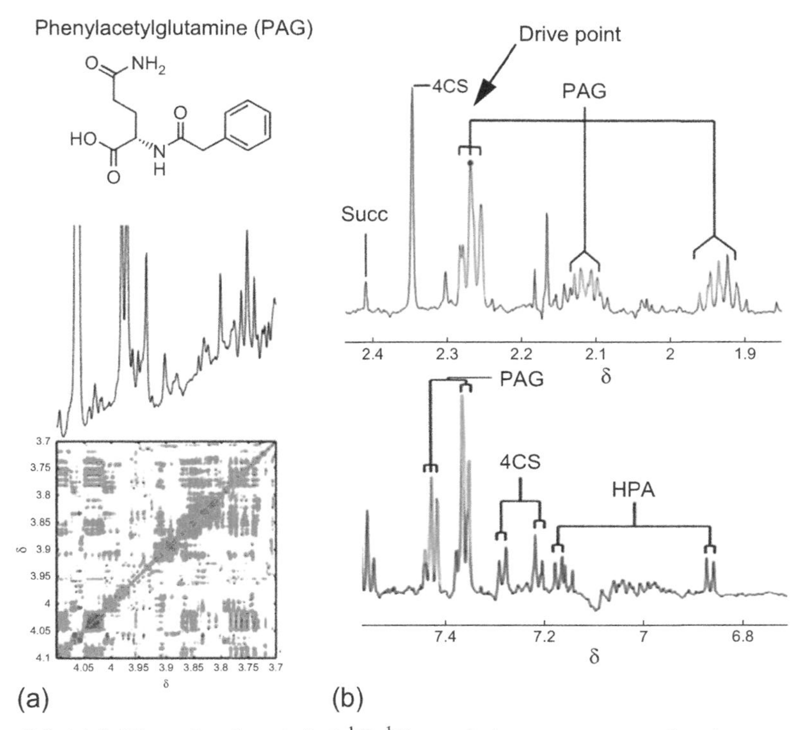

Figure 2.2 (a) 2-Dimensional statistical $^1H-^1H$ correlation spectroscopy showing connectivities and (b) 1-dimensional reconstruction of the spectrum using the phenylacetylglutamine resonance at 2.26 ppm as a drive point to identify other proton environments on the same molecule using Pearson's correlation.

statistical total correlation spectroscopy (Cloarec et al., 2005), a statistical correlation method for identifying signals relating to the same molecule or for identifying signals from molecules sharing pathway connectivities, has been developed and has shown particular utility for NMR data (Figure 2.2). These tools form part of the suite of chemometric techniques extensively used in omic analysis. These methods are briefly described in Chapter 3.

References

Adlercreutz, H., Fotsis, T., Lampe, J., Wähälä, K., Mäkelä, T., Brunow, G., Hase, T., 1993. Quantitative determination of lignans and isoflavonoids in plasma of omnivorous and vegetarian women by isotope dilution gas chromatography-mass spectrometry. Scand. J. Clin. Lab. Invest. Suppl. 215, 5–18, PubMed PMID: 8392221.

Alonso-Salces, R.M., Moreno-Rojas, J.M., Holland, M.V., Reniero, F., Guillou, C., Héberger, K., 2010. Virgin olive oil authentication by multivariate analyses of 1H NMR fingerprints and delta13C and delta2H data. J. Agric. Food Chem. 58 (9), 5586–5596. http://dx.doi.org/10.1021/jf903989b, PubMed PMID: 20373822.

Alvarez-Jubete, L., Smyth, T.J., Valverde, J., Rai, D.K., Barry-Ryan, C., 2014. Simultaneous determination of sulphoraphane and sulphoraphane nitrile in Brassica vegetables using ultra-performance liquid chromatography with tandem mass spectrometry. Phytochem. Anal. 25 (2), 141–146. http://dx.doi.org/10.1002/pca.2480, Epub 2013 Oct 16. PubMed PMID: 24449540.

Andersen, M.B., Rinnan, A., Manach, C., Poulsen, S.K., Pujos-Guillot, E., Larsen, T.M., Astrup, A., Dragsted, L.O., 2014. Untargeted metabolomics as a screening tool for estimating compliance to a dietary pattern. J. Proteome Res. 13, 1405–1418, PubMed PMID: 24444418.

Asemi, Z., Samimi, M., Tabassi, Z., Esmaillzadeh, A., 2014. The effect of DASH diet on pregnancy outcomes in gestational diabetes: a randomized controlled clinical trial. Eur. J. Clin. Nutr. 68, 490–495. http://dx.doi.org/10.1038/ejcn.2013.296, PubMed PMID: 24424076.

Bales, C.W., Kraus, W.E., 2013. Caloric restriction: implications for human cardiometabolic health. J. Cardiopulm. Rehabil. Prev. 33 (4), 201–208. http://dx.doi.org/10.1097/HCR.0b013e318295019e, PMID: 23748374; PubMed Central PMCID: PMC3696577.

Basu, S., Millett, C., 2013. Social epidemiology of hypertension in middle-income countries: determinants of prevalence, diagnosis, treatment, and control in the WHO SAGE study. Hypertension 62 (1), 18–26. http://dx.doi.org/10.1161/HYPERTENSIONAHA.113.01374.

Basu, A., Sanchez, K., Leyva, M.J., Wu, M., Betts, N.M., Aston, C.E., Lyons, T.J., 2010. Green tea supplementation affects body weight, lipids, and lipid peroxidation in obese subjects with metabolic syndrome. J. Am. Coll. Nutr. 29 (1), 31–40, PubMed PMID: 20595643.

Bertram, H.C., Hoppe, C., Petersen, B.O., Duus, J.Ø., Mølgaard, C., Michaelsen, K.F., 2007. An NMR-based metabonomic investigation on effects of milk and meat protein diets given to 8-year-old boys. Br. J. Nutr. 97 (4), 758–763, PubMed PMID: 17349089.

Bondia-Pons, I., Nordlund, E., Mattila, I., Katina, K., Aura, A.M., Kolehmainen, M., Orešič, M., Mykkänen, H., Poutanen, K., 2011. Postprandial differences in the plasma metabolome of healthy Finnish subjects after intake of a sourdough fermented endosperm rye bread versus white wheat bread. Nutr. J. 10, 116. http://dx.doi.org/10.1186/1475-2891-10-116, PubMed PMID: 22011443; PubMed Central PMCID: PMC3214176.

Brüssow, H., 2013. Microbiota and healthy ageing: observational and nutritional intervention studies. Microb. Biotechnol. 6 (4), 326–334. http://dx.doi.org/10.1111/1751-7915.12048, Epub 2013 Mar 26. Review. PubMed PMID: 23527905; PubMed Central PMCID: PMC3917467.

Cagliani, L.R., Pellegrino, G., Giugno, G., Consonni, R., 2013. Quantification of *Coffea arabica* and *Coffea canephora* var. robusta in roasted and ground coffee blends. Talanta 106, 169–173. http://dx.doi.org/10.1016/j.talanta.2012.12.003, Epub 2012.

Cajka, T., Vaclavikova, M., Dzuman, Z., Vaclavik, L., Ovesna, J., Hajslova, J., 2014. Rapid LC-MS-based metabolomics method to study the Fusarium infection of barley. J. Sep. Sci. 37, 912–919. http://dx.doi.org/10.1002/jssc.201301292, PubMed PMID: 24515453.

Caligiani, A., Coisson, J.D., Travaglia, F., Acquotti, D., Palla, G., Palla, L., Arlorio, M., 2014. Application of ^{1}H NMR for the characterisation and authentication of "Tonda Gentile Trilobata" hazelnuts from Piedmont (Italy). Food Chem. 148, 77–85. http://dx.doi.org/10.1016/j.foodchem.2013.10.001, Epub 2013 Oct 10 PubMed PMID: 24262529.

Cauchi, S., Stutzmann, F., Cavalcanti-Proença, C., Durand, E., Pouta, A., Hartikainen, A.L., Marre, M., Vol, S., Tammelin, T., Laitinen, J., Gonzalez-Izquierdo, A., Blakemore, A.I., Elliott, P., Meyre, D., Balkau, B., Järvelin, M.R., Froguel, P., 2009. Combined effects of MC4R and FTO common genetic variants on obesity in European general populations. J. Mol. Med. 87 (5), 537–546. http://dx.doi.org/10.1007/s00109-009-0451-6.

Chadeau-Hyam, M., Ebbels, T.M., Brown, I.J., Chan, Q., Stamler, J., Huang, C.C., Daviglus, M. L., Ueshima, H., Zhao, L., Holmes, E., Nicholson, J.K., Elliott, P., De Iorio, M., 2010. Metabolic profiling and the metabolome-wide association study: significance level for biomarker identification. J. Proteome Res. 9 (9), 4620–4627. http://dx.doi.org/10.1021/pr1003449, PubMed PMID: 20701291; PubMed Central PMCID: PMC2941198.

Claus, S.P., Swann, J.R., 2013. Nutrimetabonomics: applications for nutritional sciences, with specific reference to gut microbial interactions. Annu. Rev. Food Sci. Technol. 4, 381–399. http://dx.doi.org/10.1146/annurev-food-030212-182612, Epub 2013 Jan 3. Review. PubMed PMID: 23297777.

Clayton, T.A., Baker, D., Lindon, J.C., Everett, J.R., Nicholson, J.K., 2009. Pharmacometabonomic identification of a significant host-microbiome metabolic interaction affecting human drug metabolism. Proc. Natl. Acad. Sci. U. S. A. 106 (34), 14728–14733. http://dx.doi.org/10.1073/pnas.0904489106, PubMed PMID: 19667173; PubMedCentral PMCID: PMC2731842.

Cloarec, O., Dumas, M., Craig, A., Barton, R.H., Trygg, J., Hudson, J., et al., 2005. Statistical total correlation spectroscopy: an exploratory approach for latent biomarker identification from metabolic 1H NMR data sets. Anal. Chem. 77, 1282–1289.

De Guzman, J.M., Ku, G., Fahey, R., Youm, Y.H., Kass, I., Ingram, D.K., Dixit, V.D., Kheterpal, I., 2013. Chronic caloric restriction partially protects against age-related alteration in serum metabolome. Age (Dordr.) 35 (4), 1091–1104. http://dx.doi.org/10.1007/s11357-012-9430-x, PubMed PMID: 22661299; PubMed Central PMC3705111.

Dear, G.J., Plumb, R.S., Sweatman, B.C., Ayrton, J., Lindon, J.C., Nicholson, J.K., Ismail, I.M., 2000. Mass directed peak selection, an efficient method of drug metabolite identification using directly coupled liquid chromatography-mass spectrometry-nuclear magnetic resonance spectroscopy. J. Chromatogr. B Biomed. Sci. Appl. 748 (1), 281–293, PubMed PMID: 11092605.

Dragsted, L.O., 2010. Biomarkers of meat intake and the application of nutrigenomics. Meat Sci. 84 (2), 301–307. http://dx.doi.org/10.1016/j.meatsci.2009.08.028, PubMed PMID: 20374789.

Duan, Y., An, Y., Li, N., Liu, B., Wang, Y., Tang, H., 2013. Multiple univariate data analysis reveals the inulin effects on the high-fat-diet induced metabolic alterations in rat myocardium and testicles in the preobesity state. J. Proteome Res. 12 (7), 3480–3495. http://dx.doi.org/10.1021/pr400341f, PubMed PMID: 23700965.

Edmands, W.M., Beckonert, O.P., Stella, C., Campbell, A., Lake, B.G., Lindon, J.C., Holmes, E., Gooderham, N.J., 2011. Identification of human urinary biomarkers of cruciferous vegetable consumption by metabonomic profiling. J. Proteome Res. 10 (10), 4513–4521. http://dx.doi.org/10.1021/pr200326k.

Faria, A.M., Gomes-Santos, A.C., Gonçalves, J.L., Moreira, T.G., Medeiros, S.R., Dourado, L. P., Cara, D.C., 2013. Food components and the immune system: from tonic agents to allergens. Front. Immunol. 4, 102. http://dx.doi.org/10.3389/fimmu.2013.00102. eCollection 2013, PubMed PMID: 23730302. PubMed Central PMCID: PMC3656403.

Farinaro, E., Trevisan, M., Jossa, F., Panico, S., Celentano, E., Mancini, M., Zamboni, S., Dal Palú, C., Angelico, F., Del Ben, M., et al., 1991. INTERSALT in Italy: findings and community health implications. J. Hum. Hypertens. 5 (1), 15–19, PubMed PMID: 2041032.

Fearnside, J.F., Dumas, M.E., Rothwell, A.R., Wilder, S.P., Cloarec, O., Toye, A., Blancher, C., Holmes, E., Tatoud, R., Barton, R.H., Scott, J., Nicholson, J.K., Gauguier, D., 2008. Phylometabonomic patterns of adaptation to high fat diet feeding in inbred mice. PLoS One 3 (2), e1668, PMID: 18301746.

Ganesh, V., Hettiarachchy, N.S., 2012. Nutriproteomics: a promising tool to link diet and diseases in nutritional research. Biochim. Biophys. Acta 1824 (10), 1107–1117. http://dx.doi.org/10.1016/j.bbapap.2012.06.006.

Hao, J., Astle, W., De Iorio, M., Ebbels, T.M., 2012. BATMAN – An R package for the automated quantification of metabolites from nuclear magnetic resonance spectra using a Bayesian model. Bioinformatics 28 (15), 2088–2090. http://dx.doi.org/10.1093/bioinformatics/bts308, Epub 2012 May 26. PubMed PMID: 22635605.

Hardy, T.M., Tollefsbol, T.O., 2011. Epigenetic diet: impact on the epigenome and cancer. Epigenomics 3 (4), 503–518. http://dx.doi.org/10.2217/epi.11.71, Review. PubMed PMID: 22022340. PubMed Central PMCID: PMC3197720.

Heinzmann, S.S., Brown, I.J., Chan, Q., Bictash, M., Dumas, M.E., Kochhar, S., Stamler, J., Holmes, E., Elliott, P., Nicholson, J.K., 2010. Metabolic profiling strategy for discovery of nutritional biomarkers: proline betaine as a marker of citrus consumption. Am. J. Clin. Nutr. 92 (2), 436–443. http://dx.doi.org/10.3945/ajcn.2010.29672, Epub 2010 Jun 23. PubMed PMID: 20573794; PubMed Central PMCID: PMC2904656.

Heinzmann, S.S., Merrifield, C.A., Rezzi, S., Kochhar, S., Lindon, J.C., Holmes, E., Nicholson, J.K., 2012. Stability and robustness of human metabolic phenotypes in response to sequential food challenges. J. Proteome Res. 11 (2), 643–655. http://dx.doi.org/10.1021/pr2005764, Epub 2011 Dec 16. PubMed PMID: 21999107.

Holmes, E., Loo, R.L., Stamler, J., Bictash, M., Yap, I.K., Chan, Q., Ebbels, T., De Iorio, M., Brown, I.J., Veselkov, K.A., Daviglus, M.L., Kesteloot, H., Ueshima, H., Zhao, L., Nicholson, J.K., Elliott, P., 2008. Human metabolic phenotype diversity and its association with diet and blood pressure. Nature 453 (7193), 396–400. http://dx.doi.org/10.1038/nature06882. Epub 2008 Apr 20, PubMed PMID: 18425110.

Kelishadi, R., Farajian, S., 2014. The protective effects of breastfeeding on chronic non-communicable diseases in adulthood: a review of evidence. Adv. Biomed. Res. 3, 3, eCollection 2014. Review. PubMed PMID: 24600594.

Kelley, D.S., Adkins, Y., Reddy, A., Woodhouse, L.R., Mackey, B.E., Erickson, K.L., 2013. Sweet bing cherries lower circulating concentrations of markers for chronic inflammatory diseases in healthy humans. J. Nutr. 143 (3), 340–344. http://dx.doi.org/10.3945/jn.112.171371, Epub 2013 Jan 23 PubMed PMID: 23343675.

Kerckhoffs, A.P., Samsom, M., van der Rest, M.E., de Vogel, J., Knol, J., Ben-Amor, K., Akkermans, L.M., 2009. Lower Bifidobacteria counts in both duodenal mucosa-associated and fecal microbiota in irritable bowel syndrome patients. World J. Gastroenterol. 15 (23), 2887–2892, PMID: 19533811; PubMed Central PMCID:PMC2699007.

Kita, T., Asanuma, M., Miyazaki, I., Takeshima, M., 2014. Protective effects of phytochemical antioxidants against neurotoxin-induced degeneration of dopaminergic neurons. J. Pharmacol. Sci. 124 (3), 313–319, [Epub ahead of print] PubMed PMID: 24599140.

Lankinen, M., Schwab, U., Seppänen-Laakso, T., Mattila, I., Juntunen, K., Mykkänen, H., Poutanen, K., Gylling, H., Oresic, M., 2011. Metabolomic analysis of plasma metabolites that may mediate effects of rye bread on satiety and weight maintenance in postmenopausal women. J. Nutr. 141 (1), 31–36. http://dx.doi.org/10.3945/jn.110.131656, Epub 2010 Nov 17. PubMed PMID: 21084654.

Ley, R.E., Backhed, F., Turnbaugh, P., Lozupone, C.A., Knight, R.D., Gordon, J.I., 2005. Obesity alters gut microbial ecology. Proc. Natl. Acad. Sci. U. S. A. 102 (31), 11070–11075, PMID: 16033867.

Marincola, F.C., Noto, A., Caboni, P., Reali, A., Barberini, L., Lussu, M., Murgia, F., Santoru, M.L., Atzori, L., Fanos, V., 2012. A metabolomic study of preterm human and formula milk by high resolution NMR and GC/MS analysis: preliminary results. J. Matern.

Fetal Neonatal Med. 25 (Suppl. 5), 62–67. http://dx.doi.org/10.3109/14767058.2012.715436, PubMed PMID: 23025771.

Martin, F.P., Sprenger, N., Yap, I.K., Wang, Y., Bibiloni, R., Rochat, F., Rezzi, S., Cherbut, C., Kochhar, S., Lindon, J.C., Holmes, E., Nicholson, J.K., 2009. Panorganismal gut microbiome-host metabolic crosstalk. J. Proteome Res. 8 (4), 2090–2105. PMID: 19281268.

Merched, A.J., Chan, L., 2013. Nutrigenetics and nutrigenomics of atherosclerosis. Curr. Atheroscler. Rep. 15 (6), 328. http://dx.doi.org/10.1007/s11883-013-0328-6, Review. PubMed PMID: 23605288.

Merrifield, C.A., Lewis, M.C., Claus, S.P., Pearce, J.T., Cloarec, O., Duncker, S., Heinzmann, S.S., Dumas, M.E., Kochhar, S., Rezzi, S., Mercenier, A., Nicholson, J.K., Bailey, M., Holmes, E., 2013. Weaning diet induces sustained metabolic phenotype shift in the pig and influences host response to *Bifidobacterium lactis* NCC2818. Gut 62 (6), 842–851. http://dx.doi.org/10.1136/gutjnl-2011-301656, PubMed PMID: 22661492.

Montoliu, I., Genick, U., Ledda, M., Collino, S., Martin, F.P., le Coutre, J., Rezzi, S., 2013. Current status on genome-metabolome-wide associations: an opportunity in nutrition research. Genes Nutr. 8 (1), 19–27. http://dx.doi.org/10.1007/s12263-012-0313-7, PubMed PMID: 23065485; PubMed Central PMCID: PMC3534994.

Nicholson, J.K., Lindon, J.C., Holmes, E., 1999. 'Metabonomics': understanding the metabolic responses of living systems to pathophysiological stimuli via multivariate statistical analysis of biological NMR spectroscopic data. Xenobiotica 29 (11), 1181–1189, PubMed PMID: 10598751.

O'Sullivan, A., He, X., McNiven, E.M., Hinde, K., Haggarty, N.W., Lönnerdal, B., Slupsky, C. M., 2013. Metabolomic phenotyping validates the infant rhesus monkey as a model of human infant metabolism. J. Pediatr. Gastroenterol. Nutr. 56 (4), 355–363. http://dx.doi.org/10.1097/MPG.0b013e31827e1f07, PubMed PMID: 23201704.

Papoutsis, A.J., Lamore, S.D., Wondrak, G.T., Selmin, O.I., Romagnolo, D.F., 2010. Resveratrol prevents epigenetic silencing of BRCA-1 by the aromatic hydrocarbon receptor in human breast cancer cells. J. Nutr. 140 (9), 1607–1614.

Pericleous, M., Mandair, D., Caplin, M.E., 2013. Diet and supplements and their impact on colorectal cancer. J. Gastrointest. Oncol. 4 (4), 409–423. http://dx.doi.org/10.3978/j.issn.2078-6891.2013.003, Review. PubMed PMID: 24294513; PubMed Central PMCID: PMC3819783.

Praticò, G., Capuani, G., Tomassini, A., Baldassarre, M.E., Delfini, M., Miccheli, A., 2014. Exploring human breast milk composition by NMR-based metabolomics. Nat. Prod. Res. 28 (2), 95–101. http://dx.doi.org/10.1080/14786419.2013.843180, PMID: 24079341.

Preidis, G.A., Keaton, M.A., Campeau, P.M., Bessard, B.C., Conner, M.E., Hotez, P.J., 2014. The undernourished neonatal mouse metabolome reveals evidence of liver and biliary dysfunction, inflammation, and oxidative stress. J. Nutr. 144 (3), 273–281. http://dx.doi.org/10.3945/jn.113.183731, Epub 2013 Dec 31. PubMed PMID: 24381221; PubMed Central PMCID: PMC3927544.

Saulnier, D.M., Spinler, J.K., Gibson, G.R., Versalovic, J., 2009. Mechanisms of probiosis and prebiosis: considerations for enhanced functional foods. Curr. Opin. Biotechnol. 20 (2), 135–141. http://dx.doi.org/10.1016/j.copbio.2009.01.002, PubMed PMID: 19243931; PubMed Central PMCID: PMC2713183.

Schwingshackl, L., Hoffmann, G., 2014. Adherence to Mediterranean diet and risk of cancer: a systematic review and meta-analysis of observational studies. Int. J. Cancer 135, 1884–1897. http://dx.doi.org/10.1002/ijc.28824, PubMed PMID: 24599882.

Shay, C.M., Stamler, J., Dyer, A.R., Brown, I.J., Chan, Q., Elliott, P., Zhao, L., Okuda, N., Miura, K., Daviglus, M.L., Van Horn, L., 2012. Nutrient and food intakes of middle-aged adults at low risk of cardiovascular disease: the international study of macro-/micronutrients and blood pressure (INTERMAP). Eur. J. Nutr. 51 (8), 917–926. http://dx.doi.org/10.1007/00394-011-0268-2.

Solanky, K.S., Bailey, N.J., Holmes, E., Lindon, J.C., Davis, A.L., Mulder, T.P., Van Duynhoven, J.P., Nicholson, J.K., 2003. NMR-based metabonomic studies on the biochemical effects of epicatechin in the rat. J. Agric. Food Chem. 51 (14), 4139–4145, PubMed PMID: 12822959.

Sotelo, J., Slupsky, C., 2013. Metabolomics using nuclear magnetic resonance (NMR). In: Weimer, B.C., Slupsky, C. (Eds.), Metabolomics in Food and Nutrition. Woodhead Publishing Limited, Cambridge, UK.

Stella, C., Beckwith-Hall, B., Cloarec, O., Holmes, E., Lindon, J.C., Powell, J., van der Ouderaa, F., Bingham, S., Cross, A.J., Nicholson, J.K., 2006. Susceptibility of human metabolic phenotypes to dietary modulation. J. Proteome Res. 5 (10), 2780–2788, PubMed PMID: 17022649.

Strathearn, K.E., Yousef, G.G., Grace, M.H., Roy, S.L., Tambe, M.A., Ferruzzi, M.G., Wu, Q. L., Simon, J.E., Lila, M.A., Rochet, J.C., 2014. Neuroprotective effects of anthocyanin- and proanthocyanidin-rich extracts in cellular models of Parkinsońs disease. Brain Res. 1555, 60–77. http://dx.doi.org/10.1016/j.brainres.2014.01.047, pii: S0006-8993(14)00114-0. PubMed PMID: 24502982.

Turnbaugh, P.J., Hamady, M., Yatsunenko, T., Cantarel, B.L., Duncan, A., Ley, R.E., Sogin, M. L., Jones, W.J., Roe, B.A., Affourtit, J.P., Egholm, M., Henrissat, B., Heath, A.C., Knight, R., Gordon, J.I., 2009. A core gut microbiome in obese and lean twins. Nature 457 (7228), 480–484, PMID: 19043404.

Vepsäläinen, S., Koivisto, H., Pekkarinen, E., Mäkinen, P., Dobson, G., McDougall, G.J., Stewart, D., Haapasalo, A., Karjalainen, R.O., Tanila, H., Hiltunen, M., 2013. Anthocyanin-enriched bilberry and blackcurrant extracts modulate amyloid precursor protein processing and alleviate behavioral abnormalities in the APP/PS1 mouse model of Alzheimer's disease. J. Nutr. Biochem. 24 (1), 360–370. http://dx.doi.org/10.1016/j.jnutbio.2012.07.006, Epub 2012 Sep 17. PubMed PMID: 22995388.

Wachsmuth, C.J., Oefner, P.J., Dettmer, K., 2013. Equipment and metabolite identification (ID) strategies for mass-based metabolomic analysis. In: Weimer, B.C., Slupsky, C. (Eds.), Metabolomics in Food and Nutrition. Woodhead Publishing Limited, Cambridge, UK.

Wang, Y., Tang, H., Nicholson, J.K., Hylands, P.J., Sampson, J., Whitcombe, I., Stewart, C.G., Caiger, S., Oru, I., Holmes, E., 2004. Metabolomic strategy for the classification and quality control of phytomedicine: a case study of chamomile flower (*Matricaria recutita* L.). Planta Med. 70 (3), 250–255, PubMed PMID: 15114503.

Wang, Y., Lawler, D., Larson, B., Ramadan, Z., Kochhar, S., Holmes, E., Nicholson, J.K., 2007. Metabonomic investigations of aging and caloric restriction in a life-long dog study. J. Proteome Res. 6 (5), 1846–1854, PubMed PMID: 17411081.

Wiseman, H., 2000. The therapeutic potential of phytoestrogens. Expert Opin. Investig. Drugs 9 (8), 1829–1840, Review. PubMed PMID: 11060780.

Yap, I.K., Brown, I.J., Chan, Q., Wijeyesekera, A., Garcia-Perez, I., Bictash, M., Loo, R.L., Chadeau-Hyam, M., Ebbels, T., De Iorio, M., Maibaum, E., Zhao, L., Kesteloot, H., Daviglus, M.L., Stamler, J., Nicholson, J.K., Elliott, P., Holmes, E., 2010. Metabolome-wide association study identifies multiple biomarkers that discriminate north and south Chinese populations at differing risks of cardiovascular disease: INTERMAP study. J. Proteome Res. 9 (12), 6647–6654. http://dx.doi.org/10.1021/pr100798r, PubMed PMID: 20853909; PubMed Central PMCID: PMC3117148.

Zhang, Y., Yan, S., Gao, X., Xiong, X., Dai, W., Liu, X., Li, L., Zhang, W., Mei, C., 2012. Analysis of urinary metabolic profile in aging rats undergoing caloric restriction. Aging Clin. Exp. Res. 24 (1), 79–84. http://dx.doi.org/10.3275/7519, PubMed PMID: 21339700.

Chemometrics methods for the analysis of genomics, transcriptomics, proteomics, metabolomics, and metagenomics datasets

3

S.E. Richards[1], *E. Holmes*[2]
[1]Nottingham Trent University, Nottingham, United Kingdom; [2]Imperial College, London, United Kingdom

3.1 Introduction

Chemometrics is defined as a chemical discipline that uses mathematics, statistics, and formal logic to (Massart et al., 1997):

(a) design or select optimal experimental procedures,
(b) provide maximum relevant chemical information by analysing chemical data,
(c) obtain knowledge about chemical systems.

Information-rich omic technologies enable:

- the measurement of complete DNA sequences (genomics),
- the analysis of the presence and abundance of RNA transcripts (transcriptomics),
- the identification and quantification of proteins and their post-translational modifications (proteomics),
- the determination of composition and concentration changes of metabolites (metabolomics, also known as metabonomics).

Data mining over different levels of organisation (genomics, transcriptomics, proteomics, metabolomics, and metagenomics) reveals compartmentalised systems architecture in both intracellular and multicellular structures. Compartmentalised systems architecture refers to the recovery of network interactions and biochemical pathways at each level of organisation, typically without complete knowledge of the underlying systems structure (hypothesis generation). For each level of organisation and for integrative studies (the combined analysis of more than one dataset), multivariate statistical techniques are employed to extract information congruent to the research question(s) derived from the experimental design and the type of data collected.

In this chapter, we give a brief summary of the current chemometrics methods used at each level of organisation for genomics, transcriptomics, proteomics, metabolomics, and metagenomics datasets. The chemometrics methods are discussed with

Metabolomics as a Tool in Nutrition Research. http://dx.doi.org/10.1016/B978-1-78242-084-2.00003-4

respect to the fundamental research question and the experimental design employed at each level of organisation.

3.2 Unsupervised and supervised pattern recognition methods

Chemometric approaches can be organised largely into:

- unsupervised pattern recognition methods
- supervised pattern recognition methods

Unsupervised methods are those that do not require any a priori knowledge to explore multidimensional datasets with respect to a class (or group) or combined set of measured variables, such as genes, proteins, transcripts, and metabolites. Nor do these methods require information about the relation of these measured variables to a particular class (or group), such as nutritional status, country of origin, age, and gender. However, knowledge of the assumptions of the multivariate algorithms employed and a good understanding of the statistical quality of the measured variables are vital (as with all multivariate statistical approaches) to ensure high-quality modelling results. In this regard, great care and consideration should be applied when selecting data preprocessing method(s) (filtering, integration, reduction, or transformation) prior to the multivariate analyses (van den Berg et al., 2006).

Unsupervised approaches used largely in omic analyses include orthogonal decomposition methods such as:

- principal component analysis (PCA) (Jolliffe, 2005),
- trilinear decomposition methods for multiple datasets,
- parallel factor analysis (PARAFAC) (Bro, 1997a; Harshman, 1970a),
- Tucker (Tucker, 1966a).

Hierarchical clustering methods are methods in which one may obtain any number of clusters, $K, 1 \leq K \leq n$, by selecting the appropriate number of links in the dendrogram, and this is also true for non-hierarchical clustering, with the difference that the K is defined a priori by the user. A variety of dissimilarity measures (the Euclidean distance, Pearson's correlation and Spearman's rank correlation) and clustering methods (average linkage, complete linkage, single linkage, and Ward's linkage) (Dagnelie and Merckx, 1991; Mahalanobis, 1936; Ward, 1963) are available for hierarchical clustering. The result of hierarchical clustering is usually presented as a dendrogram or heat map. Correlation-based analysis includes approaches such as statistical total correlation spectroscopy (STOCSY) (Cloarec et al., 2005) and statistical heterospectroscopy (SHY) (Crockford et al., 2008).

Supervised pattern recognition or discriminant analysis methods aim at deriving classification rules that enable the user to classify new objects with unknown origin into one or several known classes. Therefore, these techniques require a priori knowledge with respect to the class (or group) membership, that is, identities of the samples or individuals with respect to their class, such as nutritional status, country of origin, and gender. However, these techniques do not require prior information to relate those groups to a measured variable such as genes, proteins, or transcripts.

The power of supervised pattern recognition methods lies in the model construction, which consists of the following steps:

(1) Selection of a training or learning set
(2) Feature or variable selection
(3) Derivation of a classification rule
(4) Validation of the classification rule

Selection of a training or learning set consists of objects of known classification for which a certain number of variables are measured. Feature or variable selection is an iterative procedure in which variables that are meaningful for the classification are retained, whilst variables with little or no discriminating (or modelling power) are omitted from the analysis. Derivation of a classification rule is dependent upon the supervised pattern recognition method selected. Validation of the classification rule is done using an independent dataset.

Supervised pattern recognition methods used in omic analyses include:

- linear discriminant analysis (Coomans et al., 1978),
- partial least squares (PLS) (Ståhle and Wold, 1987),
- non-hierarchical clustering approaches such as SIMCA (soft-independent modelling of class analogy) (Wold, 1976),
- nonlinear clustering methods such as kernel or potential density functions (Coomans and Broeckaert, 1986; Forina et al., 1987, 1991),
- neural networks (Rumelhart et al., 1986; Werbos, 1974),
- Kohonen's self-organising map (Kohonen, 1982).

Nonlinear methods such as nonlinear clustering, neural networks, and self-organising maps offer comparable or even superior classification potential; however, they do not provide transparency in terms of the discriminating signals.

3.3 Multivariate calibration methods for developing predictive models

Multivariate calibration methods are typically used for the development of semi-quantitative and quantitative models for the prediction of properties of interest. The advantage of using these methods is that the entire spectrum, that is, NMR or MS profile, can be used as a predictor rather than one variable within the measured set (i.e. one chemical shift). The incorporation of the entire spectrum tends to lead to better predictive results, although it opens up the possibility that essentially non-informative spectral regions are included in the model through chance correlations in the calibration set. Nevertheless, with multivariate data, the opportunity arises to separate the information relevant to the respective properties from non-relevant variation or random noise.

Multivariate calibration methods typically used in omic studies include:

- multivariate linear regression (Vandeginste et al., 1997),
- principal component regression (PCR) (Jeffers, 1967; Jolliffe, 2005),
- PLS (also known as projection to latent structures) (Ståhle and Wold, 1987),
- orthogonal signal correction (OSC) (Wold et al., 1998a).

Wold et al. (1998a) introduced OSC to remove the variation in the measured variables *X*, which are not correlated (or orthogonal) to the variation in predictor response *Y*. This procedure simplified and increased the robustness of the model.

Since the introduction of OSC–PLS (Beckwith-Hall et al., 2002a; Gavaghan et al., 2002a; Mao et al., 2007a; Wold et al., 1998b), several variations of the OSC–PLS procedure have been introduced, including:

- OPLS (Trygg and Wold, 2002)
- O2PLS (Trygg and Wold, 2003)

These have the same objective but utilise different methodology that results in the increased interpretability of the PLS model, with the additional benefit that the non-correlated variation can be analysed further. These techniques are also used as discriminant analysis methods in omic applications (Beckwith-Hall et al., 2002b; Gavaghan et al., 2002b; Mao et al., 2007b).

Model-free or calibration-free techniques known as self-modelling curve resolution (SMCR) consist of a family of chemometric techniques that utilise a certain mathematical decomposition to deconvolve the two-way signals from instrumentally unresolved multi-component mixtures into factors for single species. In principle, SMCR does not require a priori information concerning the data to resolve the pure variables. The only premises are a certain bilinear model for the data and some generic knowledge about the pure variable, say, non-negativity and unimodality. In common practice, these premises are naturally satisfied for two-way data obtained from multivariate measurements on mixtures with varying compositions. SMCR and multivariate curve resolution (MCR) are useful tools for exploring multi-component phenomena in complex biochemical systems (Gargallo et al., 1996; Lawton and Sylvestre, 1971; Richards et al., 2008a).

3.4 Statistical data integration methods

There are multiple ways to classify levels of data integration. Three different levels of integration are (Ebbels and Cavill, 2009)

- conceptual integration, that is, the integrative interpretation of results from multiple experiments;
- statistical integration, that is, the simultaneous multivariate analysis of data from multiple sources;
- model-based integration, that is, the construction of predictive functional networks or models from multiple experimental components.

Here, we focus on the recent developments and applications at the statistical level of data integration or data fusion (also called multiblock, multiview, or multiset data analysis) for omic applications. We will consider the challenges of data integration in the following areas:

- Across different analytic platform, that is, NMR or LC/MS
- The simultaneous analysis of biofluid or tissue sample (urine, saliva and faecal samples, liver, etc.)
- Integration of different omic experiments such as DGGE, FISH, and NMR

A detailed review of statistical integration methods for metabonomics applications is given in Richards et al. (2010).

Integration of data from multiple platforms has become a common practice in metabol(n)omics applications in spite of the challenges associated with combining data with high sample-to-variable ratios, which include differing data structure, temporal variability, instrument drift, scaling effects, missing data, heterogeneity in noise level, and high collinearity of variables, which may lead to random correlation structure. However, the potential gain in information recovery (including greater efficiencies with respect to the number of metabolites recovered), the number of samples processed (particularly in large epidemiology studies) across multiple spectroscopic and chromatographic instruments, structure elucidation, and elucidation of metabolic pathway connectivities are the main drivers to address such challenges.

3.5 Data integration: multiblock strategies

Unsupervised and supervised pattern recognition methods utilised for multiplatform analyses include multiblock strategies. These methods search for directions of similar sample distribution in the multiple dimension space defined by each measurement matrix. The contribution of each block is expressed as a measure of the extracted variability for each common dimension. The covariance and correlation structure in two-block data matrices such as (GC/MS and LC/MS) can be investigated using:

- consensus CPCA (Smilde et al., 2003)
- canonical correlation analysis (CCA) (Hotelling, 1935)

CPCA focuses on the direction describing the largest source of variance, whilst CCA identifies trends between the two datasets that are strongly correlated (Wold, 1976).

However, the number of variables in omic experiments often exceeds tens of thousands. In this case, the high dimensionality and the insufficient sample size lead to computational problems as CCA requires the computation of the inverse of the covariance matrices of X and Y. To circumvent this problem, regularised CCA (rCCA) has been recently proposed by González et al. (2009) when dealing with ill-conditioned covariance matrices by adding a regularization term on their diagonal. The proportion of the overlapping dominant sources of variance can be quantified using CPCA, validated against the matrix correlation coefficient (the RV coefficient) (Smilde et al., 2005, 2009).

Multiple factor analysis (MFA) (Escofier and Pages, 1994; Pages and Tenenhaus, 2001), a similar method to CPCA, has been applied for simultaneous analysis of ^{1}H–^{13}C heteronuclear multiple-bond connectivity, nuclear magnetic resonance spectroscopy (^{1}H–^{13}C HMBC NMR), and pyrolysis coupled with metastable atom bombardment time-of-flight mass spectrometry (Py–MAB-TOF-MS) (Dumas et al., 2005). In MFA, each block is weighted to the square root of the first eigenvalue derived from PCA of each block (Escofier and Pages, 1994; Pages and Tenenhaus, 2001) rather than the square root of the sum of squares, followed by PCA decomposition of the row augmented matrix, in CPCA. The advantage of the MFA weighting procedure is it accounts for dominant scaling effects. Furthermore, Van Deun et al. (2009) in a separate study showed that simultaneous component analysis (SCA) methods, that is, MFA, were largely dependent upon the weighting (Van Deun et al., 2009) and noise structure (van den Berg et al., 2009).

Hierarchical PCA (HPCA) (Westerhuis et al., 1998; Wold et al., 1996) has been used for the simultaneous analysis of ^{1}H NMR combined with gas chromatography/electrospray ionization time-of-flight mass spectrometry (GC–EI-TOF-MS) (Biais et al., 2009) for the global compositional analysis of melon fruit flesh extracts (Biais et al., 2009). Both HPCA and hierarchical PLS (Westerhuis et al., 1998; Wold et al., 1996) have been applied for the simultaneous analysis of LC/MS and ^{1}H NMR to classify rats dosed with citalopram (Forshed et al., 2007). Multiblock PLS algorithm (Wangen and Kowalski, 1989) has been applied to multiplatform data LC/MS and GC/MS to study the liver protection effect of traditional Chinese medicine, *fructus ligustri lucidi* (Yao et al., 2013).

Additional OPLS modelling strategies proposed for analysing multiple block spectral data include:

- hierarchical PLS (Eriksson et al., 2006)
- O2PLS

O2PLS has been used to integrate FT-NIR and GC–TOF-MS spectral data of 3000 rice FOX *Arabidopsis* lines. This analysis showed that the joint variation of predictive metabolites explained the chemical relationships between FT-NIR and GC–TOF-MS, whereas metabolite changes associated with rice gene function were determined in the unique variation (Suzuki et al., 2010).

OnPLS (Löfstedt et al., 2013) is an extension of O2PLS that decomposes a set of matrices, in either multiblock or path model analysis, such that each matrix consists of two parts:

- A globally joint part containing variation shared with all other connected matrices
- A part that contains locally joint and unique variation, that is, variation that is shared with some, but not all, other connected matrices or that is unique in a single matrix

A further extension suggested by the authors, Löfstedt et al. (2013), is to decompose the part that is not globally joint into locally joint and unique parts. To achieve this, the OnPLS method first finds and extracts a globally joint model and then applies OnPLS recursively to subsets of matrices that contain the locally joint and unique variation remaining after the globally joint variation has been extracted. This results in a set of locally joint models. This modelling strategy can be used for multiplatform, multisample, multibatch and multiomic integrative applications.

A nonlinear kernel-based classification method has been utilised to integrate GC-MS and NMR data to characterise the progression of multiple sclerosis (Smolinska et al., 2012). In order to reduce the complexities associated with high-sample-to-variable-ratio data, a feature selection method support vector machine–recursive feature elimination (SVM–RFE) was used to extract the relevant variables (Guyon et al., 2002; Hardy and Tollefsbol, 2011). The filtered GC-MS and ^{1}H NMR datasets were integrated using linear combinations of kernel matrices (Yu et al., 2011) prior to the application of PLS-DA. Smolinska et al. (2012) visualised the relative contribution of each variable to KPLS-DA model (variable importance) by applying and extending the pseudo samples principle (Krooshof et al., 2010; Postma et al., 2011) to address the issue associated with information recovery from the variable space.

A consensus (OPLS-DA) strategy for multiblock omic data has been recently developed (Boccard and Rutledge, 2013) based on the nonlinear kernel-based classification strategy by Smolinska et al. (Yu et al., 2011) that takes advantage of the easy interpretability of the OPLS-DA model with a dimensionality reduction, data reduction, and resampling steps. The method is an extension of the kernel-based approach to OPLS-DA, based on the extraction of consensus components via the decomposition of the reduced measurement matrix computed as a weighted sum of XX^T product matrices. This approach was applied in three case studies as follows: (a) fusion of mass spectrometry-based metabolomic data acquired in both negative and positive electrospray ionization modes, from leaf samples of the model plant *Arabidopsis thaliana*; (b) two-dimensional heteronuclear magnetic resonance spectroscopy for the classification of wine grape varieties based on polyphenolic extracts; and (c) a heterogeneous dataset from systems biology data related to NCI-60 cancer cell lines from different tissue origins, which include metabolomics, transcriptomics, and proteomics (Boccard and Rutledge, 2013).

Overall, consensus PCA was found to increase computational efficiency and improve prediction results when compared to multiblock PLS and data concatenation. Limitation of the method was the lack of optimization of the block weights to increase predictive power. To address this issue, the authors propose to develop a weighting scheme to account for these specific variations.

3.6 Data integration: calibration transfer methods

Calibration transfer methods (Wang et al., 1991) are important to consider as a pretreatment method for multiplatform integration, especially when transferring a study from one instrument to another or in the event of instrument failure or downtime. In large-scale studies requiring data acquisition over many months or years, study times can be reduced through data acquisition on multiple instruments and subsequent data fusion. Calibration transfer methods compensate for differences in data collected for the same samples on two or more instruments or on the same instrument at different time points.

Models based on multivariate calibration procedures such as PLS or PCR can be used to eliminate or reduce the variation in response observed between instruments. Multivariate standardised techniques such as direct standardization and reverse standardization (and their piecewise variants) use a set of transfer samples analysed on both instruments to transform the response from one instrument to another (Wang et al., 1991).

Vaughan et al. (2012) had utilised a calibration transfer method to compare the response profiles from the two LC-MS platforms and transformed the data so that both datasets could be integrated, through row-wise concatenation of pre-treated (feature selection and metabolite identification) and transformed (PLS regression) datasets. The transformed row-wise concatenated datasets were autoscaled prior to the application of PCA. It was found that the application of the calibration transform method reduced intra-sample, intra-instrumental and inter-instrumental variation and increased inter-subject variability.

3.7 Data integration: multiway/multimodal analysis methods

A number of multiway or multimodal analysis methods have been used for the full integrative modelling of multiplatform data. These techniques differ to the previously mentioned techniques in that an N-order tensor (i.e. observations $\times$ variables $\times$ time $\times \cdots$) is simultaneously decomposed/factorised without the need of first unfolding the measurement matrices prior to the analysis. An extensive review of the requirements for multiway and multiblock analysis is given in Bro (2006) and Smilde et al. (2000). These methods include but are not limited to:

- PARAFAC (Harshman, 1970b; Harshman and Lundy, 1984),
- Tucker decomposition (Kroonenberg and Deleeuw, 1980; Tenberge et al., 1987; Tucker, 1966b),
- Nway-PLS (NPLS) (Bro, 1996a),
- ANOVA–simultaneous component analysis (ASCA) with PARAFAC (an extension of ASCA to the multiway case) (Jansen et al., 2008).

Since they have been used most extensively, PARAFAC and Tucker decomposition are discussed in more detail below.

3.7.1 PARAFAC

PARAFAC is most similar to PCA since both methods provide a unique solution and are fitted in a least squares sense. However, the orthogonality and maximum variance component constraints required in PCA to obtain a unique solution are not required to obtain a unique solution in PARAFAC since the PARAFAC model is unique in itself (Bro, 1997b). The requirement and hence limitation of the PARAFAC model is that the data must be approximately low-rank trilinear to provide physically meaningful loadings (e.g. pure spectra).

PARAFAC has been applied to chromatographic studies. These include the detection of disease-resistant clones of *Eucalyptus* using a feature selection method, Fisher ratio and PARAFAC for the analysis of GC–GC–qMS. Utilising this approach, the authors were able to determine resistance biomarkers in *Eucalyptus* hybrids against rust disease (Hantao et al., 2013). PARAFAC has been applied to 2-D gas chromatography with TOF mass spectrometry (GC–GC–TOF-MS). Low levels of L-beta-methylamino-alanine (BMAA) were consistently identified in trace amounts in tissue samples that were previously undetectable in standard assays (Snyder et al., 2010).

PARAFAC has also been used in fluorescence spectroscopy excitation emission matrix (EM) measurements that were applied to human blood plasma samples from a case–control study on colorectal cancer. The combination of PARAFAC and three-way fluorescence data (EEM) was found to be particularly favourable since the parameters of the PARAFAC model could be related to estimate the relative concentration (scores) and the emission and excitation spectra (loadings) of the fluorophores in the sample. Furthermore, it was found that the discrimination results were similar whether the authors applied classification directly on the raw unfolded spectra or extracted estimates of the underlying fluorophores by use of PARAFAC. Better conditions for a chemical interpretation/understanding of the results were obtained using PARAFAC (Lawaetz et al., 2012).

PARAFAC has also been extended to two-dimensional J-resolved ^{1}H NMR data. The PARAFAC decomposition reflected the concentration, individual component spectra along the chemical shift axis and the corresponding profile along the J-coupling axis of a set of saffron samples, extracted in methanol-d_4. The PARAFAC model increased interpretability by linking the chemical shifts with the J-coupling constants (Yilmaz et al., 2011).

PARAFAC has also been utilised for lipoprotein characterization using 2-D diffusion-edited NMR spectroscopy providing chemically meaningful spectra (Dyrby et al., 2005a) and for time-resolved biomarker discovery using ^{1}H NMR (Alm et al., 2010). PARAFAC has also been applied to coeluting ^{13}C and ^{12}C isotopically labelled metabolites to improve accuracy and precision of quantitative metabolomics and ^{13}C flux analysis. The PARAFAC-based data analysis approach was used to isolate and quantify severely overlapped peaks (chromatographic resolution of ~ 0.1) from the ^{13}C-labelled cell extract internal standard from *Methylobacterium extorquens* AM1 cell cultures grown in methanol and ^{12}C-natural versions of the same metabolite from each other, background noise and overlapping interferences (such as natural ^{13}C isotopes and unknown coeluting metabolites). It was shown that the quantitative information for individual metabolites and time course analysis of isotope enrichment could be determined with high accuracy and may be of use for future dynamic ^{13}C flux studies (Yang et al., 2012).

3.7.2 Tucker decomposition

Tucker decomposition (Kroonenberg and Deleeuw, 1980; Tenberge et al., 1987; Tucker, 1966b), a generalised PCA on multiway data, has the same capabilities of PCA, that is, to compress variation, extract features and explore data. In addition to these capabilities, the presence of the core array in the Tucker decomposition allows for the interpretation of the interaction between the different components, describing the variations between the samples, and measurement on multiple variables and experiments. Furthermore, the three-way structure of the original data may allow for more direct interpretation of features common to the data (Henrion, 1994; Kroonenberg, 1983). Dyrby et al. (2005b) showed how a traditional dose–response experiment could be properly explored using Tucker3 models. Idborg et al. (2004) exemplified the use of PARAFAC and N-way partial least squares (NPLS) (Bro, 1996b) in handling metabolite screening using liquid chromatography/electrospray ionization mass spectrometry (LC/EI-MS).

Visualization of important variables in each mode (samples and measurement on multiple variables and experiments) can sometimes be difficult with these models (i.e. NPLS, Tucker and PARAFAC). An analogy to the two-way correlation loading plot to assess variable significance was considered by Lorho et al. (2006), and a generalization to the multiway case was developed using congruence loadings and applied to a metabonomics experiment using 2-D diffusion-edited NMR (Lorho et al., 2006). ASCA (Jansen et al., 2005) has been developed to increase the interpretability of a multivariate dataset in terms of the experimental design (i.e. providing a more direct answer to the experimental question at hand) and extended to the multiway case by combining ASCA with PARAFAC (PARAFASCA) (Jansen et al., 2008). This approach was used to study the time–effect of hydrazine toxicity in the composition of urine of rats evaluated by ^{1}H NMR spectroscopy. Acar et al. had completed a detailed evaluation of the limitation and advantages of data integration within the framework of coupled matrix and tensor factorization in comparison with CANDECOMP/PARAFAC(CP) models (Carroll and Chang, 1970; Harshman, 1970b).

3.8 Data integration: correlation-based approaches

Structural connectivity and biological connectivity between metabolites measured on multiple spectroscopic platforms have been achieved using correlation-based approaches, such as statistical total correlation spectroscopy (STOCSY, (Cloarec et al., 2005)). STOCSY is a correlation-based method for aiding the identification of potential biomarker molecules in metabonomics studies and adopts Pearson's or Spearman's correlation to derive a correlation matrix between each data point in a spectrum for a given set of spectra (Cloarec et al., 2005). STOCSY uses the correlation of the intensity variables in a spectrum and identifies the presence of multiple peaks from the same compound in a set of NMR spectra. Typically, excluding a high degree of signal overlap, the correlation matrix from a set of spectra containing different amounts of the same molecule shows very high correlations between the data points corresponding to the resonances of the same molecule. Furthermore, two or more molecules representing the same pathway can also show intermolecular correlations or anti-correlations because of biological covariance due to common pathway activity.

Interpretation of STOCSY outcomes in terms of clusters of metabolites with similar co-expression patterns has been recently achieved using cluster analysis statistical spectroscopy (CLASSY (Robinette et al., 2009; Wang et al., 2008)), resulting in a local–global correlation clustering scheme, unveiling pathway connectivities and variability in individual responses. The outcome of correlation and covariance analyses is used in statistical recoupling (Blaise et al., 2009) to associate regions of consecutive variables to restore spectral dependency and allows the formation of superclusters, improving the interpretability of latent variables for metabolic biomarker recovery (Blaise et al., 2009). Extensive correlation analyses on individual features or variables of interest, for example, as detected by OPLS, can be further investigated using MetaFIND (Bryan et al., 2008), which was reported to aid metabolite signature elucidation, feature discovery and inference of metabolic correlations (Bryan et al., 2008).

Alternatively, it is possible to perform HET-STOCSY (heteronuclear statistical total correlation spectroscopy) across a set of samples by using two NMR datasets of different nuclei, for example, ^{1}H and ^{31}P (Coen et al., 2007; Wang et al., 2008) or ^{19}F and ^{1}H (Keun et al., 2008). The STOCSY principle can be extended to identify correlations between NMR spectra and various types of MS data, SHY. This is particularly pertinent for nutrition research where nutrients are present in low concentrations and therefore detectable only by MS but where their metabolic effect may be detectable by NMR. The cross correlation of spectral parameters has a synergistic effect with increased information extraction, as bidirectional multivariate correlations between identified and unidentified signals can lead to mutually increased information content and significantly improved interpretability. The approach is not limited to these two platforms, and other examples include the integration of NMR and capillary electrophoresis (Garcia-Perez et al., 2010). Thus, the statistical integration of molecular profiles of the same sample using different spectroscopic platforms enables molecular biomarker identification and information recovery on metabolic pathway connectivities by the examination of different levels of the analytic platform–platform correlation matrices.

3.9 Data integration: techniques for analysing different types of genomics datasets

The emergence of high-throughput genomics datasets from different sources and platforms (e.g. gene expression, single-nucleotide polymorphisms (SNP) and copy number variation (CNV)) has greatly enhanced understanding of the interplay of these genomic factors and their influences on complex diseases. It is beneficial to explore the relationship between these different types of genomic datasets. A number of approaches have been proposed to analyse multiple genomic data, for example:

- partial least squares correlation (PLSC (Lê Cao et al., 2008))
- CCA (Hotelling, 1936)

In CCA, correlations between two datasets are determined through investigation of the canonical correlation coefficients. The canonical correlation coefficients can be calculated directly from the two datasets or from (reduced) representations such as the covariance matrices. The algorithms for both representations are based on singular value decomposition. CCA is closely related to PLSC (Wegelin, 2000), which is obtained by maximising the correlation between the linear combinations of variables from two datasets, for example, a linear combination of SNPs and a linear combination of gene expressions.

CCA has proved to be a powerful method in previous studies especially in GWAS (genome-wide association study). Peng et al. (2010) had proposed a canonical correlation-based U-statistic metric to detect SNP-based gene–gene co-association in two sample case-control datasets. They explored its type I error rate through simulations on two real datasets. In another study, Naylor et al. (2010) had implemented CCA to detect genetic associations between SNPs and gene expression levels. By this methodology, they claimed to reduce the amount of necessary comparisons.

For large-scale genomic studies, Parkhomenko et al. (2009) suggested using a sparse implementation of CCA. They divided their dataset into small subsets of variables belonging to different types and performed variable selection by maximising the correlation between these subsets. Lin et al. (2013) introduced a new group sparse CCA method (CCA-sparse group) along with an effective numerical algorithm to study the mutual relationship between two different types of genomic data (i.e. SNP and gene expression). Gumus et al. (2012) utilised CCA in searching viral integration patterns on the sequences reported by Schröder et al. (2002).

CCA-based analysis can be applied to protein datasets as well, such as for searching correlated functions between moment-based features, autocorrelation, composition, transition or distribution (Li et al., 2006; Shi et al., 2006). However, in the presence of insufficient training data, CCA tends to overfit the data. Regularised CCA (RCCA) is an improved version of CCA that tends to prevent over-fitting by using a ridge regression optimization scheme (De Bie and Be Moor, 2003). However, the regularization process required by RCCA is computationally very expensive.

The concept of "genetical genomics" (Jansen and Nap, 2001) was introduced by Jansen and Nap (2001), aiming at merging genome-wide expression profiling and genome-wide genotyping in segregating populations, using the statistical genetics used in the analysis of quantitative trait loci (QTL). A subsequent paradigm shift was introduced, known as expression QTL (eQTL) approaches (Schadt et al., 2003).

3.10 Statistical data integration of different sample types

Changes in metabolic chemistry in different body compartments caused by exposure to a biological intervention can be described as integrative metabonomics (Nicholson et al., 2002; Yap et al., 2006). Such timed profiles in multiple compartments are themselves characteristic of particular types and mechanisms. The statistical integration of multiple tissue samples can reveal metabolic information associated with, for example, the Cori cycle between the muscle and the liver or insight about renal clearance or retention from the coanalysis of plasma and urine, thus giving a more complete description of the mechanistic consequences than can be obtained from one fluid or tissue alone.

Typically for integrative metabonomics analyses, multivariate statistical models are constructed on each biofluid and (or) tissue using either unsupervised or supervised pattern recognition methods such as PCA, PLS-DA and OPLS-DA, followed by an integrated interpretation of the results from the different biological compartments. Examples of single-block analysis followed by interpretation include nutritional studies (Martin et al., 2009a) and various pre- and probiotics on gut microbiota (Claus et al., 2008; Dumas et al., 2006; Martin et al., 2008, 2009b).

However, information relating to the common systematic variance across the different compartments and the detection of inter-compartment functional relationships is hard to recover using such approaches. More recently, an integrative metabonomics approach using OSC–PLS and HPCA for the full statistical integration of the jejunum, ileum, colon, liver, spleen and kidney samples was completed in order to enhance and increase understanding of physiological and pathological consequences of a patent *Schistosoma mansoni* infection in mice (Li et al., 2009).

Spatiotemporal interorgan metabolic control functions were modelled by Montoliu et al. (2009) with various 2- and 3-way multivariate statistical approaches including PCA, multiway PCA (N-PCA) (Nomikos and MacGregor, 1994), MCR–alternating least squares (MCR–ALS) (Tauler et al., 1993) and PARAFAC to abstract the inter-compartmental functional relationships between healthy mice plasma, liver, pancreas, adrenal gland and kidney cortex. Of the multivariate approaches, MCR–ALS and PARAFAC appeared to be better adapted for stepwise variable and compartment selection for further correlation analysis because both methods provided an overview of functional relationships across matrices and enabled the characterization of compartment-specific metabolite signatures (spectrotypes (Richards et al., 2008b)). Furthermore, the spectrotypes enabled the differentiation between both specific and common biochemical profiles associated with the different biological compartments (Montoliu et al., 2009).

3.11 Statistical data integration of different molecular components in samples

Systems biology aims to combine the molecular components (transcripts, proteins and metabolites) of an organism and incorporate them into functional networks or models designed to describe its molecular connectivities and dynamic activities. On a system-wide scale, the description requires three levels of information (Albert, 2007; Grimplet et al., 2009):

(A) Identification of the components (structural annotation) and characterization of their identity (functional annotation)
(B) Identification of molecules that interact with each component
(C) Characterization of the behaviours of the transcripts, proteins and metabolites under various conditions (Gavaghan et al., 2002c)

Bioinformatics approaches in systems biology include biomarker discovery and reconstruction of regulatory signals in biological networks (see Section 3.4).

Metabolic phenotypes, or metabotypes (Blaise et al., 2007), can be analysed in a statistical genetics framework like other phenotypes, with a genetic component and an environmental component. Such framework consists of linking the genomic variation information with the metabolomic variation information using appropriate statistical tools, such as CCA. This has been used to examine the interdependent relationship between host epithelial cell gene expression and bacterial metagenomic-based profiles in healthy full-term infants in order to identify intestinal genes potentially important in microbiome regulatory pathways and the integrative gut development process in the first few months of life (Griffin et al., 2004).

Other chemometrics methods include PLS (Rantalainen et al., 2006), O2PLS (Bylesjo et al., 2007, 2009; Schwartz et al., 2012) and PARAFAC (Verouden et al., 2009). Conesa et al. (2010) evaluated Tucker3 and NPLS for analysing multi-factorial data structures to identify underlying components of variability that interconnect different blocks of omic data. These methods were used for the integration of gene expression, metabolomics and physiological data. Furthermore, Golugula et al. (2011) developed a novel efficient supervised regularised canonical correlation analysis (SRCCA) algorithm that is able to incorporate a supervised feature selection scheme to perform regularization, unlike CCA and RCCA that do not take complete advantage of class label information, when available. SRCCA was applied to the problem of predicting biochemical recurrence in prostate cancer (CaP) patients, following radical prostatectomy, by fusing histological imaging and proteomic signatures.

The use of quantitative trait locus mapping of metabolomic traits, or "mQTL", provides a very good conceptual, analytic and mathematical framework to identify genomic regions influencing metabolic profiles. This approach was introduced in plants (Keurentjes et al., 2006; Schaub et al., 2006) and in rodent genetic inter-crosses targeting type 2 diabetes (Dumas et al., 2007). Altogether, these studies apply the genetical genomics concept to metabolomic traits, or genetical metabolomics. The resulting linkage maps allowed the identification of associations between genomic sequence variants and plasma metabolites.

The mQTL approach integrates variations obtained from metabolome-wide profiling and genome-wide genotyping to identify genetic variants or *loci* influencing metabolite levels: in tissues and biofluids, if a genetic variant affects the activity of a specific enzyme, a variation in the levels of metabolic substrates or products is expected. The concept of metabolome-wide association study (MWAS) (Holmes et al., 2008) was introduced to highlight the potential of metabolomic markers in molecular epidemiology (Holmes et al., 2008).

The mQTL, GWAS and MWAS approaches have now merged in human epidemiology with several successful clinical applications (Gieger et al., 2008; Illig et al., 2010; Tanaka et al., 2009). In terms of validation of *loci*, the idea that a genome sequence variant (QTL) could directly influence simultaneously the expression of its gene (eQTL), its translation into a protein (protQTL), its effect on metabolism (mQTL) and phenotypic outcome (pQTL) provides a powerful self-validation tool (Fu et al., 2009). However, the occurrence of co-localization is very rare (<10 loci in *Arabidopsis thaliana* genome), suggesting the limits of *cis*-QTL effects. Ultimately, genetical genomic and mQTL approaches require an independent validation for any *locus* of interest identified, whether it is in an independent experimental cross for animal models (Dumas et al., 2007) or in an independent cohort for clinical applications (Illig et al., 2010).

3.12 Modelling relationships between molecular components

Metabolic pathway annotation is now part of the post-genomic knowledge compilation effort (Kanehisa and Goto, 2000), for example, mapping molecular profiles onto public databases of functional and pathway information, such as the Kyoto Encyclopaedia of Genes and Genomes (KEGG) (Kanehisa and Goto, 2000), Gene Ontology Consortium (Ashburner et al., 2000) and Interactome (Ito et al., 2001). Such databases enable the rapid development of *knowledge-based methods* for uncovering higher-order systemic operation of the cell and the organism from genomic and molecular information.

As an example, Tavazoie et al. (1999) put forward a method now known as over-representation analysis and discovered distinct expression pattern clusters in mRNA and found that they were significantly enriched for genes with similar function (Tavazoie et al., 1999). Mootha et al. (2003) introduced the concept of Gene Set Enrichment Analysis (Mootha et al., 2003; Subramanian et al., 2005), in which a set of genes involved in a signature are compared to existing knowledge about gene pathways (Curtis et al., 2005). This allows a transition between simple biological entities, such as genes, to a higher-order description, such as gene pathways, and leads to a synthetic view of the relevant biological pathways and functions affected. Gene Set Enrichment Analysis is a generic method that can be easily extended to proteomic data and metabolic profile data, or Metabolite Set Enrichment Analysis (Pontoizeau et al., in prep.).

To our knowledge, no real attempt has been made to integrate metabolomic markers to the known interactome—the rapidly growing knowledge of protein–protein interaction (PPI) networks (interactome) for human, model organisms and host–pathogen that may begin to provide network-based models for diseases (Ge et al., 2001; Ito et al., 2001; Sanchez et al., 1999). According to Sanchez et al. (1999), the total number of genes of an organism is less important than the complete repertoire of interactions potentially encoded by its genome (i.e. the interactome) (Sanchez et al., 1999). Several interactions (protein–DNA, protein–RNA and protein–protein) were initially included, but due to the presence of double-hybrid and co-immunoprecipitation assays, most of the work has focused on PPIs.

Topological properties of the entire metabolic network exhibit robustness against isolated random genetic mutations and/or metabolic perturbations. Robustness of the metabolic reaction network also depends on its high level of plasticity and regulation, which is at least part mediated by gene variants, transcriptional variation, protein abundance and modulation activity through direct molecular interactions and covalent binding (Navratil and Dumas, in prep.).

Full sequencing of various organisms now allows genome-scale metabolic reconstruction approaches. The metabolic network of organisms or tissues can then be inferred from the genome sequence. Such strategies involving network-based predictions of metabolism have been successfully applied to yeast (Dyrby et al., 2005a), and a range of other microorganisms, as well as human metabolism, are now complementary to metabolic profiling (Shlomi et al., 2008, 2009). A comprehensive review on integrated omic approaches for modelling of cellular networks is given by Joyce et al. (Joyce and Palsson, 2006).

3.13 Conclusion and future trends

The ability to generate and model rich genotypic and phenotypic data in relation to benchmark nutritional information, enabled by the advent and maturation of multiomic technologies (genomics, transcriptomics, proteomics, epigenomics, metabonomics and metagenomics) and powerful bioinformatics platforms, makes stratified and personalised nutrition a tangible proposition. New tools such as rapid evaporative ionization mass spectrometry (REIMS) will open up new possibilities in food analysis, allowing the characterization of composition within a second to minute time frame. In addition to new analytic tools in nutrimetabolomics, the creation and commercialization of databases for food components will enable the identification of adulterated products and the identification of food consumption in biofluids such as urine and serum. Harmonised instrumentation across multiple centres, for example, the six core metabolomics facilities in the United States and the National Phenome Centre in the United Kingdom, has the potential to provide a unified framework for harvesting and modelling genotypic and dynamic phenotypic datasets in relation to nutritional information. New pipelines for mathematical fusion of these information sets are required to create new systems models for the stratification of individuals in order to augment optimised nutrition, to improve food safety and to provide more holistic therapeutic management for critically ill patients.

References

Albert, R., 2007. Network inference, analysis, and modeling in systems biology. Plant Cell 19, 3327–3338.

Alm, E., Torgrip, R.J., Åberg, K.M., Schuppe-Koistinen, I., Lindberg, J., 2010. Time-resolved biomarker discovery in 1H-NMR data using generalized fuzzy Hough transform alignment and parallel factor analysis. Anal. Bioanal. Chem. 396, 1681–1689.

Ashburner, M., Ball, C.A., Blake, J.A., et al., 2000. Gene ontology: tool for the unification of biology. The Gene Ontology Consortium. Nat. Genet. 25, 25–29.

Beckwith-Hall, B.M., Brindle, J.T., Barton, R.H., et al., 2002. Application of orthogonal signal correction to minimise the effects of physical and biological variation in high resolution H-1 NMR spectra of biofluids. Analyst 127, 1283–1288.

Biais, B., Allwood, J.W., Deborde, C., et al., 2009. 1H NMR, GC-EI-TOFMS, and data set correlation for fruit metabolomics: application to spatial metabolite analysis in melon. Anal. Chem. 81, 2884–2894.

Blaise, B.J., Giacomotto, J., Elena, B., et al., 2007. Metabotyping of Caenorhabditis elegans reveals latent phenotypes. Proc. Natl. Acad. Sci. U. S. A. 104, 19808–19812.

Blaise, B.J., Shintu, L., Elena, B., et al., 2009. Statistical recoupling prior to significance testing in nuclear magnetic resonance based metabonomics. Anal. Chem. 81, 6242–6251.

Boccard, J., Rutledge, D.N., 2013. A consensus orthogonal partial least squares discriminant analysis (OPLS-DA) strategy for multiblock Omics data fusion. Anal. Chim. Acta. 769, 30–39.

Bro, R., 1996. Multiway calibration. Multilinear PLS. J. Chemom. 10, 47–61.

Bro, R., 1997. PARAFAC. Tutorial and applications. Chemometrics Intell. Lab. Syst. 38, 149–171.

Bro, R., 2006. Review on multiway analysis in chemistry—2000–2005. Crit. Rev. Anal. Chem. 36, 279–293.

Bryan, K., Brennan, L., Cunningham, P., 2008. MetaFIND: a feature analysis tool for metabolomics data. BMC Bioinform. 9, 470.

Bylesjo, M., Eriksson, D., Kusano, M., Moritz, T., Trygg, J., 2007. Data integration in plant biology: the O2PLS method for combined modeling of transcript and metabolite data. Plant J. 52, 1181–1191.

Bylesjo, M., Nilsson, R., Srivastava, V., et al., 2009. Integrated analysis of transcript, protein and metabolite data to study lignin biosynthesis in hybrid aspen. J. Proteome Res. 8, 199–210.

Carroll, J.D., Chang, J., 1970. Analysis of individual differences in multidimensional scaling via an N-way generalization of "Eckart-Young" decomposition. Psychometrika 35, 283–319.

Claus, S.P., Tsang, T.M., Wang, Y., et al., 2008. Systemic multicompartmental effects of the gut microbiome on mouse metabolic phenotypes. Mol. Syst. Biol. 4, 219.

Cloarec, O., Dumas, M., Craig, A., Barton, R.H., Trygg, J., Hudson, J., et al., 2005. Statistical total correlation spectroscopy: an exploratory approach for latent biomarker identification from metabolic 1H NMR data sets. Anal. Chem. 77, 1282–1289.

Coen, M., Hong, Y.S., Cloarec, O., et al., 2007. Heteronuclear 1H-31P statistical total correlation NMR spectroscopy of intact liver for metabolic biomarker assignment: application to galactosamine-induced hepatotoxicity. Anal. Chem. 79, 8956–8966.

Conesa, A., Prats-Montalbán, J.M., Tarazona, S., Nueda, M.J., Ferrer, A., 2010. A multiway approach to data integration in systems biology based on Tucker3 *n*PLS. Chemometrics Intell. Lab. Syst. 104, 101–111.

Coomans, D., Broeckaert, I., 1986. Potential Pattern Recognition in Chemical and Medical Decision Making. John Wiley & Sons Inc, New York.

Coomans, D., Jonckheer, M., Massart, D., Broeckaert, I., Blockx, P., 1978. The application of linear discriminant analysis in the diagnosis of thyroid diseases. Anal. Chim. Acta. 103, 409–415.

Crockford, D.J., Maher, A.D., Ahmadi, K.R., Barrett, A., Plumb, R.S., Wilson, I.D., et al., 2008. 1H NMR and UPLC-MSE statistical heterospectroscopy: characterization of drug metabolites (Xenometabolome) in epidemiological studies. Anal. Chem. 80, 6835–6844.

Curtis, R.K., Oresic, M., Vidal-Puig, A., 2005. Pathways to the analysis of microarray data. Trends Biotechnol. 23, 429–435.

Dagnelie, P., Merckx, A., 1991. Using generalized distances in classification of groups. Biom. J. 33, 683–695.

De Bie, T., De Moor, B., 2003. On the regularization of canonical correlation analysis. In: Proceedings of the Fourth International Symposium on Independent Component Analysis and Blind Source Separation, pp. 785–790.

Dumas, M.E., Canlet, C., Debrauwer, L., Martin, P., Paris, A., 2005. Selection of biomarkers by a multivariate statistical processing of composite metabonomic data sets using multiple factor analysis. J. Proteome Res. 4, 1485–1492.

Dumas, M.E., Barton, R.H., Toye, A., et al., 2006. Metabolic profiling reveals a contribution of gut microbiota to fatty liver phenotype in insulin-resistant mice. Proc. Natl. Acad. Sci. U. S. A. 103, 12511–12516.

Dumas, M.E., Wilder, S.P., Bihoreau, M.T., et al., 2007. Direct quantitative trait locus mapping of mammalian metabolic phenotypes in diabetic and normoglycemic rat models. Nat. Genet. 39, 666–672.

Dyrby, M., Petersen, M., Whittaker, A.K., Lambert, L., Nørgaard, L., Bro, R., et al., 2005a. Analysis of lipoproteins using 2D diffusion-edited NMR spectroscopy and multi-way chemometrics. Anal. Chim. Acta. 531, 209–216.

Dyrby, M., Baunsgaard, D., Bro, R., Engelsen, S.B., 2005b. Multiway chemometric analysis of the metabolic response to toxins monitored by NMR. Chemom. Intell. Lab. Syst. 76, 79–89.

Ebbels, T.M.D., Cavill, R., 2009. Bioinformatic methods in NMR-based metabolic profiling. Prog. Nucl. Magn. Reson. Spectrosc. 55, 361–374.

Eriksson, L., Toft, M., Johansson, E., Wold, S., Trygg, J., 2006. Separating Y-predictive and Y-orthogonal variation in multi-block spectral data. J. Chemometr. 20, 352–361.

Escofier, B., Pages, J., 1994. Multiple factor analysis (AFMULT package). Comput. Stat. Data Anal. 18, 121–140.

Forina, M., Lanteri, S., Armanino, C., 1987. Chemometrics in food chemistry. In: Chemometrics and Species Identification. Springer, pp. 91–143.

Forina, M., Armanino, C., Leardi, R., Drava, G., 1991. A class-modelling technique based on potential functions. J. Chemometr. 5, 435–453.

Forshed, J., Idborg, H., Jacobsson, S.P., 2007. Evaluation of different techniques for data fusion of LC/MS and 1 H-NMR. Chemom. Intell. Lab. Syst. 85, 102–109.

Fu, J., Keurentjes, J.J., Bouwmeester, H., et al., 2009. System-wide molecular evidence for phenotypic buffering in Arabidopsis. Nat. Genet. 41, 166–167.

Garcia-Perez, I., Alves, A.C., Angulo, S., et al., 2010. Bidirectional correlation of NMR and capillary electrophoresis fingerprints: a new approach to investigating Schistosoma mansoni infection in a mouse model. Anal. Chem. 82, 203–210.

Gargallo, R., Tauler, R., Cuesta-Sanchez, F., Massart, D., 1996. Validation of alternating least-squares multivariate curve resolution for chromatographic resolution and quantitation. TrAC Trends Anal. Chem. 15, 279–286.

Gavaghan, C.L., Wilson, I.D., Nicholson, J.K., 2002. Physiological variation in metabolic phenotyping and functional genomic studies: use of orthogonal signal correction and PLS-DA. FEBS Lett. 530, 191–196.

Ge, H., Liu, Z., Church, G.M., Vidal, M., 2001. Correlation between transcriptome and interactome mapping data from Saccharomyces cerevisiae. Nat. Genet. 29, 482–486.

Gieger, C., Geistlinger, L., Altmaier, E., et al., 2008. Genetics meets metabolomics: a genome-wide association study of metabolite profiles in human serum. PLoS Genet. 4, e1000282.

Golugula, A., Lee, G., Master, S.R., Feldman, M.D., Tomaszewski, J.E., Speicher, D.W., et al., 2011. Supervised regularized canonical correlation analysis: integrating histologic and proteomic measurements for predicting biochemical recurrence following prostate surgery. BMC Bioinform. 12 (483), 2105-12–2105-483.

González, I., Déjean, S., Martin, P., Gonçalves, O., Besse, P., Baccini, A., 2009. Highlighting relationships between heterogeneous biological data through graphical displays based on regularized canonical correlation analysis. J. Biol. Syst. 17, 173–199.

Griffin, J.L., Bonney, S.A., Mann, C., et al., 2004. An integrated reverse functional genomic and metabolic approach to understanding orotic acid-induced fatty liver. Physiol. Genomics 17, 140–149.

Grimplet, J., Cramer, G.R., Dickerson, J.A., et al., 2009. VitisNet: "omics" integration through grapevine molecular networks. PLoS One 4, e8365.

Gumus, E., Kursun, O., Sertbas, A., Ustek, D., 2012. Application of canonical correlation analysis for identifying viral integration preferences. Bioinformatics 28, 651–655.

Guyon, I., Weston, J., Barnhill, S., Vapnik, V., 2002. Gene selection for cancer classification using support vector machines. Mach. Learn. 46, 389–422.

Hantao, L.W., Toledo, B.R., de Lima, Ribeiro, Alves, Fabiana, Pizetta, M., Pierozzi, C.G., Furtado, E.L., et al., 2013. Comprehensive two-dimensional gas chromatography combined to multivariate data analysis for detection of disease-resistant clones of *Eucalyptus*. Talanta 116, 1079–1084.

Hardy, T.M., Tollefsbol, T.O., 2011. Epigenetic diet: impact on the epigenome and cancer. Epigenomics. 3 (4), 503–518.

Harshman, R.A., 1970. Foundations of the PARAFAC procedure: models and conditions for an" explanatory" multimodal factor analysis. UCLA Working Papers in Phonetics 16, 1.

Harshman, R.A., Lundy, M.E., 1984. The PARAFAC model for three-way factor analysis and multidimensional scaling. In: Law, H.G., Snyder, C.W., Hattie, J.A., McDonald, R.P. (Eds.), Research Methods for Multimode Data Analysis. Praeger, New York, pp. 122–215.

Henrion, R., 1994. N-way principal component analysis theory, algorithms and applications. Chemom. Intell. Lab. Syst. 25, 1–23.

Holmes, E., Loo, R.L., Stamler, J., et al., 2008. Human metabolic phenotype diversity and its association with diet and blood pressure. Nature 453, 396–400.

Hotelling, H., 1935. Canonical correlation analysis (cca). J. Educ. Psychol. 26, 139–142.

Hotelling, H., 1936. Relations between two sets of variates. Biometrika 28, 321–377.

Idborg, H., Edlund, P.O., Jacobsson, S.P., 2004. Multivariate approaches for efficient detection of potential metabolites from liquid chromatography/mass spectrometry data. Rapid Commun. Mass Spectrom. 18, 944–954.

Illig, T., Gieger, C., Zhai, G., et al., 2010. A genome-wide perspective of genetic variation in human metabolism. Nat. Genet. 42, 137–141.

Ito, T., Chiba, T., Ozawa, R., et al., 2001. A comprehensive two-hybrid analysis to explore the yeast protein interactome. Proc. Natl. Acad. Sci. U. S. A. 98, 4569–4574.

Jansen, R.C., Nap, J.P., 2001. Genetical genomics: the added value from segregation. Trends Genet. 17, 388–391.

Jansen, J.J., Hoefsloot, H.C.J., van der Greef, J., et al., 2005. ASCA: analysis of multivariate data obtained from an experimental design. J. Chemom. 19, 469–481.

Jansen, J.J., Bro, R., Hoefsloot, H.C.J., et al., 2008. PARAFASCA: ASCA combined with PARAFAC for the analysis of metabolic fingerprinting data. J. Chemom. 22, 114–121.

Jeffers, J., 1967. Two case studies in the application of principal component analysis. Appl. Stat. 16, 225–236.

Jolliffe, I., 2005. Principal Component Analysis. Wiley Online Library, New York, USA.

Joyce, A.R., Palsson, B.O., 2006. The model organism as a system: integrating 'omics' data sets. Nat. Rev. Mol. Cell Biol. 7, 198–210.

Kanehisa, M., Goto, S., 2000. KEGG: kyoto encyclopedia of genes and genomes. Nucleic Acids Res. 28, 27–30.

Keun, H.C., Athersuch, T.J., Beckonert, O., et al., 2008. Heteronuclear 19F-1H statistical total correlation spectroscopy as a tool in drug metabolism: study of flucloxacillin biotransformation. Anal. Chem. 80, 1073–1079.

Keurentjes, J.J., Fu, J., de Vos, C.H., et al., 2006. The genetics of plant metabolism. Nat. Genet. 38, 842–849.

Kohonen, T., 1982. Self-organized formation of topologically correct feature maps. Biol. Cybern. 43, 59–69.

Kroonenberg, P.M., 1983. Three-Mode Principal Component Analysis: Theory and Applications. DSWO Press, Leiden.

Kroonenberg, P.M., Deleeuw, J., 1980. Principal component analysis of 3-mode data by means of alternating least-squares algorithms. Psychometrika 45, 69–97.

Krooshof, P.W., Üstün, B., Postma, G.J., Buydens, L.M., 2010. Visualization and recovery of the (bio) chemical interesting variables in data analysis with support vector machine classification. Anal. Chem. 82, 7000–7007.

Lawaetz, A.J., Bro, R., Kamstrup-Nielsen, M., Christensen, I.J., Jørgensen, L.N., Nielsen, H.J., 2012. Fluorescence spectroscopy as a potential metabonomic tool for early detection of colorectal cancer. Metabolomics 8, 111–121.

Lawton, W.H., Sylvestre, E.A., 1971. Self modeling curve resolution. Technometrics 13, 617–633.

Lê Cao, K., Rossouw, D., Robert-Granié, C., Besse, P., 2008. A sparse PLS for variable selection when integrating omics data. Stat. Appl. Genet. Mol. Biol. 7, article 35.

Li, Z.R., Lin, H.H., Han, L.Y., Jiang, L., Chen, X., Chen, Y.Z., 2006. PROFEAT: a web server for computing structural and physicochemical features of proteins and peptides from amino acid sequence. Nucleic Acids Res. 34, W32–W37.

Li, J.V., Holmes, E., Saric, J., et al., 2009. Metabolic profiling of a Schistosoma mansoni infection in mouse tissues using magic angle spinning-nuclear magnetic resonance spectroscopy. Int. J. Parasitol. 39, 547–558.

Lin, D., Zhang, J., Li, J., Calhoun, V.D., Deng, H., Wang, Y., 2013. Group sparse canonical correlation analysis for genomic data integration. BMC Bioinform. 14, 1–16.

Löfstedt, T., Hoffman, D., Trygg, J., 2013. Global, local and unique decompositions in OnPLS for multiblock data analysis. Anal. Chim. Acta. 791, 13–24.

Lorho, G., Westad, F., Bro, R., 2006. Generalized correlation loadings. Extending correlation loadings to congruence and to multi-way models. Chemom. Intell. Lab. Syst. 84, 119–125.

Mahalanobis, P.C., 1936. On the generalized distance in statistics. Proc. Nat. Inst. Sci. (Calcutta) 2, 49–55.

Mao, H.L., Xu, M., Wang, B., et al., 2007. Evaluation of filtering effects of orthogonal signal correction on metabonomic analysis of healthy human serum H-1 NMR spectra. Acta Chim. Sin. 65, 152–158.

Martin, F.P., Wang, Y., Sprenger, N., et al., 2008. Top-down systems biology integration of conditional prebiotic modulated transgenomic interactions in a humanized microbiome mouse model. Mol. Syst. Biol. 4, 205.

Martin, F.P., Rezzi, S., Pere-Trepat, E., et al., 2009a. Metabolic effects of dark chocolate consumption on energy, gut microbiota, and stress-related metabolism in free-living subjects. J. Proteome Res. 8, 5568–5579.

Martin, F.P., Sprenger, N., Yap, I.K., et al., 2009b. Panorganismal gut microbiome-host metabolic crosstalk. J. Proteome Res. 8, 2090–2105.

Massart, D.L., Vandeginste, B., Buydens, L., De Jong, S., Lewi, P., Smeyers-Verbeke, J., 1997. Handbook of Chemometrics and Qualimetrics: Part A. Elsevier Science Pub Co, Amsterdam.

Montoliu, I., Martin, F.P., Collino, S., Rezzi, S., Kochhar, S., 2009. Multivariate modeling strategy for intercompartmental analysis of tissue and plasma 1H NMR spectrotypes. J. Proteome Res. 8, 2397–2406.

Mootha, V.K., Lindgren, C.M., Eriksson, K.F., et al., 2003. PGC-1alpha-responsive genes involved in oxidative phosphorylation are coordinately downregulated in human diabetes. Nat. Genet. 34, 267–273.
Naylor, M.G., Lin, X., Weiss, S.T., Raby, B.A., Lange, C., 2010. Using canonical correlation analysis to discover genetic regulatory variants. PLoS One 5, e10395.
Nicholson, J.K., Connelly, J., Lindon, J.C., Holmes, E., 2002. Metabonomics: a platform for studying drug toxicity and gene function. Nat. Rev. Drug Discov. 1, 153–161.
Nomikos, P., MacGregor, J.F., 1994. Monitoring batch processes using multiway principal component analysis. AICHE J. 40, 1361–1375.
Pages, J., Tenenhaus, M., 2001. Multiple factor analysis combined with PLS path modelling. Application to the analysis of relationships between physicochemical variables, sensory profiles and hedonic judgements. Chemom. Intell. Lab. Syst. 58, 261–273.
Parkhomenko, E., Tritchler, D., Beyene, J., 2009. Sparse canonical correlation analysis with application to genomic data integration. Stat. Appl. Genet. Mol. Biol. 8, 1–34.
Peng, Q., Zhao, J., Xue, F., 2010. A gene-based method for detecting gene–gene co-association in a case–control association study. Eur. J. Hum. Genet. 18, 582–587.
Postma, G., Krooshof, P., Buydens, L., 2011. Opening the kernel of kernel partial least squares and support vector machines. Anal. Chim. Acta. 705, 123–134.
Rantalainen, M., Cloarec, O., Beckonert, O., et al., 2006. Statistically integrated metabonomic-proteomic studies on a human prostate cancer xenograft model in mice. J. Proteome Res. 5, 2642–2655.
Richards, S.E., Wang, Y., Lawler, D., Kochhar, S., Holmes, E., Lindon, J.C., et al., 2008a. Self-modeling curve resolution recovery of temporal metabolite signal modulation in NMR spectroscopic data sets: application to a life-long caloric restriction study in dogs. Anal. Chem. 80, 4876–4885.
Richards, S.E., Wang, Y., Lawler, D., et al., 2008b. Self-modeling curve resolution: a new approach to recovering temporal metabolite signal modulation in NMR spectroscopic data: application to a life-long caloric restriction study in dogs. Anal. Chem. 80, 4876–4885.
Richards, S.E., Dumas, M.E., Fonville, J.M., Ebbels, T., Holmes, E., Nicholson, J.K., 2010. Intra-and Inter-omic fusion of metabolic profiling data in a systems biology framework. Chemometrics Intell. Lab. Syst. 104, 121–131.
Robinette, S.L., Veselkov, K.A., Bohus, E., et al., 2009. Cluster analysis statistical spectroscopy using nuclear magnetic resonance generated metabolic data sets from perturbed biological systems. Anal. Chem. 81, 6581–6589.
Rumelhart, D., Hinton, G., Williams, R., 1986. Learning internal representations by error propagation. In: Rumelhart, D.E., McClelland, J.L. (Eds.), Parallel Distributed Processing. Foundations. MIT Press, Cambridge, MA.
Sanchez, C., Lachaize, C., Janody, F., et al., 1999. Grasping at molecular interactions and genetic networks in Drosophila melanogaster using FlyNets, an Internet database. Nucleic Acids Res. 27, 89–94.
Schadt, E.E., Monks, S.A., Drake, T.A., et al., 2003. Genetics of gene expression surveyed in maize, mouse and man. Nature 422, 297–302.
Schaub, J., Schiesling, C., Reuss, M., Dauner, M., 2006. Integrated sampling procedure for metabolome analysis. Biotechnol. Prog. 22, 1434–1442.
Schröder, A.R., Shinn, P., Chen, H., Berry, C., Ecker, J.R., Bushman, F., 2002. HIV-1 integration in the human genome favors active genes and local hotspots. Cell 110, 521–529.
Schwartz, S., Friedberg, I., Ivanov, I.V., Davidson, L.A., Goldsby, J.S., Dahl, D.B., et al., 2012. A metagenomic study of diet-dependent interaction between gut microbiota and host in infants reveals differences in immune response. Genome Biol. 13, r32.

Shi, J., Zhang, S., Liang, Y., Pan, Q., 2006. Prediction of protein subcellular localizations using moment descriptors and support vector machine. In: Pattern Recognition in Bioinformatics. Springer, New York, pp. 105–114.

Shlomi, T., Cabili, M.N., Herrgard, M.J., Palsson, B.O., Ruppin, E., 2008. Network-based prediction of human tissue-specific metabolism. Nat. Biotechnol. 26, 1003–1010.

Shlomi, T., Cabili, M.N., Ruppin, E., 2009. Predicting metabolic biomarkers of human inborn errors of metabolism. Mol. Syst. Biol. 5, 263.

Smilde, A.K., Westerhuis, J.A., Boque, R., 2000. Multiway multiblock component and covariates regression models. J. Chemometr. 14, 301–331.

Smilde, A.K., Westerhuis, J.A., de Jong, S., 2003. A framework for sequential multiblock component methods. J. Chemometr. 17, 323–337.

Smilde, A.K., van der Werf, M.J., Bijlsma, S., van der Werff-van der Vat, B.J., Jellema, R.H., 2005. Fusion of mass spectrometry-based metabolomics data. Anal. Chem. 77, 6729–6736.

Smilde, A.K., Kiers, H.A., Bijlsma, S., Rubingh, C.M., van Erk, M.J., 2009. Matrix correlations for high-dimensional data: the modified RV-coefficient. Bioinformatics 25, 401–405.

Smolinska, A., Blanchet, L., Coulier, L., Ampt, K.A., Luider, T., Hintzen, R.Q., et al., 2012. Interpretation and visualization of non-linear data fusion in kernel space: study on metabolomic characterization of progression of multiple sclerosis. PLoS One 7, e38163.

Snyder, L.R., Hoggard, J.C., Montine, T.J., Synovec, R.E., 2010. Development and application of a comprehensive two-dimensional gas chromatography with time-of-flight mass spectrometry method for the analysis of l-β-methylamino-alanine in human tissue. J. Chromatogr. A 1217, 4639–4647.

Ståhle, L., Wold, S., 1987. Partial least squares analysis with cross-validation for the two-class problem: a Monte Carlo study. J. Chemometr. 1, 185–196.

Subramanian, A., Tamayo, P., Mootha, V.K., et al., 2005. Gene set enrichment analysis: a knowledge-based approach for interpreting genome-wide expression profiles. Proc. Natl. Acad. Sci. U. S. A. 102, 15545–15550.

Suzuki, M., Kusano, M., Takahashi, H., Nakamura, Y., Hayashi, N., Kobayashi, M., et al., 2010. Rice-Arabidopsis FOX line screening with FT-NIR-based fingerprinting for GC-TOF/MS-based metabolite profiling. Metabolomics 6, 137–145.

Tanaka, T., Shen, J., Abecasis, G.R., et al., 2009. Genome-wide association study of plasma polyunsaturated fatty acids in the InCHIANTI Study. PLoS Genet. 5, e1000338.

Tauler, R., Kowalski, B., Fleming, S., 1993. Multivariate curve resolution applied to spectral data from multiple runs of an industrial-process. Anal. Chem. 65, 2040–2047.

Tavazoie, S., Hughes, J.D., Campbell, M.J., Cho, R.J., Church, G.M., 1999. Systematic determination of genetic network architecture. Nat. Genet. 22, 281–285.

Tenberge, J.M.F., Deleeuw, J., Kroonenberg, P.M., Tenberge, J.M.F., Deleeuw, J., Kroonenberg, P.M., 1987. Some additional results on principal components-analysis of 3-mode data by means of alternating least-squares algorithms. Psychometrika 52, 183–191.

Trygg, J., Wold, S., 2002. Orthogonal projections to latent structures (O-PLS). J. Chemom. 16, 119–128.

Trygg, J., Wold, S., 2003. O2-PLS, a two-block (X-Y) latent variable regression (LVR) method with an integral OSC filter. J. Chemom. 17, 53–64.

Tucker, L.R., 1966. Some mathematical notes on three-mode factor analysis. Psychometrika 31, 279–311.

van den Berg, R.A., Hoefsloot, H.C.J., Westerhuis, J.A., Smilde, A.K., van der Werf, M.J., 2006. Centering, scaling, and transformations: improving the biological information content of metabolomics data. BMC Genomics 7, 142.

van den Berg, R.A., Van Mechelen, I., Wilderjans, T.F., et al., 2009. Integrating functional genomics data using maximum likelihood based simultaneous component analysis. BMC Bioinform. 10, 1–12.

Van Deun, K., Smilde, A.K., van der Werf, M.J., Kiers, H.A., Van Mechelen, I., 2009. A structured overview of simultaneous component based data integration. BMC Bioinform. 10, 246.

Vandeginste, B., Massart, D., Buydens, L., De Jong, S., Lewi, P., Smeyers-Verbeke, J., 1997. Handbook of Chemometrics and Qualimetrics: Data Handling in Science and Technology: Parts A and B. In: Elsevier, Amsterdam.

Vaughan, A.A., Dunn, W.B., Allwood, J.W., Wedge, D.C., Blackhall, F.H., Whetton, A.D., et al., 2012. Liquid chromatography–mass spectrometry calibration transfer and metabolomics data fusion. Anal. Chem. 84, 9848–9857.

Verouden, M.P.H., Notebaart, R.A., Westerhuis, J.A., et al., 2009. Multi-way analysis of flux distributions across multiple conditions. J. Chemom. 23, 406–420.

Wang, Y., Veltkamp, D.J., Kowalski, B.R., 1991. Multivariate instrument standardization. Anal. Chem. 63, 2750–2756.

Wang, Y., Cloarec, O., Tang, H., et al., 2008. Magic angle spinning NMR and 1H-31P heteronuclear statistical total correlation spectroscopy of intact human gut biopsies. Anal. Chem. 80, 1058–1066.

Wangen, L., Kowalski, B., 1989. A multiblock partial least squares algorithm for investigating complex chemical systems. J. Chemometr. 3, 3–20.

Ward Jr., J.H., 1963. Hierarchical grouping to optimize an objective function. J. Am. Stat. Assoc. 58, 236–244.

Wegelin, J.A., 2000. A Survey of partial least squares (PLS) methods, with emphasis on the two-block case. Technical Report, University of Washington.

Werbos, P., 1974. Beyond Regression: New Tools for Prediction and Analysis in the Behavioral Sciences. Harvard University Press, Cambridge, MA.

Westerhuis, J.A., Kourti, T., MacGregor, J.F., 1998. Analysis of multiblock and hierarchical PCA and PLS models. J. Chemom. 12, 301–321.

Wold, S., 1976. Pattern recognition by means of disjoint principal components models. Pattern Recogn. 8, 127–139.

Wold, S., Kettaneh, N., Tjessem, K., 1996. Hierarchical multiblock PLS and PC models for easier model interpretation and as an alternative to variable selection. J. Chemom. 10, 463–482.

Wold, S., Antti, H., Lindgren, F., Öhman, J., 1998a. Orthogonal signal correction of near-infrared spectra. Chemometrics Intell. Lab. Syst. 44, 175–185.

Wold, S., Anttil, H., Lindgren, F., Ohman, J., 1998b. Orthogonal signal correction of near-infrared spectra. Chemom. Intell. Lab. Syst. 44 (175), 185.

Yang, S., Nadeau, J.S., Humston-Fulmer, E.M., Hoggard, J.C., Lidstrom, M.E., Synovec, R.E., 2012. Gas chromatography–mass spectrometry with chemometric analysis for determining ^{12}C and ^{13}C labeled contributions in metabolomics and ^{13}C flux analysis. J. Chromatogr. A 1240, 156–164.

Yao, W., He, M., Jiang, Y., Zhang, L., Ding, A., Hu, Y., 2013. Integrated LC/MS and GC/MS metabolomics data for the evaluation of protection function of fructus ligustri lucidi on mouse liver. Chromatographia 76, 1171–1179.

Yap, I.K., Clayton, T.A., Tang, H., et al., 2006. An integrated metabonomic approach to describe temporal metabolic disregulation induced in the rat by the model hepatotoxin allyl formate. J. Proteome Res. 5, 2675–2684.

Yilmaz, A., Nyberg, N.T., Jaroszewski, J.W., 2011. Metabolic profiling based on two-dimensional J-resolved 1H NMR data and parallel factor analysis. Anal. Chem. 83, 8278–8285.

Yu, S., Tranchevent, L., Moor, B., Moreau, Y., 2011. Kernel-Based Data Fusion for Machine Learning: Methods and Applications in Bioinformatics and Text Mining. Springer, Berlin.

Part Two

Applications in nutrition research

Application of lipidomics in nutrition research

X. Han[1], Y. Zhou[2]
[1]Sanford-Burnham Medical Research Institute, Orlando, FL, USA; [2]Institute for Nutritional Sciences, Shanghai Institutes for Biological Sciences, P.R. China

4.1 Introduction

Lipidomics, which studies cellular lipids (i.e. the lipidome) in a large scale, has emerged as a rapidly expanding research field under the umbrella of systems biology. Researchers in lipidomics determine the structures, functions, interactions, and dynamics of cellular lipids, identify their cellular localisation (i.e. subcellular membrane compartments and domains); and measure the dynamic changes that occur during physiological and pathophysiological perturbations. Lipidomics plays an important role in nutritional research. In this chapter, the current status of the platforms for lipidomics analysis is summarised, and the applications of lipidomics for nutritional research are briefly discussed.

4.2 Lipids

Lipids are a complex mixture of metabolites, which have recently been classified into eight categories: fatty acyls, glycerolipids, glycerophospholipids, sphingolipids, sterol lipids, prenol lipids, saccharolipids, and polyketides (Fahy et al., 2005). Fatty acyls are structurally the most simple category that includes various classes of fatty acids, eicosanoids, docosanoids, fatty alcohols, fatty aldehydes, fatty esters, fatty amides, fatty nitriles, fatty ethers, and hydrocarbons. Fatty acids are the basic building blocks of more complex lipids, such as glycerolipids. Glycerolipids include monoacylglycerol, diacylglycerol, and triacylglycerol (TAG) species. These neutral lipids have a glycerol backbone with fatty acid chains linked to the hydroxyl groups of glycerol. It should be pointed out that fatty alcohols linked by an ether bond are also found in these neutral lipids in low abundance (Bartz et al., 2007).

Glycerophospholipids are key components of cellular membranes, although they are involved in metabolism and signalling. The complexity of glycerophospholipids can be illustrated with the classes (different headgroups), subclasses (different linkages of an aliphatic chain to the hydroxyl group of glycerol at the first position based on stereospecific numbering system (i.e. *sn*-1)), and individual molecular species (different aliphatic chain structures) (Figure 4.1). Based on its name, individual molecular species in this category of lipids contain three components: "glycero-" (i.e. at least one

Metabolomics as a Tool in Nutrition Research. http://dx.doi.org/10.1016/B978-1-78242-084-2.00004-6

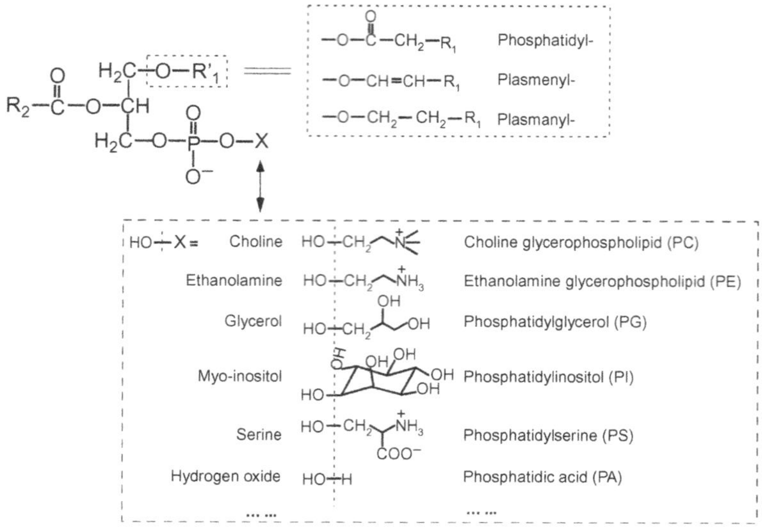

Figure 4.1 General structural features of glycerophospholipids.

glycerol molecule is centred in each individual species), "phospho-" (i.e. at least one phosphodiester is linked to a hydroxyl group of glycerol at the *sn*-3 position), and one or two aliphatic chains that are connected to the *sn*-1, *sn*-2, or both hydroxyl groups of glycerol. As we know, there are over 10 varieties of the moieties (X) esterified with the phosphate (i.e. over 10 different classes) (Figure 4.1) and over 30 kinds of possible aliphatic chains containing different numbers of carbon atoms (i.e. chain length), different degrees of unsaturation, and different locations of these double bonds. In addition, there exist three different linkages of the aliphatic chain with the hydroxyl group of glycerol at the *sn*-1 position (i.e. three different subclasses). Accordingly, we can easily estimate that the possible numbers of individual molecular species in the category of glycerophospholipids should be approximately 30,000. In practise, mass spectrometric analysis has detected the presence of large numbers of individual lipid species (e.g. plasmalogen, cardiolipin, and TAG) (Han et al., 2013; Kiebish et al., 2010; Yang et al., 2007).

Sphingolipid is another category of complex cellular lipids that contain a common structural feature, a sphingoid base backbone. The majority of the sphingolipid species can be represented by a general structure with three building blocks (Figure 4.2). The building block X represents a different polar moiety (linked to the oxygen at the C1 position of the sphingoid base). These polar moieties include hydrogen, phosphoethanolamine, phosphocholine, galactose, glucose, lactose, sulphated galactose, and other complex sugar groups, corresponding to ceramide, ceramide phosphoethanolamine, sphingomyelin, galactosylceramide, glucosylceramide, lactosylceramide, sulphatide, and other glycosphingolipids such as gangliosides, respectively (Figure 4.2). The building block Y represents a fatty acid, which is acylated to the primary amine at the C2 position of the sphingoid base. A variety of fatty acids including those

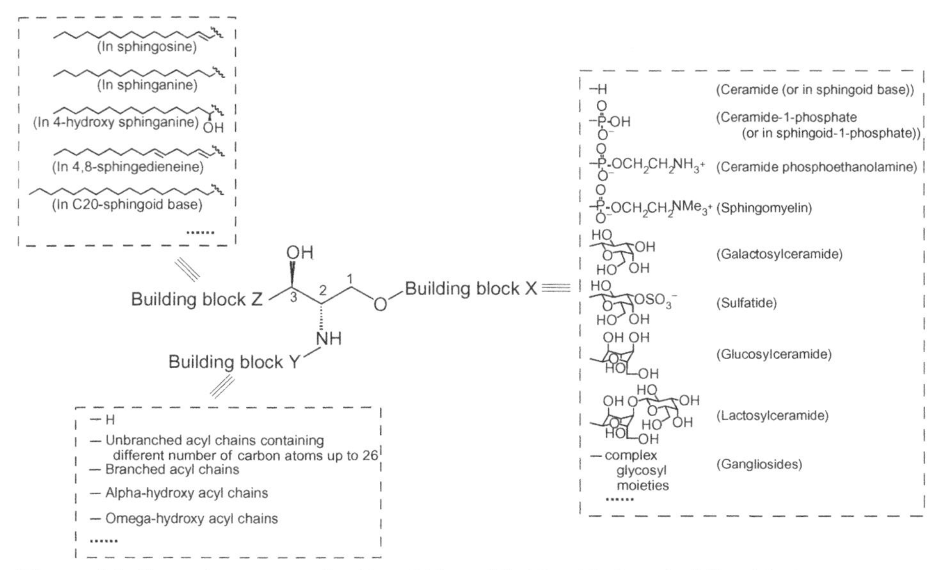

Figure 4.2 General structure of sphingoid-based lipids with three building blocks. Reprinted from Han et al. (2012) with permission from Wiley Periodicals, Inc., Copyright 2011.

containing a hydroxyl group (usually located at the alpha or omega position) (Figure 4.2) can occupy this position. The building block Z represents the aliphatic chain present in all sphingoid bases, which is linked through a carbon–carbon bond to the C3 position. This aliphatic chain varies by length, the degree of unsaturation, the presence of a branch in the chain, and the presence of additional hydroxyl group(s) (Figure 4.2). Hundreds of thousands of possible sphingolipid species can be constructed from the combination of these three building blocks (Yang et al., 2009a).

Sterols are a class of lipids containing a common steroid core of a fused four-ring structure with a hydrocarbon side chain and an alcohol group. Cholesterol is the primary sterol lipid in mammals and is an important constituent of cellular membranes. Oxidisation and/or metabolism of cholesterol yields numerous oxysterols, steroids, bile acids, etc., many of which are important signalling molecules in biological systems. Cholesterol esters esterified with a variety of fatty acids are enriched in lipoprotein particles such as low-density lipoproteins (LDL) and very low-density lipoproteins (VLDL).

Lipids play distinct and critical roles in nutrition and health. They are the crucial components of cellular membranes, which constitute an impermeable barrier of cellular compartments and provide appropriate motifs for membrane protein function. Lipids serve as an energy storage depot. Many lipids serve as active second messengers. While many lipids can be endogenously synthesised in the human body, certain essential fatty acids such as linoleic acid and α-linolenic acid, must be obtained from the diet because they cannot be synthesised from other simple precursors in the diet (Holman, 1960; Simopoulos, 2000). The lipids obtained from diet are in the intact forms of triacylglycerols, cholesterol and its esters, glycerophospholipids, and sphingolipids. These lipids are absorbed as chylomicron in the intestine and processed into lipoprotein particles (i.e. VLDL and LDL) in the liver. The fatty acid building blocks as well as other small constituents are released to serve as nutrients from these particles by a variety of enzymes such as lipases. The cells absorb the produced fatty acids and deliver them to mitochondria to produce ATP through coordinate machinery operation of fatty acid β-oxidation and respiratory chain. Accordingly, dietary lipids are important components of nutrition.

However, excessive intake of dietary lipids (and energy in general) leads to membrane lipid abnormality, intracellular lipid accumulation, and altered lipid signals (Sack, 2013). The combination of these abnormalities ultimately leads to cell dysfunction and subsequently organ function disorder. Therefore, lipid disorder is closely associated with many pathophysiological complications, such as heart disease, high blood pressure, gestational and type 2 diabetes, inflammatory bowel disease, Alzheimer's disease, depression and multiple sclerosis (Han, 2005; Qi, 2012).

4.3 Lipidomics

Lipidomics is an analytical chemistry-based research field that studies cellular lipidomes (i.e. all cellular lipids) on a large scale and at the intact molecular level (Blanksby and Mitchell, 2010; Dennis, 2009; Griffiths and Wang, 2009; Gross and Han, 2011; Han and Gross, 2003; Han et al., 2012; Shevchenko and Simons, 2010; Wenk, 2005). The research in this field involves precisely identifying the structures of cellular lipid species including the number of atoms, the number and location of double bonds, individual aliphatic chains, and the regiospecificity of each isomer, etc; accurately quantifying individual identified lipid species for pathway analysis; comparably profiling the lipid samples for biomarker discovery; and determining the nutritional status and interactions of individual lipid species with other lipids, proteins, and metabolites *in vivo*. The analysis of lipid structures, mass levels, cell functions, and interactions in a spatial and temporal fashion provides the dynamic changes of lipids during physiological (e.g. nutritional) or pathological perturbations. Accordingly, lipidomics plays an essential role in defining the biochemical mechanisms underlying lipid-related disease processes through identification of alterations in cellular lipid signalling, metabolism, trafficking, and homeostasis.

The typical lipidomics workflow in lipidomics consists of three main components including (1) sampling and lipid sample preparation, (2) lipid analysis, and (3) data processing and bioinformatics. These components are briefly and separately discussed in the remaining parts of this section.

4.3.1 Sampling and lipid sample preparation

Sampling is a primary component for a successful lipidomics analysis and should be strictly controlled under identical conditions as possible. Blood cell contamination should be eliminated if one is sampling for plasma or serum, which can be generally achieved through gentle spinning down the blood cells of freshly collected blood. Blood contamination should be eliminated for tissue sampling from blood-containing organs through perfusion. It is suggested to freeze-clamp the entire available organ or tissue and then pulverise the tissue wafers into a fine powder with a stainless-steel mortar and pestle at the temperature of liquid nitrogen prior to weighing a few milligrams of tissue sample. This could eliminate the organ inhomogeneity to a certain degree. If sampling is the particular section of an organ (e.g. the brain), criteria for determination of sample representation should be established and care should be taken during dissection (Han, 2010).

The amount of sample necessary to perform the analysis of a cellular lipidome is dependent on the analytical instrument available and the choice of a method. For example, when using multi-dimensional MS-based shotgun lipidomics (MDMS-SL) with a triple quadrupole mass spectrometer (Vantage, Thermo Fisher Scientific) with a TriVersa NanoMate device (Advion BioScience Ltd., Ithaca, NY) for sample injection, the required starting material is approximate 10 mg of wet tissue, one million of cells, 100 μL of plasma, or 200 μg of protein of a membrane fraction (Cheng et al., 2007). With such a sample size, the platform enables one to analyse over 30 lipid classes and 2000 individual molecular species following multiplexed sample processing (Yang et al., 2009a).

Lipid extraction is one of the key steps to the successful analyses of cellular lipidomes by mass spectrometry in general and in particular when using direct infusion. Traditionally, lipid samples from biological sources are extracted using a mixture of chloroform and methanol based on the Folch method (Folch et al., 1957), the modified method of Bligh and Dyer (Christie and Han, 2010), or other solvent combinations (Matyash et al., 2008). Internal standards should be spiked into the samples at the earliest step possible in order to minimise concerns regarding incomplete recovery. Different solvent systems may have distinct extraction recoveries for various lipid classes and molecular species.

During the extraction, a salt should be used that matches the adducts preferred for mass spectrometric analysis. Acidic extraction conditions can lead to destruction of plasmalogens, so the usage of acid(s) during extraction should be used with caution. The presence of detergents may complicate the analysis of individual lipid species by mass spectrometry resulting from extensive ion suppression and may also affect the column separation of lipids. Thus, detergents should be avoided in sample preparation when possible. If present, great care needs to be exercised in removing as much of the detergent as possible. It should be noted that many researchers use solid-phase extraction chromatography procedures to prepare a fraction of particular lipids for mass spectrometric analysis (Christie and Han, 2010).

4.3.2 Lipid analysis

Lipid analysis is the core of lipidomics. Many types of advanced instruments and technologies could be applied for this purpose. Historically, gas chromatography, liquid chromatography, fluorescence spectroscopy, nuclear magnetic resonance spectroscopy, etc., have been widely used for lipid analysis (Feng and Prestwich, 2006). Nowadays, due to the advances in its technologies for sensitivity, mass resolution, mass accuracy, and speed, mass spectrometry is an essential tool for lipid analysis in lipidomics.

Two types of analytics are commonly applied in lipidomics: (i) *hypothesis-driven* targeted analysis and (ii) a comprehensive, *hypothesis-generating*, non-targeted analysis. In the targeted analysis, only a defined group of lipids, usually one or a few lipid classes, is analysed with a targeted analytical protocol. While this approach allows very sensitive and robust determination of the selected lipid species, it gives relatively limited information about the global lipidome. The non-targeted approaches aim to cover molecular lipids across a wide range of lipid classes in a single analysis.

There are two major complimentary approaches in mass spectrometry-based lipidomics. One is developed after direct infusion, which has been referred to as shotgun lipidomics, whereas the other uses liquid chromatographic separations prior to mass spectrometric analysis. As briefly described below, LC-MS approaches are more suitable for targeted analysis, particularly for minor lipid classes, while shotgun lipidomics could be applied for both types of analyses.

4.3.2.1 Shotgun lipidomics

Shotgun lipidomics was originally defined as a strategy for global analysis of a cellular lipidome directly from the lipid extract of a biological sample in a high-throughput manner (Han and Gross, 2005a). Nowadays, shotgun lipidomics is generally discussed in terms of the methodologies for lipid analysis based on direct infusion. Shotgun lipidomics exploits the chemical and physical properties of lipids to facilitate the high-throughput global analysis of a cellular lipidome directly from organic extracts of biological samples (Han and Gross, 2005a). In shotgun lipidomics, a mass spectrum displaying molecular ions of individual molecular species of a lipid class of interest can be acquired at a constant concentration of the lipid solution without a time restriction. This unique feature allows researchers to perform precursor-ion scans of particular fragment ions and/or neutral loss scans of desired neutrally lost fragments for individual molecular species of a lipid class or a category of lipid classes for their identification and quantitation without the time constraints. Unfortunately, this approach is not ideal for the analysis of poorly ionised lipids in low abundance as a result of ion suppression. Another limitation of this method is its inability to distinguish isomeric species when their fragmentation patterns are identical.

There are at least three different platforms of shotgun lipidomics in practise including (1) profiling of lipid molecular species of a class by scanning a characteristic fragment diagnostic of the class (Brugger et al., 1997; Welti and Wang, 2004), (2) identification and quantification of individual lipid molecular species by using tandem mass spectrometry employing high-mass-accuracy/high-mass-resolution mass spectrometers (Ejsing et al., 2006; Ekroos et al., 2002; Schwudke et al., 2006, 2007; Stahlman et al., 2009), and (3) identification and quantification of individual lipid molecular species by multi-dimensional mass spectrometry-based shotgun lipidomics (MDMS-SL) (Han and Gross, 2001, 2005b; Han et al., 2004b, 2012).

Since naturally occurring lipids are composed of known building blocks (see above), MDMS-SL analyses those building blocks that are characteristic of individual molecular species of a lipid class of interest (i.e. building blocks of the class of interest). A typical example is the analysis of lysophosphatidylcholine (LPC) species including regioisomers even though LPC species are minor in lipid extract and the mass spectrometric analysis is ion suppressed by the co-existing abundant lipid species such as phosphatidylcholine (PC). The fragmentation patterns of sodiated LPC species (i.e. $[M+Na]^{+}$) after collision-induced dissociation contain multiple abundant and informative fragments corresponding to the building blocks of these species. These include the neutral losses of trimethylamine (i.e. $[M+Na\text{-}59]^{+}$) and sodium cholinephosphate (i.e. $[M+Na\text{-}205]^{+}$) as well as the ions corresponding to choline (i.e. *m/z* 104) and sodiated five-membered cyclophosphane (i.e. *m/z* 147) (Han and Gross, 1996). The aliphatic substituent can be derived from the *m/z* value after identification of its linkage to a glycerol backbone. Importantly, the intensity ratio of the choline (i.e. *m/z* 104) and sodiated five-membered cyclophosphane (i.e. *m/z* 147) ions was determined as 3.5 for the *sn*-1 acyl species and 0.125 for *sn*-2 acyl species (Han and Gross, 1996; Yang et al., 2009b). Accordingly, two-dimensional MS analyses of these building blocks identify individual LPC species from their sodium adducts including the location of the aliphatic chain in any extract from a biological sample. It should be noted that without addition of any modifiers to an infusion solution, sodium adducts of LPC species are always prominently detected. Figure 4.3 shows a two-dimensional spectrum for identification of LPC species. The spectrum consists of five scans in the positive-ion mode acquired in the mass region of *m/z* 400–600 after direct infusion of a diluted lipid extract of rabbit myocardium. These scans include a full-MS scan, a neutral loss scan of 59 amu (NLS59), a neutral loss scan of 205 amu (NLS205), a precursor-ion scan of 104 Thomson (PIS104), and a precursor-ion scan of 147 Thomson (PIS147). NLS59 could be used to "filter" the low-abundant LPC species in this mass range and identify the fatty aliphatic chains in these "isolated" species (Yang et al., 2009b). LPC species were further confirmed by NLS205, which is specific to sodiated LPC species in this mass region. Significant changes to an intensity ratio of an LPC species to the selected internal standard in NLS59 in comparison to that of the counterpart in NLS205 identified the species as an ether-linked LPC species (Yang et al., 2009a,b). For example, the intensities of both ions at *m/z* 502 and 504 are markedly reduced in NLS205 relative to those in NLS59, indicating that these ions are ether-linked LPC species. Finally, the intensity ratio of ions at *m/z* 104 and 147 (which could be determined from PIS104 and PIS147 of each species) identifies the regiospecificity of LPC species (Han and Gross, 1996). From the two-dimensional MS analyses (Figure 4.3), 19 LPC species were identified and quantified in extracts of rabbit myocardium after discriminating the regioisomers (Yang et al., 2009b).

4.3.2.2 LC-MS for lipid analysis

LC-MS analysis of lipids is largely dependent on column separation. Numerous column types including normal-phase, reverse-phase, HILIC, ion exchange, and affinity have been employed for this purpose (Guo and Lankmayr, 2010). The major advantage of LC-MS analysis is to use chromatographic separation to simplify the complex lipid extracts. For example, a normal-phase column could be applied for resolving a

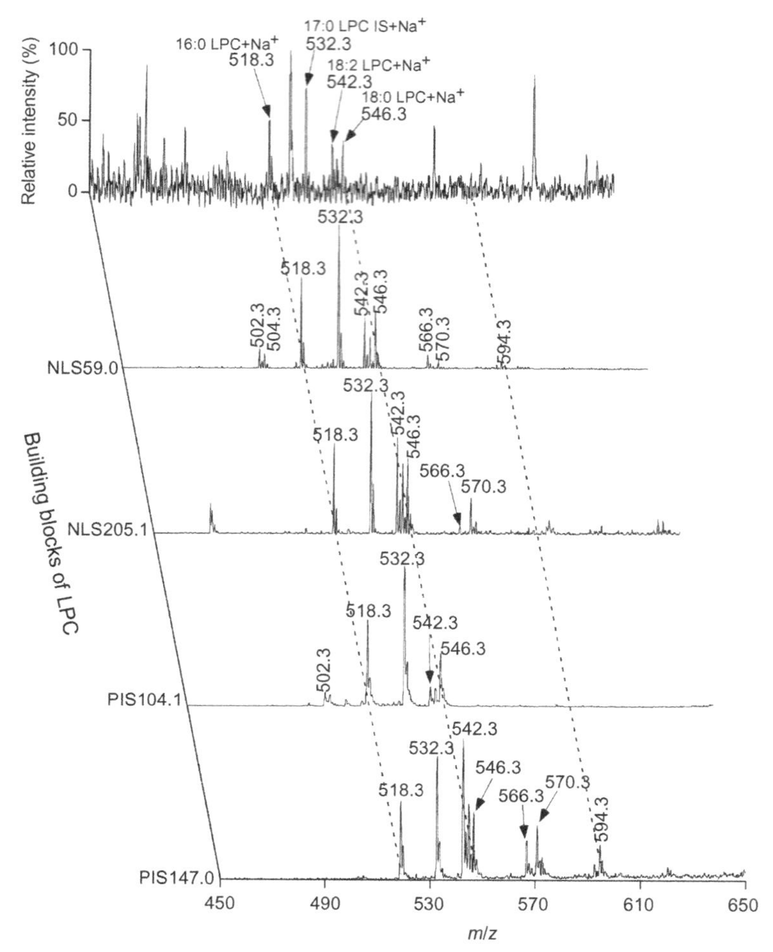

Figure 4.3 Representative two-dimensional mass spectrometric analyses of lysophosphatidylcholine molecular species in lipid extracts of rabbit myocardium. Modified from Yang et al. (2009b) with permission from Elsevier B.V., Copyright 2009.

lipid mixture to individual lipid class, or a reverse-phase column may be used to separate lipid species based on their different hydrophobicities. Of course, no single column is able to totally resolve a biological lipid extract into single species. Thus, combinations of different types of columns have been explored for two-dimensional or multi-dimensional separations either online or offline (Guo and Lankmayr, 2010). Generally, offline separation approaches (including step fractionations) are broadly used for enrichment and analysis of lipid classes that are not easily ionised or are present in low abundances.

In contrast to shotgun lipidomics, in LC-MS analysis, lipid concentrations are constantly changing, and identification and quantification of lipid species have to be done in a very limited time frame. These features make the LC-MS-based methodology for the analysis of lipid species distinct from those in shotgun lipidomics. In the analysis of lipids by LC-MS, single/multiple reaction monitoring (SRM/MRM) becomes the preferred method for the detection of a particular species since it can be done in a very short time frame. To achieve MRM detection, pre-determination of individual lipid species at a certain elution time is required. This approach is unable to conduct global analysis of individual lipid species for any sample without pre-determination. Moreover, this approach only determines a body of species containing the pair of transition ions. Alternatively, global lipid analysis by LC-MS could be conducted by using single-ion monitoring (SIM) in which any ion of interest could be extracted from the total ion chromatograph. To reduce any artificial ion extraction, very high-mass-accuracy/high-mass-resolution instrumentation is always required. This approach determines the entire body of lipid species having identical molecular weight. The third approach for lipid analysis by LC-MS is data-dependent analysis of ions. Although this is an ideal approach for identification and quantification of individual lipid species, the short elution time does not allow one to extensively identify all ions detected. When the elution time is narrow, as is observed in UPLC, it is more difficult to attain extensive identification. Finally, it should be noted that the changing concentration may result in ion suppression and subsequent artefacts during quantification.

4.3.3 Data processing and bioinformatics

Large amounts of data are generated in lipidomics. It is fortunate that all the areas of data processing and bioinformatics for lipidomics, including automated data processing, statistical analysis of datasets, and pathway and network analysis, have made great advances.

For automation of data processing, generation of libraries and/or databases that contain information about the structures, masses, isotope patterns, and MS/MS spectra in different ionisation modes of lipids, along with possible LC retention times, is critical. This approach is analogous to the libraries of GC-MS spectra, which can be used to search a compound of interest after GC-MS analysis. Currently, the most comprehensive libraries/databases that contain these types of information include the ones generated by the LIPID MAPS consortium (http://www.lipidmaps.org) (Sud et al., 2007) as well as the METLIN created at the Scripps Research Institute (http://metlin.scripps.edu). The website developed by the group of Dr. Taguchi in Japan (http://lipidsearch.jp/LipidNavigator.htm) enables investigators to search a lipid species based on different parameters, including fragmentation patterns. It should be noted that shotgun lipidomics identifies lipid species *in situ* and that a theoretical database constructed based on the building blocks of individual lipid classes is sufficient (Yang et al., 2009a).

There are a few programs and/or software packages that perform multiple data-processing steps such as spectral filtering, peak detection, alignment, normalisation, baseline correction, and exploratory data analysis and visualisation for the requirements of LC-MS methods (Fahy et al., 2007; Forrester et al., 2004; Hartler et al., 2011;

Hermansson et al., 2005; Hubner et al., 2009; Laaksonen et al., 2006; Sysi-Aho et al., 2007; Yang et al., 2011). These programs were developed and largely depend on the elution times and the determined masses of individual ions. The algorithm called LipidQA or LipidBlast (Kind et al., 2013; Song et al., 2007, 2009) is designed after the same line of reasoning as a search of the GC-MS library and contains many product-ion spectra. With these tools, one can potentially identify a lipid species with a match of a fragmentation pattern of the species along with other available information manually or automatically. Unfortunately, identification of the eluted species is complicated when there is incomplete resolution of individual species of a class. In this case, either an improvement of the resolution of individual species or train for the analysis of the product-ion spectra acquired from standard isomeric/isobaric mixtures will be necessary.

Similarly, there are multiple programs and/or software packages that were developed based on the principles of shotgun lipidomics, including LIMSA (Haimi et al., 2006), LipidProfiler (Ejsing et al., 2006), LipidInspector (Schwudke et al., 2006), AMDMS-SL (Yang et al., 2009a), and LipidXplorer (Herzog et al., 2012). The LIMSA software package, which is available through the website (www.helsinki.fi/science/lipids/software.html), serves as an interface to process data from individual full-MS and tandem-MS spectra. The software package LipidView, offered by AB SCIEX, which was developed in the line of LipidProfiler and LipidXplorer, deals with the multiple PIS and NLS data or others acquired with those instruments with high-mass accuracy/high-mass resolution (e.g. Q-TOF and Orbitrap). The AMDMS-SL program was developed in order to identify and quantify individual lipid species from the data obtained from MDMS-based shotgun lipidomics.

The next step in bioinformatics is to perform statistical comparisons between datasets. To this end, any commercially available software (e.g. SAS, NCSS, IBM SPSS Statistics, and SIMCA-P) can be used for biostatistical analyses such as principal component analysis (PCA), multivariate analysis of variance (MANOVA), and partial least square (PLS) regression. For example, the application of PCA, PLS, and fuzzy c-means clustering for data analysis of metabolomics has found that use of a proper statistical analysis method is essential to improve visualisation, accurate classification, and outlier estimation (Li et al., 2009).

Despite the development of numerous pathway analysis tools (van Iersel et al., 2008; Wheelock et al., 2009), their application for the analysis of altered lipids resulting from different states due to physical, pathophysiological, or pathological changes remains a challenge since no good models are available for the analysis. Different models have been applied for the analysis of certain pathways in a network (Cowart et al., 2010; Dhingra et al., 2007; Fahy et al., 2007; Kapoor et al., 2008; Kiebish et al., 2010; Merrill et al., 2009; Zarringhalam et al., 2012). The LIPID MAPS consortium has comprehensively reconstructed lipid pathways based on both experimental data and data from literature by using tools such as VANTED (Junker et al., 2006) and Pathway Editor (Byrnes et al., 2009). The uses of the VANTED platform in lipidomics have been reviewed extensively (Wheelock et al., 2009). The Pathway Editor allows *de novo* pathway creation and downloading of LIPID MAPS and KEGG lipid metabolic pathways, as well as retrieval of measured time-dependent changes to lipid metabolism components (Byrnes et al., 2009). A quantitative dynamic model of C_{16}-branch of sphingolipid metabolism developed by Gupta et al. (2011) is a clear example of integration of lipidomics and transcriptomics data towards a systems biology approach for understanding sphingolipid biology. Yetukuri et al. (2007) developed a lipid pathway reconstruction method based on lipidomics and transcriptomics data. Similar studies are expected in the future for other lipids. Very recently, we have developed and validated a novel bioinformatic approach to assess the differential contributions of the known synthesis pathways to TAG pools through simulation of TAG ion profiles determined by shotgun lipidomics (Han et al., 2013). This can be used to assess the changes of TAG biosynthesis pathways induced by nutrition.

4.4 Lipidomics in nutrition research

It is well known that diet may directly be associated with metabolic dysfunction such as the "metabolic syndrome" (Moller and Kaufman, 2005; Unger and Scherer, 2010). However, the connections of specific diets with health outcomes remain elusive. Metabolic regulation is different from person to person and at different ages. An optimal diet for one individual is not necessarily ideal for the other. Accordingly, the primary goal of nutrition research is to understand the link between specific diets and health outcomes and to optimise dietary nutrition for human well-being, thereby delaying or preventing diet-related diseases. Although genetics is an important factor for metabolic syndromes, dietary habits and nutrition are a key modifiable factor contributing to these diseases. The lipidome is sensitive to many pathogenically relevant factors such as host genotype, gut microbiota, and diet (see Murphy and Nicolaou, 2013 for recent review). Lipidomics is therefore considered a powerful platform to study the contributions of genes, diet, nutrients, and human metabolism for health and disease. Specifically, lipidomics is important for nutritional research in (1) the monitoring of individual nutritional status; (2) the follow-up of compliance, progress, and success of dietary guidance and intervention; (3) the identification of side effects, unexpected metabolic responses, or lack of response to specific dietary changes; (4) the recognition of metabolic shifts in individuals due to environmental changes or lifestyle modifications; and (5) the normal progression of ageing and maturation (Stella et al., 2006). Lipidomics can also be applied for food research, such as the development of food products and evaluation of food quality, functionality, bioactivity, and toxicity through monitoring the lipid changes.

4.4.1 Lipidomics in the determination of the effects of specific diets or challenge tests

Lipidomics has been widely applied to determine the changes of lipidomes in response to caloric restriction. For example, utilising shotgun lipidomics, it was demonstrated that modest caloric restriction (i.e. overnight fasting) results in accelerated phospholipid hydrolysis, membrane remodelling, and triglyceride accumulation in murine myocardium (Han et al., 2004a). After brief periods of fasting (4 and 12 h) substantial decreases occurred in the choline and ethanolamine glycerophospholipid pools in mouse myocardium (collectively, a decrease of 39 nmol phospholipid/mg protein after 12-h fasting representing ~25% of total phospholipid mass). The study also shows that aliphatic chain length shortening is present in the major phospholipid classes further reducing endogenous myocardial energy stored in phospholipid aliphatic chains and altering the physical properties of myocardial membranes. In contrast to reduction of phospholipid mass, myocardial triacylglycerol content is not decreased during fasting, but increases nearly threefold during 12 h of re-feeding and returns to baseline levels after 24 h of re-feeding. Other examined lipid classes are not changed during fasting. In contrast to myocardium, no decreases in phospholipid mass are found, but a dramatic decrease of triacylglycerol mass is manifest after 12 h of fasting in skeletal muscle. These results identify phospholipids as a rapidly mobilisable energy source during modest caloric deprivation in murine myocardium, while triacylglycerols are a major source of energy reserve in skeletal muscle. However, shotgun lipidomics analysis of the lipidome of mouse cerebral cortex after chronic caloric restriction only demonstrates the alterations in sulphatide homeostasis (Kiebish et al., 2012).

A 6-month caloric restriction (25 %) study revealed significantly larger differences of fasting-to-postprandial acylcarnitine concentrations manifest in individuals with caloric restriction compared to controls since acylcarnitine accumulation is toxic (Huffman et al., 2012). The study also reveals that the observed differences are related to improvements in insulin sensitivity (Huffman et al., 2012).

Targeted lipidomics analysis of plasma samples from impaired glucose-tolerant individuals after an oral glucose tolerance test compared to controls has shown a correlation between significant changes in bile acids and glucose homeostasis (Shaham et al., 2008). This finding indicates that lipidomic profiling of lipid changes might be used to predict diabetes and guide its treatment.

Lipidomic profiles have been determined for subjects with myocardial infarction or unstable ischaemic attack after dietary intervention including either fatty fish or lean fish for 8 weeks (Lankinen et al., 2009; Schwab et al., 2008). It has been found that numerous lipid species including ceramides, LPCs, diacylglycerols, PCs, and lysophosphatidylethanolamines are significantly decreased in the group fed the fatty fish diet, whereas cholesterol esters and specific long-chain TAGs are significantly increased in the group fed the lean fish diet (Lankinen et al., 2009). The decrease in LPC and ceramide content in the fatty fish group might be related to the anti-inflammatory effects of *n*-3 polyunsaturated fatty acids, since both LPC and ceramide are the major bioactive lipid components involving inflammation (Aiyar et al., 2007).

Lipidomics profiling has been used to determine the effects of plant sterols on lipid metabolism (Szymanska et al., 2012) since it is well known that plant sterol intervention could lead to reduction of both total cholesterol and LDL cholesterol (De Smet et al., 2012). Healthy mildly hypercholesterolaemic subjects consumed two plant sterol-enriched yoghurt drinks containing different fat contents for 4 weeks and lipidomics analysis of serum samples was performed (Szymanska et al., 2012). It has been found that both drinks resulted in the reduction of both total and LDL cholesterol levels (Noakes et al., 2005). In addition, the low-fat drink resulted in a reduction of the levels of several sphingomyelins. This reduction, which correlates well with the reduction of LDL cholesterol, could be due to the co-localisation of sphingomyelins and cholesterol on the surface layer of LDL lipoproteins.

Lipidomics has also been used to determine the effects of probiotic intervention on global lipidomic profiles in humans (Kekkonen et al., 2008). Decreased mass levels of LPC species, sphingomyelins, and several PC species were detected after exposure to probiotic lactobacillus rhamnosus GG bacteria for 3 weeks. These changes may be due to the metabolic events behind the beneficial effects of lactobacillus rhamnosus GG on gut barrier function (Ng et al., 2009).

4.4.2 Lipidomics in the investigation of metabolic syndrome and associated diseases

The origin of metabolic syndrome is multifactorial. In addition to the genetic variation, environmental factors, such as nutrition, dietary patterns, and lifestyles, play a key role in its development. This could be represented from the study of monozygotic twins discordant for obesity, which is independent of genetic factors (Wopereis et al., 2009). The study demonstrated that obesity was related to distinct changes of the global serum lipid profile (Wopereis et al., 2009). In comparison to nonobese co-twins, increased levels of LPCs (which are bioactive lipids associated with pro-inflammatory and proatherogenic conditions (Yan et al., 2005)) and decreased levels of ether phospholipids (which are known to exert antioxidative properties (Engelmann, 2004)) are manifest in obese co-twins. Importantly, these lipid changes are well correlated with insulin resistance, a metabolic characteristic of acquired obesity in these healthy adult twins. The authors have therefore pointed out that proper management of obesity, with a new generation of therapies targeted to the lipid metabolism pathways, will most likely correct these abnormalities, and favourably modify the risk, course, and outcome of diabetes and cardiovascular diseases. Further lipidomic analyses of adipose tissue in the same twin population have provided molecular mechanisms underpinning the acquired obesity (Pietilainen et al., 2011). It has been found that the obese twin individuals possessed increased levels of palmitoleic acid and arachidonic acid in their adipose tissue. A comprehensive analysis of fatty acid composition of erythrocyte in middle-aged and older Chinese individuals revealed higher levels of docosahexaenoic acid (DHA), but neither eicosapentaenoic acid (EPA) nor docosapentaenoic acid (DPA) was significantly associated with lower odds of metabolic syndrome or elevated blood pressure and triglycerides (Zhang et al., 2012).

Tetra18:2 cardiolipin (CL) depletion occurred at the very early stages of type I diabetic model mice induced by streptozotocin (Han et al., 2005, 2007). CL species are extensively remodelled at very early stages, leading to a diversified molecular species profile (Han et al., 2007). Fatty acyl contents of 18:2 and 18:1 in CL, particularly the former, are dramatically decreased; in contrast, the content of 22:6 is substantially increased (Figure 4.4). Therefore, the CL species containing fatty acyl chain longer

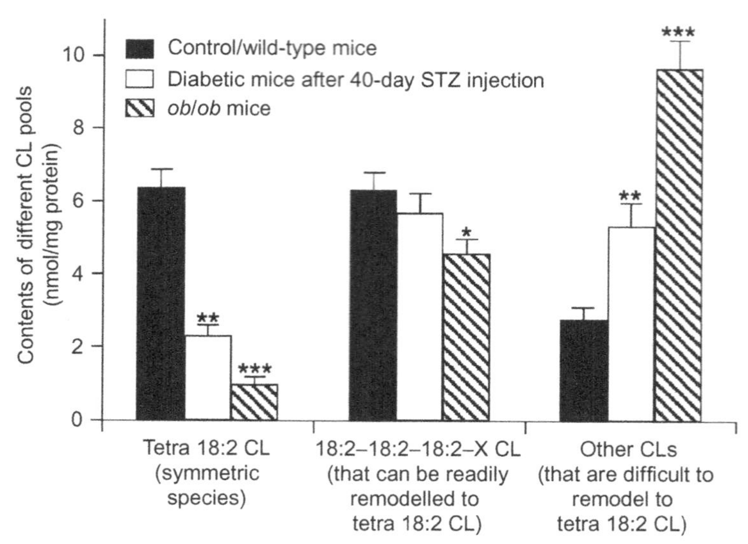

Figure 4.4 The contents of different cardiolipin pools including symmetric, modestly symmetric (i.e. that can be readily remodelled to symmetric ones), and highly asymmetric (i.e. that are difficult to remodel to symmetric ones) cardiolipin species. STZ, streptozotocin; X, one of any fatty acyl chains other than 18:2. $*p<0.01$; $**p<0.001$; $***p<0.0001$. Data are obtained from Han et al. (2007).

than 18 carbon atoms are drastically increased including 18:2–22:6–22:6–22:6, 18:2–20:3–22:6–22:6, and 18:2–18:2–22:6–22:6, as well as 18:2–18:2–18:2–20:3. Similar to the type I diabetic model, changes of CL species are also manifest in mouse heart of type II diabetes (e.g. insulin-resistant, leptin-deficient *ob/ob* mice) (Han et al., 2007). These kinds of CL profiles are ubiquitously present in other mouse heart of type II diabetes mellitus such as high-fat-induced, *db/db*, or protein kinase AKT2 knockout model (X. Han, unpublished data). We believe that the extensive CL remodelling in diabetic myocardium should have sequentially impacts on mitochondrial dysfunction and cardiac dysfunction.

It is important to recognise that mitochondrial and peroxisomal phospholipases are key players in the regulation of cellular bioenergetics and signalling (Gadd et al., 2006; Kinsey et al., 2007). Mice deficient in phospholipase $A_2\gamma$ (iPLA$_2\gamma^{-/-}$) are resistant to high-fat-diet-induced weight gain, hyperinsulinaemia, and insulin (Mancuso et al., 2010). Shotgun lipidomics of adipose tissue from wild-type mice demonstrated a twofold increase in TAG content after being fed a high-fat diet as compared to iPLA$_2\gamma^{-/-}$ mice fed either a standard chow or a high-fat diet. In addition, shotgun lipidomics of skeletal muscle has revealed a decreased CL content with an altered molecular species composition in iPLA$_2\gamma^{-/-}$ mice, thereby identifying for the first time the mechanism underlying mitochondrial uncoupling in this experimental model (Mancuso et al., 2010). Tissue macrophage inflammatory pathways have also been shown to contribute to obesity-associated insulin resistance (Xu et al., 2003).

Hypertension is recognised to be related, among other factors, to unhealthy dietary habits such as excessive intake of calories, alcohol, and salt (Srinath Reddy and Katan, 2004). Large population-based cohort studies have shown that dyslipidaemia plays a key role in the development of hypertension (Dutro et al., 2007). Lipidomics analysis has revealed that lipid metabolism in hypertensive subjects is clearly different from that in controls, with PC and TAG levels being higher in patient plasma (Hu et al., 2011). It has been found that the levels of TAG species containing two or three saturated fatty acyl chains were significantly higher in hypertensive subjects, which suggested their potential role in lipotoxicity (Hu et al., 2011). In addition, a large number of neutral lipid species were significantly elevated in patients, but drastically reduced after treatment with antihypertensive agents.

4.4.3 Lipidomics to control food quality

Lipidomics is also a powerful tool for controlling food quality and detecting fraud in food products. The specificity and sensitivity of MS-based methods are officially recognised by international quality system control agencies for the detection of fraud and bad practises in food manipulation (Aiello et al., 2011). The term "foodomics" has been coined to define studies in the food and nutrition domains through the application of advanced "omics" technologies to improve the health and well-being of consumers (Cifuentes, 2009). The MS-based strategies for foodomics have recently been reviewed (Herrero et al., 2012).

TAG species present in oils and fats are important constituents of the human diet, largely depending on the degree of fatty acyl saturation. To this end, both MDMS shotgun lipidomics and multistage tandem mass spectrometric approaches could be used to characterise those species in complex mixtures (Han et al., 2004b; Hsu and Turk, 1999; Lin and Arcinas, 2008).

Changes in phospholipid composition during storage are one of the most important changes affecting the freshness of fish, with oxidation and hydrolysis of phospholipids being the main reasons for quality deterioration. Shotgun lipidomics has been used for effective analyses of phospholipids from fish muscle stored at room temperature (Wang and Zhang, 2011). For example, some phosphatidylethanolamine species that are present in low concentrations in fresh samples are increased during storage. Those authors have suggested that those species may come from microbiome breeding in the muscle, a phenomenon that has not been identified previously (Wang and Zhang, 2011), implying its potential relevance as a marker of fish quality. MALDI-TOF/MS has also been applied for the characterisation of crude lipid extracts of several dietary products including cow milk, soymilk, and chicken egg (Calvano et al., 2010).

4.5 Conclusion and future trends

Lipidomics has been increasingly utilised in nutritional research. The available analytical methodologies have already allowed lipid analysis in a high-throughput, effective, and sensitive fashion. The major obstruction of lipidomics platforms for application in nutritional research is the bioinformatics tools for interpretation of lipidomic data at the biological, biophysical, and physiological levels.

In nutritional research, lipidomics allows effective and sensitive measurements of markers of complex pathological states related to altered lipid homeostasis and metabolism induced by nutritional interventions or changes of the caloric intake. In the future, lipidomics should allow development of more personalised approaches for dietary guidance and provide tools for shifting the focus of clinical nutrition research from disease treatment and management to disease prevention. Lipidomics could also be applied to identify clinical endpoints of a dietary intervention as well as novel biomarkers, which could be utilised to validate health claims of functional and health-promoting dietary components. In food development, lipidomics could be used to monitor the bioactivity and bioavailability of food products to optimise their dietary value and evaluate their health effects and safety. Taken together, lipidomics should play an important role in nutritional research in all aspects.

Acknowledgement

This work was partially supported by National Institute of General Medical Sciences Grant R01 GM105724 and intramural institutional research funds.

References

Aiello, D., De Luca, D., Gionfriddo, E., Naccarato, A., Napoli, A., Romano, E., Russo, A., Sindona, G., Tagarelli, A., 2011. Review: multistage mass spectrometry in quality, safety and origin of foods. Eur. J. Mass Spectrom. (Chichester, Eng) 17, 1–31.

Aiyar, N., Disa, J., Ao, Z., Ju, H., Nerurkar, S., Willette, R.N., Macphee, C.H., Johns, D.G., Douglas, S.A., 2007. Lysophosphatidylcholine induces inflammatory activation of human coronary artery smooth muscle cells. Mol. Cell. Biochem. 295, 113–120.

Bartz, R., Li, W.H., Venables, B., Zehmer, J.K., Roth, M.R., Welti, R., Anderson, R.G., Liu, P., Chapman, K.D., 2007. Lipidomics reveals that adiposomes store ether lipids and mediate phospholipid traffic. J. Lipid Res. 48, 837–847.

Blanksby, S.J., Mitchell, T.W., 2010. Advances in mass spectrometry for lipidomics. Annu Rev Anal Chem (Palo Alto, Calif) 3, 433–465.

Brugger, B., Erben, G., Sandhoff, R., Wieland, F.T., Lehmann, W.D., 1997. Quantitative analysis of biological membrane lipids at the low picomole level by nano-electrospray ionization tandem mass spectrometry. Proc. Natl. Acad. Sci. U. S. A. 94, 2339–2344.

Byrnes, R.W., Cotter, D., Maer, A., Li, J., Nadeau, D., Subramaniam, S., 2009. An editor for pathway drawing and data visualization in the Biopathways Workbench. BMC Syst. Biol. 3, 99.

Calvano, C.D., Carulli, S., Palmisano, F., 2010. 1H-pteridine-2,4-dione (lumazine): a new MALDI matrix for complex (phospho)lipid mixtures analysis. Anal. Bioanal. Chem. 398, 499–507.

Cheng, H., Jiang, X., Han, X., 2007. Alterations in lipid homeostasis of mouse dorsal root ganglia induced by apolipoprotein E deficiency: a shotgun lipidomics study. J. Neurochem. 101, 57–76.

Christie, W.W., Han, X., 2010. Lipid Analysis: Isolation, Separation, Identification and Lipidomic Analysis. The Oily Press, Bridgwater, England.

Cifuentes, A., 2009. Food analysis and foodomics. J. Chromatogr. A 1216, 7109.

Cowart, L.A., Shotwell, M., Worley, M.L., Richards, A.J., Montefusco, D.J., Hannun, Y.A., Lu, X., 2010. Revealing a signaling role of phytosphingosine-1-phosphate in yeast. Mol. Syst. Biol. 6, 349.

De Smet, E., Mensink, R.P., Plat, J., 2012. Effects of plant sterols and stanols on intestinal cholesterol metabolism: suggested mechanisms from past to present. Mol. Nutr. Food Res. 56, 1058–1072.

Dennis, E.A., 2009. Lipidomics joins the omics evolution. Proc. Natl. Acad. Sci. U. S. A. 106, 2089–2090.

Dhingra, S., Freedenberg, M., Quo, C.F., Merrill Jr., A.H., Wang, M.D., 2007. Computational modeling of a metabolic pathway in ceramide de novo synthesis. Conf. Proc. IEEE Eng. Med. Biol. Soc. 2007, 1405–1408.

Dutro, M.P., Gerthoffer, T.D., Peterson, E.D., Tang, S.S., Goldberg, G.A., 2007. Treatment of hypertension and dyslipidemia or their combination among US managed-care patients. J. Clin. Hypertens (Greenwich) 9, 684–691.

Ejsing, C.S., Duchoslav, E., Sampaio, J., Simons, K., Bonner, R., Thiele, C., Ekroos, K., Shevchenko, A., 2006. Automated identification and quantification of glycerophospholipid molecular species by multiple precursor ion scanning. Anal. Chem. 78, 6202–6214.

Ekroos, K., Chernushevich, I.V., Simons, K., Shevchenko, A., 2002. Quantitative profiling of phospholipids by multiple precursor ion scanning on a hybrid quadrupole time-of-flight mass spectrometer. Anal. Chem. 74, 941–949.

Engelmann, B., 2004. Plasmalogens: targets for oxidants and major lipophilic antioxidants. Biochem. Soc. Trans. 32, 147–150.

Fahy, E., Subramaniam, S., Brown, H.A., Glass, C.K., Merrill Jr., A.H., Murphy, R.C., Raetz, C. R., Russell, D.W., Seyama, Y., Shaw, W., Shimizu, T., Spener, F., van Meer, G., VanNieuwenhze, M.S., White, S.H., Witztum, J.L., Dennis, E.A., 2005. A comprehensive classification system for lipids. J. Lipid Res. 46, 839–861.

Fahy, E., Cotter, D., Byrnes, R., Sud, M., Maer, A., Li, J., Nadeau, D., Zhau, Y., Subramaniam, S., 2007. Bioinformatics for lipidomics. Methods Enzymol. 432, 247–273.

Feng, L., Prestwich, G.D., 2006. Functional Lipidomics. CRC Press Taylor & Francis Group, Boca Raton, FL.

Folch, J., Lees, M., Sloane Stanley, G.H., 1957. A simple method for the isolation and purification of total lipides from animal tissues. J. Biol. Chem. 226, 497–509.

Forrester, J.S., Milne, S.B., Ivanova, P.T., Brown, H.A., 2004. Computational lipidomics: a multiplexed analysis of dynamic changes in membrane lipid composition during signal transduction. Mol. Pharmacol. 65, 813–821.

Gadd, M.E., Broekemeier, K.M., Crouser, E.D., Kumar, J., Graff, G., Pfeiffer, D.R., 2006. Mitochondrial iPLA2 activity modulates the release of cytochrome c from mitochondria and influences the permeability transition. J. Biol. Chem. 281, 6931–6939.

Griffiths, W.J., Wang, Y., 2009. Mass spectrometry: from proteomics to metabolomics and lipidomics. Chem. Soc. Rev. 38, 1882–1896.

Gross, R.W., Han, X., 2011. Lipidomics at the interface of structure and function in systems biology. Chem. Biol. 18, 284–291.

Guo, X., Lankmayr, E., 2010. Multidimensional approaches in LC and MS for phospholipid bioanalysis. Bioanalysis 2, 1109–1123.

Gupta, S., Maurya, M.R., Merrill Jr., A.H., Glass, C.K., Subramaniam, S., 2011. Integration of lipidomics and transcriptomics data towards a systems biology model of sphingolipid metabolism. BMC Syst. Biol. 5, 26.

Haimi, P., Uphoff, A., Hermansson, M., Somerharju, P., 2006. Software tools for analysis of mass spectrometric lipidome data. Anal. Chem. 78, 8324–8331.

Han, X., 2005. Lipid alterations in the earliest clinically recognizable stage of Alzheimer's disease: implication of the role of lipids in the pathogenesis of Alzheimer's disease. Curr. Alzheimer. Res. 2, 65–77.

Han, X., 2010. Multi-dimensional mass spectrometry-based shotgun lipidomics and the altered lipids at the mild cognitive impairment stage of Alzheimer's disease. Biochim. Biophys. Acta 1801, 774–783.

Han, X., Gross, R.W., 1996. Structural determination of lysophospholipid regioisomers by electrospray ionization tandem mass spectrometry. J. Am. Chem. Soc. 118, 451–457.

Han, X., Gross, R.W., 2001. Quantitative analysis and molecular species fingerprinting of triacylglyceride molecular species directly from lipid extracts of biological samples by electrospray ionization tandem mass spectrometry. Anal. Biochem. 295, 88–100.

Han, X., Gross, R.W., 2003. Global analyses of cellular lipidomes directly from crude extracts of biological samples by ESI mass spectrometry: a bridge to lipidomics. J. Lipid Res. 44, 1071–1079.

Han, X., Gross, R.W., 2005a. Shotgun lipidomics: electrospray ionization mass spectrometric analysis and quantitation of the cellular lipidomes directly from crude extracts of biological samples. Mass Spectrom. Rev. 24, 367–412.

Han, X., Gross, R.W., 2005b. Shotgun lipidomics: multi-dimensional mass spectrometric analysis of cellular lipidomes. Expert Rev. Proteomics 2, 253–264.

Han, X., Cheng, H., Mancuso, D.J., Gross, R.W., 2004a. Caloric restriction results in phospholipid depletion, membrane remodeling and triacylglycerol accumulation in murine myocardium. Biochemistry 43, 15584–15594.

Han, X., Yang, J., Cheng, H., Ye, H., Gross, R.W., 2004b. Towards fingerprinting cellular lipidomes directly from biological samples by two-dimensional electrospray ionization mass spectrometry. Anal. Biochem. 330, 317–331.

Han, X., Yang, J., Cheng, H., Yang, K., Abendschein, D.R., Gross, R.W., 2005. Shotgun lipidomics identifies cardiolipin depletion in diabetic myocardium linking altered substrate utilization with mitochondrial dysfunction. Biochemistry 44, 16684–16694.

Han, X., Yang, J., Yang, K., Zhao, Z., Abendschein, D.R., Gross, R.W., 2007. Alterations in myocardial cardiolipin content and composition occur at the very earliest stages of diabetes: a shotgun lipidomics study. Biochemistry 46, 6417–6428.

Han, X., Yang, K., Gross, R.W., 2012. Multi-dimensional mass spectrometry-based shotgun lipidomics and novel strategies for lipidomic analyses. Mass Spectrom. Rev. 31, 134–178.

Han, R.H., Wang, M., Fang, X., Han, X., 2013. Simulation of triacylglycerol ion profiles: bioinformatics for interpretation of triacylglycerol biosynthesis. J. Lipid Res. 54, 1023–1032.

Hartler, J., Trotzmuller, M., Chitraju, C., Spener, F., Kofeler, H.C., Thallinger, G.G., 2011. Lipid data analyzer: unattended identification and quantitation of lipids in LC-MS data. Bioinformatics 27, 572–577.

Hermansson, M., Uphoff, A., Kakela, R., Somerharju, P., 2005. Automated quantitative analysis of complex lipidomes by liquid chromatography/mass spectrometry. Anal. Chem. 77, 2166–2175.

Herrero, M., Simo, C., Garcia-Canas, V., Ibanez, E., Cifuentes, A., 2012. Foodomics: MS-based strategies in modern food science and nutrition. Mass Spectrom. Rev. 31, 49–69.

Herzog, R., Schuhmann, K., Schwudke, D., Sampaio, J.L., Bornstein, S.R., Schroeder, M., Shevchenko, A., 2012. LipidXplorer: a software for consensual cross-platform lipidomics. PLoS One 7, e29851.

Holman, R.T., 1960. Essential fatty acids in nutrition and metabolism. Arch. Intern. Med. 105, 33–38.
Hsu, F.-F., Turk, J., 1999. Structural characterization of triacylglycerols as lithiated adducts by electrospray ionization mass spectrometry using low-energy collisionally activated dissociation on a triple stage quadrupole instrument. J. Am. Soc. Mass Spectrom. 10, 587–599.
Hu, C., Kong, H., Qu, F., Li, Y., Yu, Z., Gao, P., Peng, S., Xu, G., 2011. Application of plasma lipidomics in studying the response of patients with essential hypertension to antihypertensive drug therapy. Mol. Biosyst. 7, 3271–3279.
Hubner, G., Crone, C., Lindner, B., 2009. lipID—a software tool for automated assignment of lipids in mass spectra. J. Mass Spectrom. 44, 1676–1683.
Huffman, K.M., Redman, L.M., Landerman, L.R., Pieper, C.F., Stevens, R.D., Muehlbauer, M. J., Wenner, B.R., Bain, J.R., Kraus, V.B., Newgard, C.B., Ravussin, E., Kraus, W.E., 2012. Caloric restriction alters the metabolic response to a mixed-meal: results from a randomized, controlled trial. PLoS One 7, e28190.
Junker, B.H., Klukas, C., Schreiber, F., 2006. VANTED: a system for advanced data analysis and visualization in the context of biological networks. BMC Bioinformatics 7, 109.
Kapoor, S., Quo, C.F., Merrill Jr., A.H., Wang, M.D., 2008. An interactive visualization tool and data model for experimental design in systems biology. Conf. Proc. IEEE Eng. Med. Biol. Soc. 2008, 2423–2426.
Kekkonen, R.A., Sysi-Aho, M., Seppanen-Laakso, T., Julkunen, I., Vapaatalo, H., Oresic, M., Korpela, R., 2008. Effect of probiotic Lactobacillus rhamnosus GG intervention on global serum lipidomic profiles in healthy adults. World J. Gastroenterol. 14, 3188–3194.
Kiebish, M.A., Bell, R., Yang, K., Phan, T., Zhao, Z., Ames, W., Seyfried, T.N., Gross, R.W., Chuang, J.H., Han, X., 2010. Dynamic simulation of cardiolipin remodeling: greasing the wheels for an interpretative approach to lipidomics. J. Lipid Res. 51, 2153–2170.
Kiebish, M.A., Young, D.M., Lehman, J.J., Han, X., 2012. Chronic caloric restriction attenuates a loss of sulfatide content in the PGC-1α-/-mouse cortex: a potential lipidomic role of PGC-1α in neurodegeneration. J. Lipid Res. 53, 273–281.
Kind, T., Liu, K.H., Lee do, Y., Defelice, B., Meissen, J.K., Fiehn, O., 2013. LipidBlast in silico tandem mass spectrometry database for lipid identification. Nat. Methods 10, 755–758.
Kinsey, G.R., McHowat, J., Beckett, C.S., Schnellmann, R.G., 2007. Identification of calcium-independent phospholipase A2gamma in mitochondria and its role in mitochondrial oxidative stress. Am. J. Physiol. Renal. Physiol. 292, F853–F860.
Laaksonen, R., Katajamaa, M., Paiva, H., Sysi-Aho, M., Saarinen, L., Junni, P., Lutjohann, D., Smet, J., Van Coster, R., Seppanen-Laakso, T., Lehtimaki, T., Soini, J., Oresic, M., 2006. A systems biology strategy reveals biological pathways and plasma biomarker candidates for potentially toxic statin-induced changes in muscle. PLoS One 1, e97.
Lankinen, M., Schwab, U., Erkkila, A., Seppanen-Laakso, T., Hannila, M.L., Mussalo, H., Lehto, S., Uusitupa, M., Gylling, H., Oresic, M., 2009. Fatty fish intake decreases lipids related to inflammation and insulin signaling—a lipidomics approach. PLoS One 4, e5258.
Li, X., Lu, X., Tian, J., Gao, P., Kong, H., Xu, G., 2009. Application of fuzzy c-means clustering in data analysis of metabolomics. Anal. Chem. 81, 4468–4475.
Lin, J.T., Arcinas, A., 2008. Analysis of regiospecific triacylglycerols by electrospray ionization-mass spectrometry(3) of lithiated adducts. J. Agric. Food Chem. 56, 4909–4915.
Mancuso, D.J., Sims, H.F., Yang, K., Kiebish, M.A., Su, X., Jenkins, C.M., Guan, S., Moon, S. H., Pietka, T., Nassir, F., Schappe, T., Moore, K., Han, X., Abumrad, N.A., Gross, R.W., 2010. Genetic ablation of calcium-independent phospholipase A2gamma prevents obesity and insulin resistance during high fat feeding by mitochondrial uncoupling and increased adipocyte fatty acid oxidation. J. Biol. Chem. 285, 36495–36510.

Matyash, V., Liebisch, G., Kurzchalia, T.V., Shevchenko, A., Schwudke, D., 2008. Lipid extraction by methyl-tert-butyl ether for high-throughput lipidomics. J. Lipid Res. 49, 1137–1146.

Merrill Jr., A.H., Stokes, T.H., Momin, A., Park, H., Portz, B.J., Kelly, S., Wang, E., Sullards, M.C., Wang, M.D., 2009. Sphingolipidomics: a valuable tool for understanding the roles of sphingolipids in biology and disease. J. Lipid Res. 50 (Suppl), S97–S102.

Moller, D.E., Kaufman, K.D., 2005. Metabolic syndrome: a clinical and molecular perspective. Annu. Rev. Med. 56, 45–62.

Murphy, S.A., Nicolaou, A., 2013. Lipidomics applications in health, disease and nutrition research. Mol. Nutr. Food Res. 57, 1336–1346.

Ng, S.C., Hart, A.L., Kamm, M.A., Stagg, A.J., Knight, S.C., 2009. Mechanisms of action of probiotics: recent advances. Inflamm. Bowel Dis. 15, 300–310.

Noakes, M., Clifton, P.M., Doornbos, A.M., Trautwein, E.A., 2005. Plant sterol ester-enriched milk and yoghurt effectively reduce serum cholesterol in modestly hypercholesterolemic subjects. Eur. J. Nutr. 44, 214–222.

Pietilainen, K.H., Rog, T., Seppanen-Laakso, T., Virtue, S., Gopalacharyulu, P., Tang, J., Rodriguez-Cuenca, S., Maciejewski, A., Naukkarinen, J., Ruskeepaa, A.L., Niemela, P.S., Yetukuri, L., Tan, C.Y., Velagapudi, V., Castillo, S., Nygren, H., Hyotylainen, T., Rissanen, A., Kaprio, J., Yki-Jarvinen, H., Vattulainen, I., Vidal-Puig, A., Oresic, M., 2011. Association of lipidome remodeling in the adipocyte membrane with acquired obesity in humans. PLoS Biol. 9, e1000623.

Qi, L., 2012. Gene-diet interactions in complex disease: current findings and relevance for public health. Curr. Nutr. Rep. 1, 222–227.

Sack, M., 2013. Obesity and cardiac function—the role of caloric excess and its reversal. Drug Discov. Today Dis. Mech. 10, e41–e46.

Schwab, U., Seppanen-Laakso, T., Yetukuri, L., Agren, J., Kolehmainen, M., Laaksonen, D.E., Ruskeepaa, A.L., Gylling, H., Uusitupa, M., Oresic, M., 2008. Triacylglycerol fatty acid composition in diet-induced weight loss in subjects with abnormal glucose metabolism—the GENOBIN study. PLoS One 3, e2630.

Schwudke, D., Oegema, J., Burton, L., Entchev, E., Hannich, J.T., Ejsing, C.S., Kurzchalia, T., Shevchenko, A., 2006. Lipid profiling by multiple precursor and neutral loss scanning driven by the data-dependent acquisition. Anal. Chem. 78, 585–595.

Schwudke, D., Liebisch, G., Herzog, R., Schmitz, G., Shevchenko, A., 2007. Shotgun lipidomics by tandem mass spectrometry under data-dependent acquisition control. Methods Enzymol. 433, 175–191.

Shaham, O., Wei, R., Wang, T.J., Ricciardi, C., Lewis, G.D., Vasan, R.S., Carr, S.A., Thadhani, R., Gerszten, R.E., Mootha, V.K., 2008. Metabolic profiling of the human response to a glucose challenge reveals distinct axes of insulin sensitivity. Mol. Syst. Biol. 4, 214.

Shevchenko, A., Simons, K., 2010. Lipidomics: coming to grips with lipid diversity. Nat. Rev. Mol. Cell Biol. 11, 593–598.

Simopoulos, A.P., 2000. Human requirement for N-3 polyunsaturated fatty acids. Poult. Sci. 79, 961–970.

Song, H., Hsu, F.F., Ladenson, J., Turk, J., 2007. Algorithm for processing raw mass spectrometric data to identify and quantitate complex lipid molecular species in mixtures by data-dependent scanning and fragment ion database searching. J. Am. Soc. Mass Spectrom. 18, 1848–1858.

Song, H., Ladenson, J., Turk, J., 2009. Algorithms for automatic processing of data from mass spectrometric analyses of lipids. J. Chromatogr. B 877, 2847–2854.

Srinath Reddy, K., Katan, M.B., 2004. Diet, nutrition and the prevention of hypertension and cardiovascular diseases. Public Health Nutr. 7, 167–186.

Stahlman, M., Ejsing, C.S., Tarasov, K., Perman, J., Boren, J., Ekroos, K., 2009. High throughput oriented shotgun lipidomics by quadrupole time-of-flight mass spectrometry. J. Chromatogr. B 877, 2664–2672.

Stella, C., Beckwith-Hall, B., Cloarec, O., Holmes, E., Lindon, J.C., Powell, J., van der Ouderaa, F., Bingham, S., Cross, A.J., Nicholson, J.K., 2006. Susceptibility of human metabolic phenotypes to dietary modulation. J. Proteome Res. 5, 2780–2788.

Sud, M., Fahy, E., Cotter, D., Brown, A., Dennis, E.A., Glass, C.K., Merrill Jr., A.H., Murphy, R.C., Raetz, C.R., Russell, D.W., Subramaniam, S., 2007. LMSD: LIPID MAPS structure database. Nucleic Acids Res. 35, D527–D532.

Sysi-Aho, M., Katajamaa, M., Yetukuri, L., Oresic, M., 2007. Normalization method for metabolomics data using optimal selection of multiple internal standards. BMC Bioinformatics 8, e93.

Szymanska, E., van Dorsten, F.A., Troost, J., Paliukhovich, I., van Velzen, E.J., Hendriks, M. M., Trautwein, E.A., van Duynhoven, J.P., Vreeken, R.J., Smilde, A.K., 2012. A lipidomic analysis approach to evaluate the response to cholesterol-lowering food intake. Metabolomics 8, 894–906.

Unger, R.H., Scherer, P.E., 2010. Gluttony, sloth and the metabolic syndrome: a roadmap to lipotoxicity. Trends Endocrinol. Metab. 21, 345–352.

van Iersel, M.P., Kelder, T., Pico, A.R., Hanspers, K., Coort, S., Conklin, B.R., Evelo, C., 2008. Presenting and exploring biological pathways with PathVisio. BMC Bioinformatics 9, 399.

Wang, Y., Zhang, H., 2011. Tracking phospholipid profiling of muscle from Ctennopharyngodon idellus during storage by shotgun lipidomics. J. Agric. Food Chem. 59, 11635–11642.

Welti, R., Wang, X., 2004. Lipid species profiling: a high-throughput approach to identify lipid compositional changes and determine the function of genes involved in lipid metabolism and signaling. Curr. Opin. Plant Biol. 7, 337–344.

Wenk, M.R., 2005. The emerging field of lipidomics. Nat. Rev. Drug Discov. 4, 594–610.

Wheelock, C.E., Goto, S., Yetukuri, L., D'Alexandri, F.L., Klukas, C., Schreiber, F., Oresic, M., 2009. Bioinformatics strategies for the analysis of lipids. Methods Mol. Biol. 580, 339–368.

Wopereis, S., Rubingh, C.M., van Erk, M.J., Verheij, E.R., van Vliet, T., Cnubben, N.H., Smilde, A.K., van der Greef, J., van Ommen, B., Hendriks, H.F., 2009. Metabolic profiling of the response to an oral glucose tolerance test detects subtle metabolic changes. PLoS One 4, e4525.

Xu, H., Barnes, G.T., Yang, Q., Tan, G., Yang, D., Chou, C.J., Sole, J., Nichols, A., Ross, J.S., Tartaglia, L.A., Chen, H., 2003. Chronic inflammation in fat plays a crucial role in the development of obesity-related insulin resistance. J. Clin. Invest. 112, 1821–1830.

Yan, S., Chai, H., Wang, H., Yang, H., Nan, B., Yao, Q., Chen, C., 2005. Effects of lysophosphatidylcholine on monolayer cell permeability of human coronary artery endothelial cells. Surgery 138, 464–473.

Yang, K., Zhao, Z., Gross, R.W., Han, X., 2007. Shotgun lipidomics identifies a paired rule for the presence of isomeric ether phospholipid molecular species. PLoS One 2, e1368.

Yang, K., Cheng, H., Gross, R.W., Han, X., 2009a. Automated lipid identification and quantification by multi-dimensional mass spectrometry-based shotgun lipidomics. Anal. Chem. 81, 4356–4368.

Yang, K., Zhao, Z., Gross, R.W., Han, X., 2009b. Systematic analysis of choline-containing phospholipids using multi-dimensional mass spectrometry-based shotgun lipidomics. J. Chromatogr. B 877, 2924–2936.

Yang, K., Fang, X., Gross, R.W., Han, X., 2011. A practical approach for determination of mass spectral baselines. J. Am. Soc. Mass Spectrom. 22, 2090–2099.

Yetukuri, L., Katajamaa, M., Medina-Gomez, G., Seppanen-Laakso, T., Vidal-Puig, A., Oresic, M., 2007. Bioinformatics strategies for lipidomics analysis: characterization of obesity related hepatic steatosis. BMC Syst. Biol. 1, 12.

Zarringhalam, K., Zhang, L., Kiebish, M.A., Yang, K., Han, X., Gross, R.W., Chuang, J., 2012. Statistical analysis of the processes controlling choline and ethanolamine glycerophospholipid molecular species composition. PLoS One 7, e37293.

Zhang, G., Sun, Q., Hu, F.B., Ye, X., Yu, Z., Zong, G., Li, H., Zhou, Y., Lin, X., 2012. Erythrocyte n-3 fatty acids and metabolic syndrome in middle-aged and older Chinese. J. Clin. Endocrinol. Metab. 97, E973–E977.

Analysing human metabolic networks using metabolomics: understanding the impact of diet on health

5

N. Poupin, F. Jourdan
Institut National de la Recherche Agronomique (INRA), Paris, France

5.1 Introduction

Metabolism is often investigated on the scale of metabolic pathways. But metabolic shifts can result from processes spanning several pathways. To investigate these global responses to stress, untargeted approaches are used to record qualitative and quantitative data on biochemical entities (e.g. metabolites) belonging to several metabolic functions. The bioinformatics solution we present in this chapter is designed to interpret these datasets (focusing on metabolome) in order to understand the metabolic modulations that may occur in response to changes in environmental conditions (e.g. nutritional changes).

Considered globally, human metabolic functions are achieved through thousands of biochemical reactions that turn substrate metabolites into products. These output molecules can then be processed by one or several reactions, thus creating cascade of reactions. Taken together, these metabolic reactions create a large molecular web called a metabolic network. When used most directly, metabolic networks provide a mechanistic interpretation of *in vivo* or *in vitro* biomarker metabolites by identifying which reactions connect them. This metabolic network mapping has proved to be a way to simultaneously interpret post-genomic and metabolomics data (Deo et al., 2010; Zelezniak et al., 2010).

Metabolic networks can also be used to identify metabolites contained in raw metabolomics data. In fact, taking into account all reactions can help analysts reduce the size of the potential metabolome by keeping only biologically relevant molecules. On the contrary, metabolites that cannot be synthesised or consumed by any reaction are expected to occur in the samples.

These genome-scale metabolic network approaches have been successfully applied in several studies on human metabolism. For instance, they have been used to predict and confirm biomarkers for inborn metabolic errors (Shlomi et al., 2009), and these networks are also exploited more and more frequently in cancer research to decipher the metabolic shifts specific to cancerous cells (Folger et al., 2011). Based on these observations, networks can then be used to guide research towards new and relevant therapeutic targets (Frezza et al., 2011). The network structure can also help to detect

Metabolomics as a Tool in Nutrition Research. http://dx.doi.org/10.1016/B978-1-78242-084-2.00005-8

potentially off-target drug effects by simulating the global impacts of a metabolic drug. Metabolic network reconstructions can also be built for human parasites (e.g. Leishmania major, the organism that causes cutaneous leishmaniasis in mammalian hosts; Chavali et al., 2008) and used as the basis for identifying weak points in the system that can serve as potential drug targets (Rahman and Schomburg, 2006).

In the nutrition field, the combined use of metabolic networks and metabolomics is particularly well suited to exploring how some particular diets (through imbalanced nutrient composition, excess or deficiency in some compound, etc.) may modulate the use or activity of metabolic pathways in the cell and alter metabolic homeostasis. This approach should help identify cellular and molecular mechanisms associated with metabolic diseases or specific dietary conditions; for instance, it might elucidate the link between diet and cellular mechanisms involved in the development of diseases such as diabetes or obesity.

This chapter first describes how metabolic networks are defined and built. We then focus on metabolic networks for human studies and point out databases and file formats available to access this knowledge. In the process, we show how metabolomics data can be imported into these networks. In the following sections, we describe different approaches to metabolic modelling, focusing on graph modelling, and we finally present how these graphs can be mined to determine which metabolic subnetworks are related to the investigated perturbation.

5.2 Metabolic network reconstruction

5.2.1 Genome-based reconstruction method

Genome-scale metabolic networks were first built for microorganisms and model organisms such as *Escherichia coli* or yeast, and several releases of these networks now allow a more accurate image of these organisms' metabolisms (Orth et al., 2011; Price et al., 2004). With sequencing technologies becoming more rapid, it is now possible to access genomic information for a large range of organisms. A bioinformatics generic approach was thus proposed to reconstruct metabolic networks based on genomic data (Thiele and Palsson, 2010a), and this approach is now applied to a large range of eukaryotic and prokaryotic organisms.

The first step of the reconstruction process consists of listing potential metabolic reactions based on the genomic information of an organism. Computational methods are used to retrieve the proteins (enzymes) that can be produced based on the gene sequences. Then enzymatic activities are associated with one or several enzymes, using EC numbers. These numbers are four-digit codes that describe enzymatic activities (e.g. EC number 6.2.1.30 corresponds to the phenylacetyl-CoA ligase). Databases such as Enzyme (Bairoch, 2000) or Brenda (Schomburg et al., 2004) are subsequently used to find the metabolic reactions (substrates, reaction, products) corresponding to these EC numbers.

This first draft reconstruction often contains false positives (reactions that should not be in the network) and false negatives (missing reactions) (Ginsburg, 2006).

Methods are designed to fill these gaps and remove wrong annotations. It can be achieved by checking for reactions that, if they are added, will complete a pathway. This "pathway holes" search is implemented using the Pathway Tools software (Karp et al., 2011). Another option consists of checking whether specific compounds can be produced given the stoichiometric parameters available in the reconstruction (DeJongh et al., 2007).

To validate a reconstruction, metabolic scenarios are tested. A reconstruction is considered to be valid if the network is able to fulfil some known metabolic functions, meaning that a set of metabolic reactions allows synthesising a metabolite B from a metabolite A (e.g. generation of energy via oxidative phosphorylation). When information in the draft reconstruction is sufficient, the ability of the network to generate biomass (essential molecules necessary for cell growth) can also be tested using flux-balance analysis (FBA) methods (Raman and Chandra, 2009). This validation step requires knowledge of the stoichiometry of the reactions and the ability to translate the network structure into a stoichiometric matrix to allow for flux calculation. Finally, the total inhibition of particular reactions can be tested and compared to experimentally known effects (Chang et al., 2010; Shlomi et al., 2009; Shlomi et al., 2008).

The compartmentalisation of metabolic reactions is a challenging problem that was not faced in most microorganisms' reconstructions. Methods have been developed for retrieving this information from genomic data by identifying gene synteny or targeting signals (Shatkay et al., 2007). The network structure and the related flux of molecules also strongly constrain reaction localisation: when some of the reaction localisations are known, researchers can use this information to infer the localisation of other ones (Mintz-Oron et al., 2009).

5.2.2 Biochemical reconstruction

Many enzymatic functions are not associated with genes, and some functions are not yet associated with enzymes. This lack of association can explain the fact that the size of the network metabolome does not necessarily fit the size of the metabolome observed in metabolomics samples. Indeed, the Human Metabolome Database currently contains 40,153 metabolites (version 3.0) (Wishart et al., 2013), and the latest version of the human network contains 2626 unique metabolites (Thiele et al., 2013). For instance, metabolites coming from food intake (food metabolome) remain largely unspecified in genome-scale networks. Chemoinformatics methods, based on informatics and chemistry, enable metabolic network reconstructions without genetic information through retrosynthetic biology. They can, given an exogenous compound, find a biosynthetic path allowing connections between this compound and the rest of the network (Carbonell et al., 2011). Another way to connect the observed metabolites to the metabolic network consists of building *ab initio* networks (Breitling et al., 2006b; Jourdan et al., 2008). This method is based on high-resolution mass spectrometry metabolomics data, which can now be generated. Given two metabolites A and B, of molecular weight w_A and w_B, respectively, we can compute the difference $w_X = |w_A - w_B|$ and check whether it corresponds to a known biochemical transformation. For instance, a carboxylation reaction will be associated with a mass difference of 43.98983, which corresponds to the molecular weight of CO_2. These chemoinformatics approaches are not yet implemented in the reconstruction pipelines. But they open a new field in network reconstruction, and the growing activity in metabolomics and the development of high- and ultra-high-resolution spectrometric methods will allow the generalisation of these approaches.

5.2.3 Manual curation

Nevertheless, fully automatic reconstruction is not possible, and a long and tedious process of manual curation is required to produce a relevant genome-scale metabolic network reconstruction. Thiele and Palsson formalised this curation through "jamborees" during which specific annotation tasks are assigned to curators over the course of a few days of meetings (Thiele and Palsson, 2010b). To facilitate this collaborative annotation, some tools are available. For instance, Pathway Tools software allows metabolic network reconstruction and manual curation of all genes, protein reactions, and metabolites contained in a BioCyc database (Karp et al., 2011). Organism-specific BioCyc databases were created that way and are available online (e.g. HumanCyc, EcoC, etc.). They are classified based on their level of annotation: tier 1 means intensively curated (HumanCyc is part of this group; Romero et al., 2005), tier 2 means that the database is under curation, and tier 3 means that the database is only the output of an automatic reconstruction (Caspi et al., 2012). Other software suites offer manual curation of reconstructed networks (Forth et al., 2010; May et al., 2013).

Manual annotation may be more or less supported by experimental evidence. In order to keep track of this level of information, a confidence score was introduced for each reaction. These scores are 0 (not evaluated), 1 (no evidence is available, but the reaction is required for modelling), 2 (evidence for gene function or indirect evidence for biochemical reaction based on physiological data), 3 (direct and indirect evidence for gene function), and 4 (direct evidence for gene product function and biochemical reaction) (Thiele and Palsson, 2010a).

All together genome-scale metabolic network reconstruction takes between 6 months and 1 year. Moreover, as for genome annotation, networks are regularly updated based on new experimental evidences and the results of new bioinformatics methods. Finally, it may lead to alternative efforts, especially for model organisms, as it will be discussed for the human network in the following section.

5.3 Human metabolic networks

5.3.1 Human metabolic databases and genome-scale networks

The human genome has been available and fully annotated since 2004 (Lander et al., 2004), and information on genes related to metabolic functions is gathered in databases such as Entrez Gene (Maglott et al., 2005). Based on this knowledge, databases storing metabolic reactions started providing access to human metabolic pathways. Within KEGG, researchers can retrieve a list of all enzymatic reactions for which corresponding genes are found in human genome (Kanehisa et al., 2008). A dedicated BioCyc database called HumanCyc, which relates human metabolic pathways to the human genome, was also released and is still maintained (Romero et al., 2005). The Reactome database aims to gather all human metabolic reactions (Joshi-Tope et al., 2005). Since their first releases, these databases are regularly updated based on manual curation, cross-referencing with other databases, and bibliographic knowledge (Croft et al., 2013).

Since 2007, research groups have been working on building genome-scale networks based on these lists of reactions. Unlike databases, these networks are available in single files and can be directly used to perform computations. More than 1500 data from the literature were used to build the first genome-scale reconstruction of the human metabolic network (Recon1), which contained 1496 genes and 3744 metabolic reactions (Duarte et al., 2007). Other human genome-scale networks were built using alternative approaches (Gille et al., 2010; Hao et al., 2010; Ma et al., 2007) (see Table 5.1 for a detailed comparison). In this chapter, we focus on the Recon initiative, whose latest release (Recon2) compiles the data available in the other reconstructions and results in a network containing 1789 genes, 7440 reactions, and 2626 metabolites (Thiele et al., 2013). These models describe the global metabolic capacities of the organism. But tissues and cell lines may have different metabolic behaviours, meaning different network structures. Methods are currently developed to identify these metabolic specificities.

5.3.2 *Tissue-specific metabolic networks*

More recently, efforts have been made to develop cell- or tissue-specific networks that include only the reactions that are known or strongly suspected to be active in a specific tissue or cell type. Most of the reconstructions of human tissue- or cell type-specific networks are derived from Recon1 (Duarte et al., 2007), which constitutes a basis for the list of network components (compartments, metabolites, and reactions) that could be included in tissue-specific networks. Reactions from this initial global network are removed, kept, or modulated (directionality, stoichiometry, compartmentalisation may be adjusted) based on the literature about tissue-specific metabolic functions and on high-throughput data (transcriptomic, metabolomic, proteomic) obtained in cell- or tissue-specific contexts. Additional metabolites or reactions may also be added if information strongly supporting their presence is reported in the literature. For instance, in the small intestine metabolic network reconstruction, 312 reactions that were not present in Recon1 were added (Sahoo and Thiele, 2013). These reactions are mostly transport reactions that allow accounting for enterocytes-specific transport systems.

These tissue- or cell type-specific networks aim at reproducing the major metabolic functions known to be performed by the tissue, thus accounting for the metabolic specificity of the tissue. For instance, the hepatic-specific network developed from Recon1 is able to produce urea, whereas other cell-specific networks are not (Thiele et al., 2013). Such networks allow for the prediction of specific metabolic behaviours of various tissues and are expected to have better explanatory and predictive power than global reconstructions (Vlassis et al., 2014). This step is thus necessary to investigate the specific metabolic and regulation processes of tissues and potential effects of specific metabolic diseases.

Table 5.1 **Genome-scale networks**

Year	Name	Recon-struction	Data/databases used	Genes	Unique metabolites	Reactions	Compartments	Format	Validation	Reference
2007	Recon1	Manual	KEGG, now EntrezGene, GeneCards, LIGAND, BRENDA + biological evidence from literature	1496	1509	3744	Cytoplasm/ExS/ mitochondrion/ GA/ER/lysosome/ peroxysome/ nucleus	SBML	288 simulated metabolic functions	Duarte et al. (2007)
2007	EHMN	Manual	KEGG, Uniprot, HGNC, now EntrezGene, Ensembl, GeneCards + literature information on human reactions	2322	2715	2824	No	SBML	Essentiality of some nutrients (EAA, *n*-3 and *n*-6 FA, and vitamins)	Ma et al. (2007)
2010	EHMN	Manual	Gene ontology (for protein location information)	2322	2651	4229	Cytosol/ExS/ mitochondrion/GA/ ER/lysosome/ peroxysome/ nucleus	SBML	68 simulated metabolic processes	Hao et al. (2010)
2012	iHuman 1512	Manual	Recon1 + EHMN + KEGG and HumanCyc databases	1512	3397	4144	Cytoplasm/ExS/ mitochondrion/GA/ ER/lysosome/ peroxysome/ nucleus	SBML		Agren et al. (2012)
2013	Recon2	Manual	Recon1, HepatoNet1, EHMN + literature information	1789	2626	7440	Cytoplasm/ExS/ mitochondrion/GA/ ER/lysosome/ peroxysome/ nucleus	SBML xls Matlab	354 simulated metabolic functions	Thiele et al. (2013)

EAA, essential amino acids; ER, endoplasmic reticulum; FA, fatty acids; GA, golgi apparatus; SBML, systems biology markup language.

Tissue-specific metabolic network reconstruction can be performed either manually or automatically. A manual reconstruction consists of a thorough literature search for all metabolic pathways that have been shown to occur in the considered tissue, using literature-based knowledge of tissue-specific reactions, information on gene annotation from databases such as Entrez Gene (Maglott et al., 2005), and information on proteins from databases such as UniProt (The UniProt Consortium, 2013) or Brenda (Schomburg et al., 2004, 2013). Computational methods then quickly and automatically build tissue- or cell type-specific networks. In these methods, the first step consists in identifying a set of reactions that are likely to be active in the considered context, based mainly on evidence from context-specific gene-expression data. Then, different algorithms heuristically prune the initial global network in order to extract a subnetwork that includes as many of these reactions as possible, while constituting a well-connected and biologically consistent network. The underlying hypothesis is that there is a strong correlation between measured gene expression and network-predicted reaction activity, so that the reaction activity in a specific context can be inferred from measured gene expression for the associated enzyme in this context, which may be untrue in the case of posttranscriptional regulation. This reconstruction may not be possible for all kinds of tissues or cells since the availability of comprehensive proteomic and transcriptomic datasets for specific cell-types or tissues may be limited.

Cell type- or tissue-specific genome-scale metabolic networks have been manually reconstructed for hepatocytes (Bordbar et al., 2011a; Gille et al., 2010), SI enterocyte (Sahoo and Thiele, 2013), adipocytes (Bordbar et al., 2011a; Mardinoglu et al., 2013), neuronal cells (Lewis et al., 2010), erythrocytes (Bordbar et al., 2011b), myocite (Bordbar et al., 2011a), and fibroblast (Vo et al., 2007). Besides, computational methods have been applied to the global human metabolic network reconstruction Recon1 to derive specific metabolic networks for numerous human cell-types and cancer cell-types (Agren et al., 2012; Thiele et al., 2013). A review of developed tissue- or cell-specific genome-scale metabolic networks is given in Figure 5.1.

In the field of nutrition, such tissue-specific network reconstruction may be useful for investigating specific modulations that occur in diet-related diseases, as well as the impact of diet on tissue metabolism. A network metabolic reconstruction of the small intestine enterocyte predicted changes in metabolite fluxes involved in metabolic syndrome under an average American diet compared to a balanced diet (higher secretion fluxes of cholesterol polyesters, triglycerides, and glucose in the extracellular space) (Sahoo and Thiele, 2013). A developed adipocyte model (Mardinoglu et al., 2013) was used to understand the mechanistic changes in adipocyte metabolism in response to obesity, and it enabled identifying metabolites that correspond to up- or down-regulated genes in obese subjects and that could be used as biomarkers for altered metabolism in these subjects (e.g. the increased level of androsterone in plasma). This model also supported the prediction that some metabolic fluxes linked to mitochondrial dysfunction (uptake of glucose, fatty acids (FAs), oxidative phosphorylation, mitochondrial and perixomal B-oxidation, FA metabolism, and TCA cycle) were changed in obese subjects, and that these changes likely result from transcriptional down-regulation. Such models can also be used to detect potential therapeutic targets: for instance, the adipocyte network predicted a lower mitochondrial acetyl-CoA production in obese subjects, and suggested that it could be increased by supplementation of β-alanine.

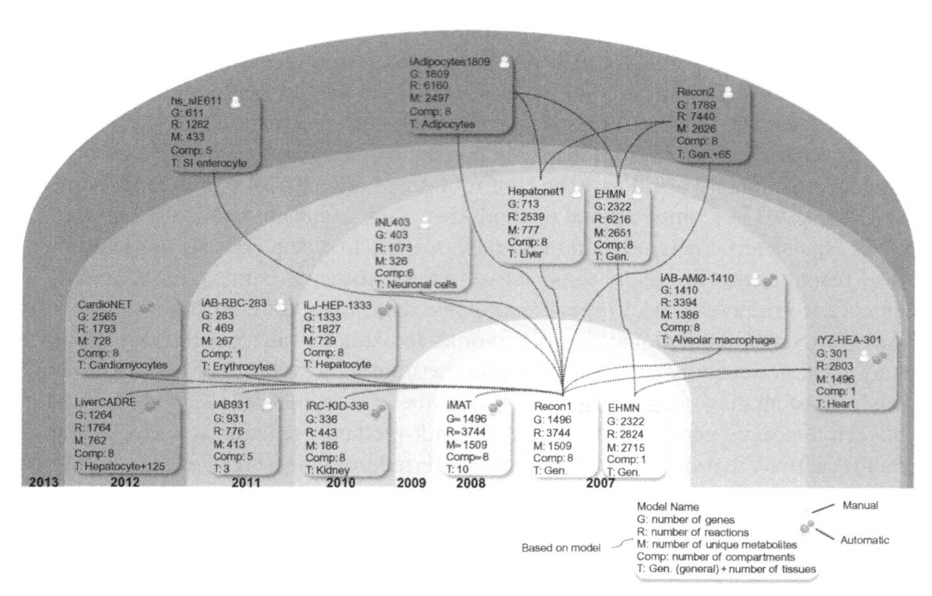

Figure 5.1 Human genome-scale networks, overview, and chronology. Human genome-scale networks evolution from 2007 to 2013. For each network, the number of genes, reactions, unique metabolites (not taking into account compartments), and compartments are provided. "T" specifies if the network corresponds to a tissue or the general organism (Gen.). If the authors presented several tissue networks, the number of these networks is provided. Networks are linked when one network was built based on a previous one.

5.3.3 Limitations

Even if genome-scale networks aim to be as complete as possible by performing gap-filling methods, reactions are still missing, and consequently, metabolites may not be found in these knowledge sources. The first reason for this absence of reactions is that reactions leading to the synthesis of these compounds are not annotated in the genome. These orphan metabolic reactions (Lespinet and Labedan, 2005) represent 23% of the activities classified by the Enzymatic Commission (EC) (Yamada et al., 2012). Moreover, some metabolites are mentioned by families (or generic function) like "an alcohol". This is particularly the case for lipids. For instance, the reactions required for long-chain fatty acid biosynthesis are described, but the large variety of compounds that can be generated using these reactions are not all mentioned. This is an issue when attempting to interpret metabolomics data related to these compounds.

These missing reactions also have impacts on the structure of the network. They may contain dead-end metabolites (metabolites that can only be produced or consumed in the network) or blocked reactions (reactions that cannot carry a nonzero flux in the network because of missing substrates, products, or cofactors, or because they involve dead-end metabolites).

Constant improvement of network annotation allows improving network structures, implying more reliable bioinformatics analysis. To perform these computations, it is necessary to have access to these networks in program-readable files via dedicated exchange formats.

5.3.4 Exchange formats

Databases provide easy access to information, but they cannot be easily used directly by bioinformatics programs. KEGG provides KGML files (requires a paid license since 2012) for pathways. HumanCyc and all BioCyc databases have their own formats for databases (PGDBs), but they require using Pathway Tools software (Karp et al., 2011). Nevertheless, Pathway Tools software allows exporting in Systems Biology Markup Language (SBML) format, which is now becoming the standard for genome-scale metabolic networks.

SBML follows the markup language formalism, as do many resources on the web (e.g. HTML files) (Hucka et al., 2003). This format allows both having human- and computer-readable flat files. SBML, like all markup language structures, is hierarchically organised. The SBML document constitutes the root level, which contains four subsections (see Figure 5.2 "network" inset). The first one describes the units used in the network, the second contains the list of compartments, the third contains the list of all metabolites, and the fourth provides the list of all reactions.

All metabolites, called "species" are referenced by an ID (see Figure 5.2 "Metabolite" inset). Note that, when metabolites are localised in several cellular compartments, a species is created for each localisation, resulting in several IDs for the same metabolite (e.g. species in Figure 5.2 is located in cytoplasm). Other pieces of information are provided, such as a standard name or compound charge status. A "notes" section then allows the addition of miscellaneous information, such as formula or InChI code. The drawback is that these "notes" are not standard and may not be found in other networks. Finally, metabolite annotations can be added by following semantic web (rdf) convention.

Reactions are also described by an ID, a standard name, and additional notes (see Figure 5.2 "Reaction" inset). These notes often contain the pathways involving the reaction (SUBSYSTEM), the EC number, the genes associated with the reaction, the annotation confidence score, and sometimes external references such as Pubmed identifiers. The "reaction" section then contains a list of reactants and a list of products identified by species identifiers. Finally, kinetic and flux values can be set in a specific subsection.

The advantage of this format is that it can be extended by redefining the structure of the hierarchy (e.g. by adding a new subsection). The main drawback is that information contained in the "notes" sections, which is important in systems biology (e.g. gene identifiers), does not follow the same format in all networks.

Finally, web servers such as MetExplore (Cottret et al., 2010) or BIGG (Schellenberger et al., 2010) are importing these files in databases that can then be requested like other metabolic databases.

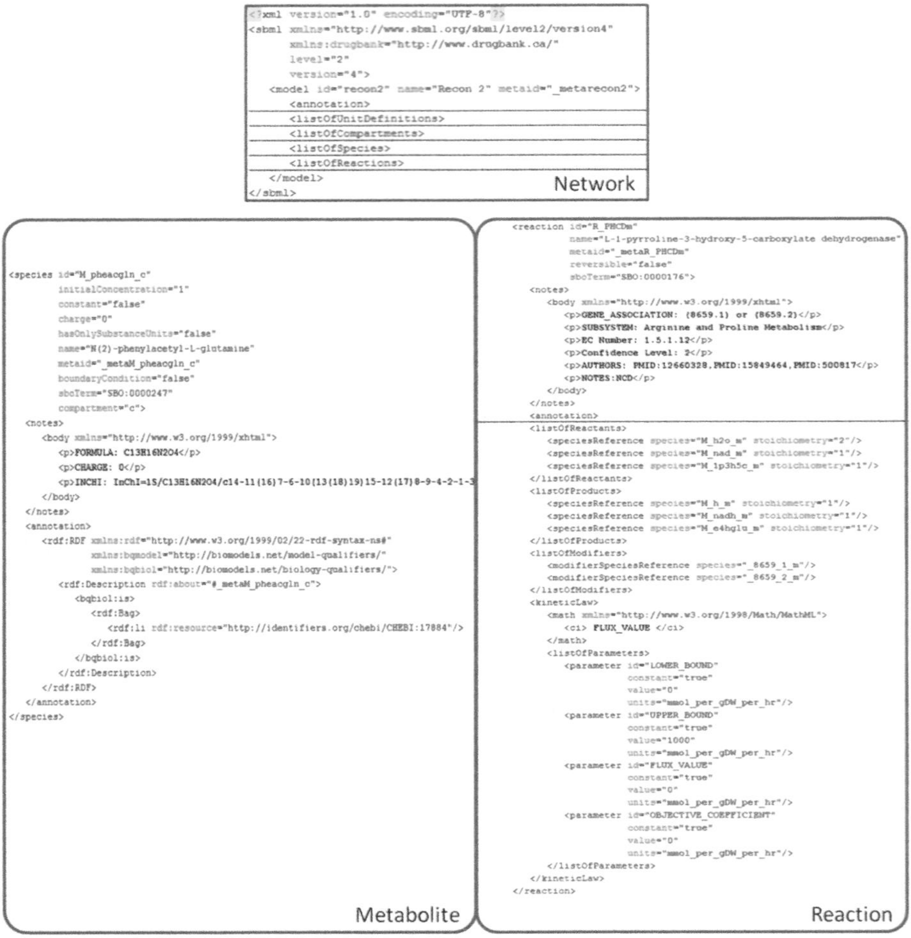

```
<?xml version="1.0" encoding="UTF-8"?>
<sbml xmlns="http://www.sbml.org/sbml/level2/version4"
      xmlns:drugbank="http://www.drugbank.ca/"
      level="2"
      version="4">
   <model id="recon2" name="Recon 2" metaid="_metarecon2">
      <annotation>
      <listOfUnitDefinitions>
      <listOfCompartments>
      <listOfSpecies>
      <listOfReactions>
   </model>
</sbml>
```

Network

```
<species id="M_pheacgln_c"
         initialConcentration="1"
         constant="false"
         charge="0"
         hasOnlySubstanceUnits="false"
         name="N(2)-phenylacetyl-L-glutamine"
         metaid="_metaM_pheacgln_c"
         boundaryCondition="false"
         sboTerm="SBO:0000247"
         compartment="c">
   <notes>
      <body xmlns="http://www.w3.org/1999/xhtml">
         <p>FORMULA: C13H16N2O4</p>
         <p>CHARGE: 0</p>
         <p>INCHI: InChI=1S/C13H16N2O4/c14-11(16)7-6-10(13(18)19)15-12(17)8-9-4-2-1-3
      </body>
   </notes>
   <annotation>
      <rdf:RDF xmlns:rdf="http://www.w3.org/1999/02/22-rdf-syntax-ns#"
               xmlns:bqmodel="http://biomodels.net/model-qualifiers/"
               xmlns:bqbiol="http://biomodels.net/biology-qualifiers/">
         <rdf:Description rdf:about="#_metaM_pheacgln_c">
            <bqbiol:is>
               <rdf:Bag>
                  <rdf:li rdf:resource="http://identifiers.org/chebi/CHEBI:17884"/>
               </rdf:Bag>
            </bqbiol:is>
         </rdf:Description>
      </rdf:RDF>
   </annotation>
</species>
```

Metabolite

```
<reaction id="R_PHCDm"
          name="L-1-pyrroline-3-hydroxy-5-carboxylate dehydrogenase"
          metaid="_metaR_PHCDm"
          reversible="false"
          sboTerm="SBO:0000176">
   <notes>
      <body xmlns="http://www.w3.org/1999/xhtml">
         <p>GENE_ASSOCIATION: (8659.1) or (8659.2)</p>
         <p>SUBSYSTEM: Arginine and Proline Metabolism</p>
         <p>EC Number: 1.5.1.12</p>
         <p>Confidence Level: 2</p>
         <p>AUTHORS: PMID:12660328,PMID:15849464,PMID:500817</p>
         <p>NOTES:NCD</p>
      </body>
   </notes>
   <annotation>
   <listOfReactants>
      <speciesReference species="M_h2o_m" stoichiometry="2"/>
      <speciesReference species="M_nad_m" stoichiometry="1"/>
      <speciesReference species="M_1p3h5c_m" stoichiometry="1"/>
   </listOfReactants>
   <listOfProducts>
      <speciesReference species="M_h_m" stoichiometry="1"/>
      <speciesReference species="M_nadh_m" stoichiometry="1"/>
      <speciesReference species="M_e4hglu_m" stoichiometry="1"/>
   </listOfProducts>
   <listOfModifiers>
      <modifierSpeciesReference species="_8659_1_m"/>
      <modifierSpeciesReference species="_8659_2_m"/>
   </listOfModifiers>
   <kineticLaw>
      <math xmlns="http://www.w3.org/1998/Math/MathML">
         <ci> FLUX_VALUE </ci>
      </math>
      <listOfParameters>
         <parameter id="LOWER_BOUND"
                    constant="true"
                    value="0"
                    units="mmol_per_gDW_per_hr"/>
         <parameter id="UPPER_BOUND"
                    constant="true"
                    value="1000"
                    units="mmol_per_gDW_per_hr"/>
         <parameter id="FLUX_VALUE"
                    constant="true"
                    value="0"
                    units="mmol_per_gDW_per_hr"/>
         <parameter id="OBJECTIVE_COEFFICIENT"
                    constant="true"
                    value="0"
                    units="mmol_per_gDW_per_hr"/>
      </listOfParameters>
   </kineticLaw>
</reaction>
```

Reaction

Figure 5.2 Systems biology markup language (SBML) file structure. The "Network" inset shows the overall hierarchical structure of the SBML file. The "Metabolite" inset describes the information available for each metabolite (species), and the "Reaction" inset shows the data structure for reactions.

5.4 Linking metabolomics data and metabolic network elements

5.4.1 Metabolomics dataset

In this section and the following ones, we use an experiment performed by O'Sullivan et al., 2011 as a benchmark. The aim of this work was to use untargeted metabolomics in order to assess dietary intake patterns. Three distinct dietary patterns were characterised in the study population on the basis of the relative contribution of different nutrient groups: two of them resembled healthy type diets (groups 1 and 2, with high intakes of fruits, vegetables, fish, and wholegrain bread), whereas the other one displayed characteristics of a typical unhealthy diet (group 3, with high intakes of meat products and white bread and low intakes of fruits and vegetables). Results show that these three distinct dietary patterns were reflected in plasma and urine metabolomics, with, for instance, higher plasma levels of some polyunsaturated and monounsaturated fatty acids in the third group and higher urinary concentrations of glycine and phenylacetylglutamine in the first group. In order to go further in the biological interpretation of these patterns, authors identified metabolites specifically linked to each dietary group. They especially identified *O*-acetylcarnitine and phenylacetylglutamine as potential biomarkers for red-meat and vegetable consumption levels, respectively. Then they proposed a mechanistic interpretation of the metabolic pathways potentially involved in these diet-induced changes in the metabolomic profiles. In this section, we show how we can use this list of metabolites (see first column of Table 5.2) and the human metabolic network to automatically find the metabolic reactions affected by these diet changes, and consequently, we raise similar conclusions.

5.4.2 Metabolite identifiers

Interpreting metabolomics data in the context of metabolic networks first requires establishing a correspondence (mapping) between experimentally identified metabolites and those in the network. For instance, glycine is referred to by the identifier "M_gly" in the Recon2 metabolic network. Moreover, metabolic networks such as Recon2 contain compartments, making it necessary to specify the localisation of the metabolite: "M_gly_c" for glycine in cytoplasm. To facilitate reading, we focus on cytoplasm metabolism in the following discussion and do not use the localisation suffix.

Network identifiers and experimentalist naming conventions are subjective and often vary. In order to automatically cross-reference these identifiers, researchers would need to develop a universal way to refer to a given metabolite. But even if several identifiers are available, none is shared by all metabolic network databases. Some of these identifiers are based on the chemical structure of the molecule (InChi, mol, SMILES), and others are database-related identifiers (KEGG, BioCyc, HMDB, Reactome; Croft et al., 2013). The network description sometimes contains possible alternative identifiers, but as shown in Table 5.2, these cross-references are not always available.

To overcome this mapping challenge, methods and services are developed in order to provide ways to index the different identifiers corresponding to the same metabolite (e.g. Chemical Translation Service provided by Oliver Fiehn's laboratory). But most of them do not take into account network identifiers. To solve this issue, the MetaNetX web server is using chemical information on molecules to build a synonym table between databases and networks (Ganter et al., 2013). For a given compound, the server retrieves related metabolites from HMDB, ChEBI, and PubChem databases and from KEGG, MetaCyc, Seed, and BIGG genome-scale networks. Nevertheless, not all human metabolic networks are available in this database. Finally, there is no cross-link to nutrition-related databases such as FooDB.

Table 5.2 **Metabolites identified in metabolomics and corresponding identifiers in databases and models**

Metabolite identifiers in O'Sullivan et al. (2011)	Recon2	HumanCyc	KEGG	Reactome	Hepatonet1	EHMN
Glycine	M_gly	GLY	C00037	114750	HC00045	C00037
O-Acetylcarnitine	M_acrn	*O*-Acetylcarnitine	NF	390287	HC00966	C02571
Phenylacetylglutamine	M_pheacgln	CPD-1097	C04148	177152	NF	NF
Acetoacetate	M_acac	3-Ketobutyrate	C00164	29666	HC00159	C00164
N, *N*-Dimethylglycine	M_dmgly	Dimethyl-glycine	C01026	1614585	NF	C01026
Trimethylamine oxide	NF	NF	NF	140963	NF	NF

5.4.3 *Metabolite mapping using exact masses*

With the increase in mass spectrometer resolution, it is now possible to detect masses up to a few parts per million (ppm). Hence, from one mass, it is now generally possible to find one formula (Breitling et al., 2006a). This new technological improvement is used to perform mapping based on exact mass (Cottret et al., 2010; Wägele et al., 2012). Nevertheless, exact-mass mapping has to be taken with care because it will not distinguish isomers, such as sugars in the glycolysis pathway, and may result in false positive mappings. Fully automatic mapping based on identifiers or masses thus poses a challenging problem, especially when dealing with several metabolic networks and several metabolomics datasets. Even if tools are available to help build synonym tables, it is often necessary to manually search good identifiers in the network by searching a database such as HumanCyc or browsing the SBML file of the network. Given that genome-scale metabolic networks are used more and more often to interpret metabolomics data, reflections on identifiers are ongoing. These efforts will probably lead to a standardisation of network descriptions that will be translated in the SBML file format structure.

5.5 Metabolism modelling, from pathways to network

5.5.1 *Pathway analysis and its limitation in global approaches*

Biomarkers may take part in several metabolic functions (pathways). A large variety of tools are available that, when given a list of metabolites, retrieve a list of pathways in which these metabolites are involved. If quantitative values are associated with metabolites, it is then possible to perform pathway enrichment analysis (see Khatri et al., 2012). This approach computes the statistical significance of each pathway based on metabolomics data.

A convenient way to interpret data involves visualising metabolites in metabolic pathway maps. KEGG and BioCyc provide tools for generating these kinds of representations (Arakawa et al., 2005; Kanehisa et al., 2012; Paley and Karp, 2006). Figures 5.3–5.5 show the results of this visualisation using the O'Sullivan dataset. Figure 5.3 presents the KEGG visualisation in which the identified metabolites are highlighted in red within the global map of all metabolic pathways and more specifically within the "glycine, serine, and threonine metabolism" pathway (Figure 5.4). KEGG provides generic maps for metabolic pathways. Organism-specific pathways are shown by highlighting the annotated reactions in green to indicate pathways active in the organism. For instance, Figure 5.4 shows green-highlighted reactions involved in human glycine, serine, and threonine metabolism. Figure 5.5 shows a cellular overview diagram of human metabolic pathways, as described in HumanCyc. Contrary to KEGG, this diagram only shows reactions that can occur in the human organism. Highlighted nodes also correspond to biomarker metabolites. It should be noted that there are more nodes highlighted than biomarkers in the O'Sullivan dataset. This discrepancy is due to the fact that the representation used is a combination of all pathways and a metabolite may occur in several of these pathways.

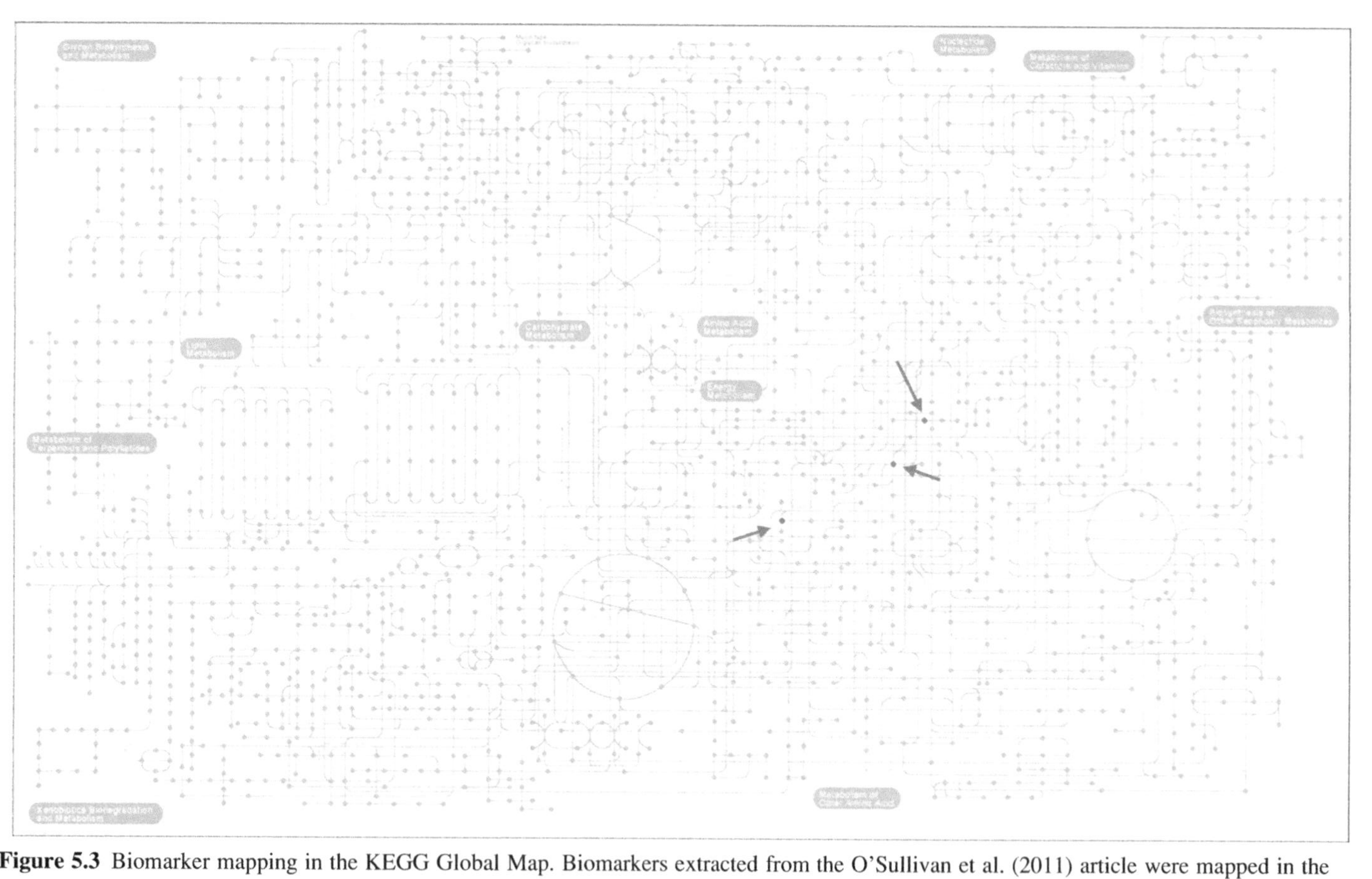

Figure 5.3 Biomarker mapping in the KEGG Global Map. Biomarkers extracted from the O'Sullivan et al. (2011) article were mapped in the overview diagram provided by KEGG for all metabolic pathways. Dots identified by arrows correspond to biomarkers.

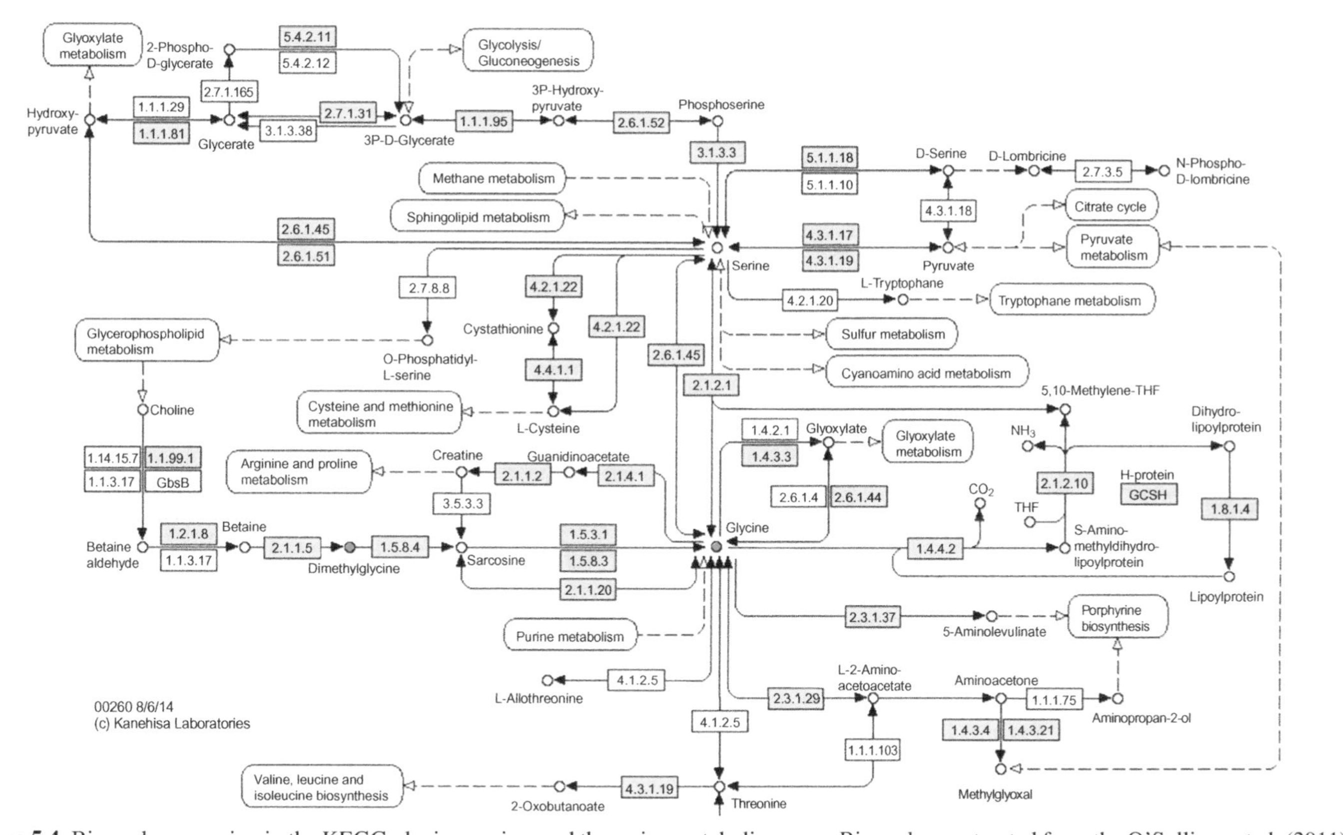

Figure 5.4 Biomarker mapping in the KEGG glycine, serine, and threonine metabolism map. Biomarkers extracted from the O'Sullivan et al. (2011) article were mapped on the glycine, serine, and threonine metabolism pathway. Shaded reactions correspond to reactions that are catalysed by enzymes with associated genes identified in the human genome. The two metabolites (circles) that are filled and identified by arrows correspond to biomarkers.

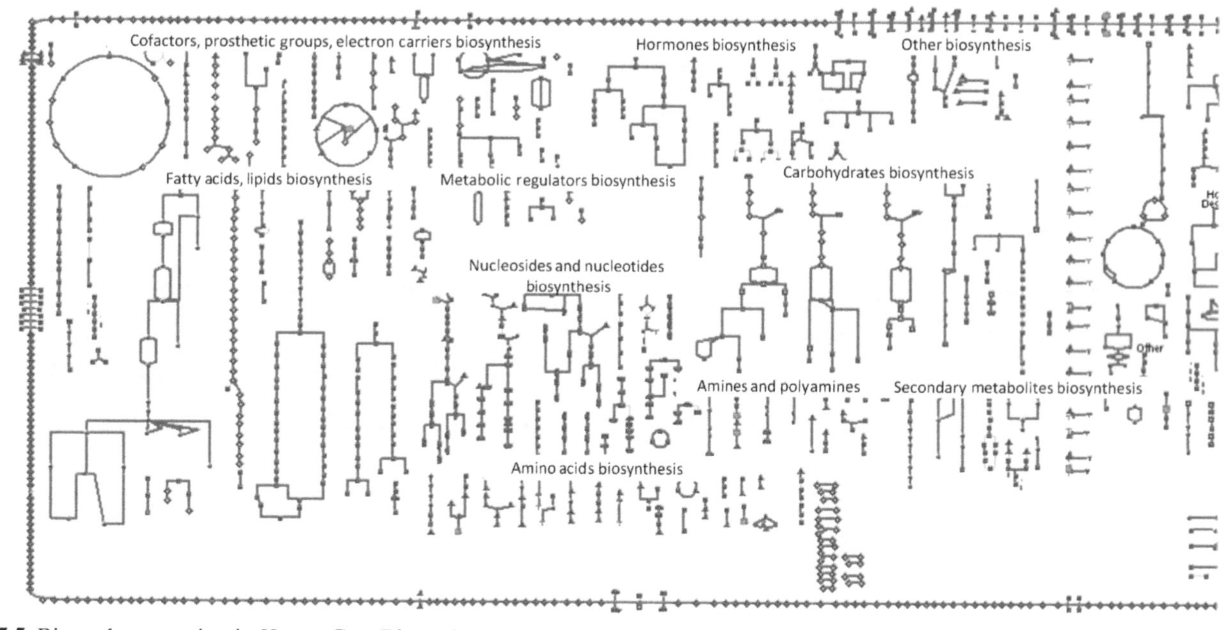

Figure 5.5 Biomarker mapping in HumanCyc. Biomarkers extracted from the O'Sullivan et al. (2011) article were mapped on the HumanCyc cellular overview diagram. This diagram gathers all metabolic pathways in the database. Shaded nodes correspond to biomarkers. Note that there are many nodes highlighted because biomarkers appear in several metabolic pathways.

In pathway-oriented visualisation approaches, such as those used with KEGG and HumanCyc, it is difficult to get a complete picture of all the reactions that can consume or produce a given compound. For instance, only some of the reactions involving glycine are depicted on KEGG pathway "glycine, serine, and threonine metabolism" (central node on Figure 5.4), whereas the KEGG database connects this compound to 34 pathways and potentially 61 reactions. Moreover, the other metabolites identified in the experiment are found in many other pathways. This exemplifies the limitation of pathway-oriented analysis for untargeted global studies. We thus need a method that allows the detection of a process that spans several metabolic pathways. Networks will be the solution because they gather all metabolic pathways into a single object.

5.5.2 Overview of metabolic modelling

The most faithful simulations of metabolism predict metabolite concentrations over time. To do so, they must model the reaction kinetics and define the initial concentration of each metabolite in the model. The definition of both parameters requires time-consuming experiments and cannot be transposed from one organism to another. Moreover, to simulate these models, it is necessary to solve large systems of ordinary differential equations, which require time and computational resources. Hence, these highly informative methods are only used on a small scale (few reactions and metabolites).

The reaction kinetics are the main limitation to expanding models to genome-scale networks because they allow changes in metabolite concentrations and require differential equations to be solved. Nevertheless, if metabolite concentrations are assumed to be constant, then the problem can be stated as a set of linear equations. Each equation, which corresponds to the mass-balance equation of a metabolite, sums the consumption and production rates of the given metabolite through all the implied reactions, taking into account the stoichiometry. Under these steady-state constraints, the full system can be solved using linear programming, even when dealing with thousands of reactions. The computation provides a value for each reaction that corresponds to its metabolic flux (conversion rate of metabolites through a reaction). The steady-state assumption was introduced by Schuster and Schuster (1993) and first used to identify all possible minimal metabolic functions (elementary modes) that a biological system can perform at steady state (Schuster and Hilgetag, 1994; Schuster et al., 2000). Metabolic network complexity and redundancy imply that millions of elementary modes can be found for a network containing only 106 reactions and 89 metabolites, as with *E. coli* central carbon metabolism (Terzer and Stelling, 2008).

To lower the number of solutions, constraints are added based on the assumption that metabolism is optimised to fulfil biological objectives such as growth. Methods were developed to find feasible metabolic flux distributions that, at steady states, will maximise these biological objective functions, while ensuring mass balance. The usual biological objectives are maximisation of the biomass production rate and maximisation of the energy production rate. These FBA methods were first used in microbiology (Price et al., 2004; Schellenberger et al., 2011) and are now applied to solve human metabolism questions (Mo and Palsson, 2009). However, defining the objective function is challenging because it is highly dependent on the studied organism. An additional way to lower the number of possible solutions is to predefine boundaries on reaction fluxes (i.e. to set upper and lower limits for fluxes). All these information elements are available in recently published networks, but they still need to be tuned according to the organism, tissue, or cell line.

Another strong requirement is to define what occurs inside and outside the system. In fact, only metabolites within the system will be constrained to be at steady state. From a global perspective, the need to determine the reactions inside and outside a system requires researchers to list all the exchange reactions and thus to have a clear view of transporters, which are not evident when dealing with humans. These constraint-based methods still require many parameters, and their prediction power is highly sensitive to the quality of the network topology. Defining all these parameters is a challenging problem when dealing with human cells, and, as yet, such approaches have rarely been applied for investigating the impact of the diet on metabolism. For these reasons, we focus on a more descriptive approach based on graph modelling.

5.5.3 Graph-based modelling

A network is a structure in which elements (nodes) are connected by links (edges). The mathematical formalism for this kind of objects is a graph made of a set of nodes N and edges E. This model has been used to solve everyday life problems since the eighteenth century, when it was first used by Leonhard Euler to solve the Königsberg's Bridges problem (Euler, 1741). A large range of methods (algorithms) has been developed since Euler's time to find information in large graphs, such as a minimal sequence of edges connecting two nodes (shortest path problem). Many of these methods have been successfully applied to biological networks at different scales: organisms (e.g. food webs), cells (e.g. neural networks), molecular networks (e.g. protein–protein interactions), and even intra-molecular networks (e.g. *de novo* assembly of new-generation sequencing data).

The first challenge in graph modelling involves choosing which elements will be mapped to nodes and what will be the links corresponding to edges. For metabolic networks, several options are possible and will result in different graph types (Cottret and Jourdan, 2010; Lacroix et al., 2008). Figure 5.6 displays examples of different possible graphs built from the same initial list of reactions (panel 1). In a metabolite graph, nodes correspond to metabolites, and two nodes are connected if they are the substrate and product of the same reaction (see Figure 5.6, panels 2 and 3). Conversely, a reaction graph assigns reactions to nodes and connects two reactions if at least one product of the first reaction is the substrate of the second (see Figure 5.6, panels 4 and 5). The enzyme network follows the same definition as the reaction network. A bipartite graph contains two kinds of nodes: reactions and metabolites. The edges connect reaction nodes to the corresponding substrate and product nodes (see Figure 5.6, panel 6). Finally, the hypergraph model contains metabolite nodes and a reaction is modelled by a single hyperedge that connects all of its substrate nodes to all of its product nodes.

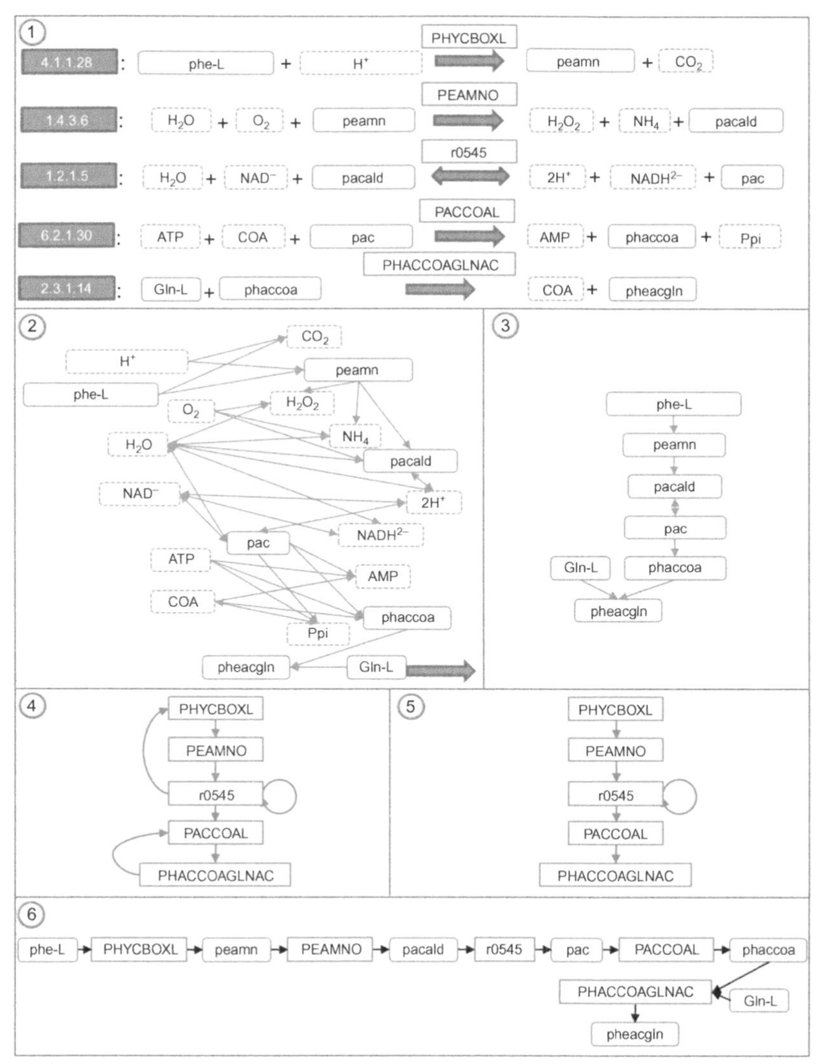

Figure 5.6 Metabolic graph models. Panel 1 presents a list of reactions extracted from Recon2 v01. These reactions were selected because, according to the O'Sullivan et al. (2011) article, they may be involved in the metabolic response to changes in fruit and vegetable intakes. The following abbreviations are used for metabolites: phe-L (L-phenylalanine), peamn (2-phenylethanaminium), pacald (phenylacetaldehyde), pac (phenylacetate), COA (Coenzyme A), Ppi (diphosphate), phaccoa (phenylacetyl-CoA), gln-L (L-glutamine), pheacgln (*N*(2)-phenylacetyl-L-glutamine). The following abbreviations are used for reactions: PHYCBOXL (L-Phenylalanine carboxylase), PEAMNO (Phenethylamine oxidase), r0545 (Phenylacetaldehyde: NAD^+ oxidoreductase), PACCOAL (phenylacetate-CoA ligase), PHACCOAGLNAC (Phenylacetyl-CoA: L-glutamine alpha-*N*-phenylacetyltransferase). The metabolites represented by dashed lines are considered to be side compounds and used for filtering. Panel 2 shows the metabolite graph that accounts for all reactions and metabolites. Panel 3 also presents a metabolite graph with all reactions, but this graph does not account for side compounds. Panel 4 corresponds to a reaction graph with all metabolites, and panel 5 presents a reaction graph built using a reaction list, without taking into account side compounds. Finally, panel 6 shows a bipartite graph based on the filtered list of metabolites.

Choosing the right graph model is important because, even if the list of reactions is the same, it may end up producing different graph structures (Cottret and Jourdan, 2010; Lacroix et al., 2008). The reaction graph is often used to study the evolution of metabolism (Lacroix et al., 2006). The metabolite graph is used to investigate paths between metabolites (Antonov et al., 2009). The bipartite graph has the advantage of providing an unbiased model of the network because it keeps the information on substrates and products. However, this graph is more difficult to handle from an algorithmic point of view because problems are then equivalent to hypergraph problems. A way to maintain the bipartite-modelling level of information, while avoiding these algorithmic problems, involves using the bipartite graph and applying graph algorithms without taking into account the co-substrate information.

Reversibility of reactions can be modelled using graph formalism. In that case, graph is oriented by defining the source and target for edges (arcs). Given that some reactions may be reversible and others may only occur in one direction, the graph may contain both oriented and non-oriented edges. Reversibility of reactions is strongly linked to environmental conditions. In fact, a reaction may occur in one direction in a specific condition (e.g. microorganism growing on a specific carbon source) and in another direction when external conditions change. Thus, graph-orientation quality depends on the level of annotation of the metabolic network.

A graph is well suited for understanding the overall structure (topology) of a network. For instance it is possible to identify weak points (Albert et al., 2000) that may have a strong impact on the metabolism of the organism when targeted by a drug. The challenge is to translate the notion of the weak point into a local topological property. To this end, the notion of the choke point was introduced in parasitology: these nodes are the only reactions that produce or consume a metabolite. If they are therapeutically inhibited, they induce accumulation or deprivation of a specific metabolite, resulting in potentially lethal impacts on parasite metabolism (Rahman and Schomburg, 2006).

One of the main issues when developing algorithms for metabolic graphs is the presence of ubiquitous compounds, such as water, that are involved in many reactions. Because they are connected by many edges (high degree), these ubiquitous compounds may be selected by graph algorithms as interesting elements, although they are not relevant from a biological point of view. For example, Figure 5.6 (panel 2) shows a metabolite graph that accounts for side compounds, while Figure 5.6 (panel 3) shows a graph built without them. It is obvious that the linear structure underlying this pathway is better shown after filtering. Note that, as shown by Figure 5.6 (panels 4 and 5), filtering also has impacts on the reaction graph. The challenge is then to filter these artificial hubs before performing computations (Cottret and Jourdan, 2010). This filtering can be done by automatically removing nodes with the highest degrees or by using a database of known ubiquitous compounds. Tools such as MetExplore (Cottret et al., 2010) also allow manual definition of these lists and the creation of resulting graphs. Another solution consists of avoiding these nodes during computation, as shown in the next section for path-search algorithms.

5.6 Subnetwork extraction between identified metabolites

5.6.1 *Finding reaction paths between biomarkers*

As stated earlier, metabolomics identifies metabolites that may occur in different parts of the network. Moreover, because networks contain thousands of elements, it is not possible to visually retrieve the cascade of reactions connecting these nodes (see Figure 5.7). It is thus necessary to develop algorithms that automatically extract a subset of reactions that creates a subnetwork connecting the interesting metabolites. A large variety of methods can be used to perform this subnetwork extraction (Faust and Van Helden, 2012; Milreu et al., 2014). The common idea is to retrieve paths between elements of interest. In metabolomics we focus on paths between metabolites. Nevertheless, these methods can also be applied to reactions and even to other kinds of biological networks. A metabolic path $p(u,v)$ between two metabolites u and v is defined as the set of nodes that have to be traversed to go from u to v. Given that the graph is directed, paths $p(u,v)$ and $p(v,u)$ may be different, and thus, they must both be accounted for in our computation. It is possible to add weight to each node or edge belonging to the path. Then we can decide to select paths with the lightest weight (lightest path). This option was successfully used to avoid unrealistic paths going through water or other side compounds. These nodes are given an heavy weight, meaning that the algorithm avoids them during the computation (Croes et al., 2005). This approach can be improved by incorporating the information on molecular function group transfers between substrates and products of reactions, as

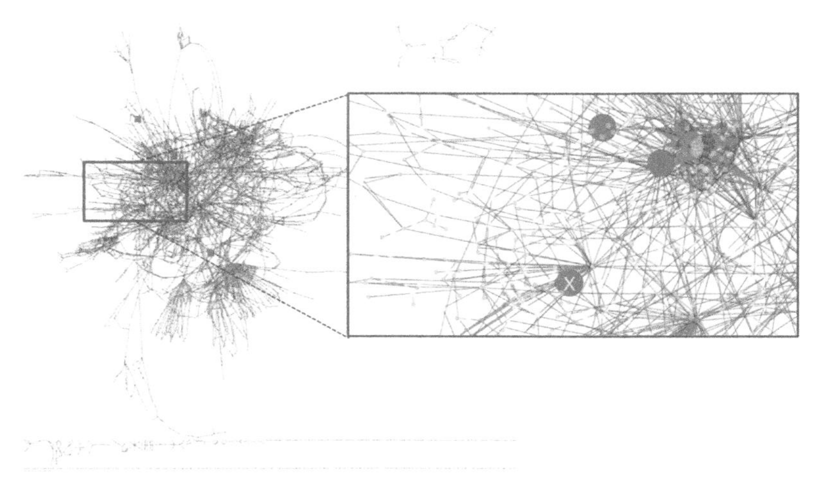

Figure 5.7 Biomarker mapping in a human genome-scale metabolic network. The bipartite graph without side compounds was built based on Recon2 v01. Larger shaded nodes are biomarkers identified in the O'Sullivan et al. (2011) article. The right inset shows a zoom-in view of the network. The selected node (large node marked X) is glycine metabolite. All edges connected to glycine correspond to reactions that can consume or produce this metabolite.

described by Faust et al. using KEGG RPAIR data (Faust et al., 2009). Unfortunately, this last information is not available in all networks. For instance, it is currently not available for the Recon2 network.

The type of graph model used is also important. In fact, with the bipartite graph, each reversible reaction is split by creating new reaction nodes. One node models the reaction in one direction, and the other models the reaction going in the opposite direction. This process has the advantage of taking into account the reversibility of reactions. Nevertheless, a path may go through a reaction in one direction and then through it again in the opposite one, creating unwanted cycles. To avoid this situation, it is necessary to add a checking step in the algorithm for the bipartite graph, which is not the case for the metabolite graph for instance.

Once the directed paths are computed between each pair of biomarkers, they are all merged in a single subnetwork. The size of this subnetwork is strongly related with the size of the input list of biomarkers. In fact, a large number of biomarkers will induce a lot of paths that may cover most of the reactions of the original network. To overcome this issue, Antonov et al. (2009) proposed using a threshold on maximum path length. This threshold is increased one by one, and a subnetwork is computed at each step. The final, selected subnetwork is the minimal network that connects all the biomarkers. The quality of a subnetwork can be evaluated by testing the null hypothesis, or estimating the probability of obtaining this resulting subnetwork or a subnetwork of similar quality from a random set of biomarkers (Antonov et al., 2009). Nevertheless, because this approach is mainly used for a small set of biomarkers, a manual inspection of results is still possible (Jourdan et al., 2010).

5.6.2 Retrieving and improving a biological interpretation of biomarkers

O'Sullivan et al. (2011) have identified potential metabolomic biomarkers of specific dietary intakes. For instance, they reported a positive association between urinary phenylacetylglutamine concentration and vegetable intake. Although this work was done mainly with a fingerprinting objective, the authors provide an interpretation of the significant changes in phenylacetylglutamine concentration observed in biofluids. Figure 5.8(b) shows this interpretation. Based on the list of biomarkers quoted in the article, a subnetwork was extracted from Recon2, using the MetExplore web server (Cottret et al., 2010). The first step consisted of mapping the metabolite biomarkers on the network. Phenylacetate was added to the search list of metabolites because it was considered to be an intake metabolite coming mainly from plant food sources. We focused on Recon2 cytoplasm metabolism and filtered out ubiquitous metabolites (water, carbon dioxide, ammonium, etc.). The network was imported into Cytoscape visualisation software (Shannon et al., 2003), and finally, via a plugin we implemented in Cytoscape, we created the subnetwork. The automatic outcome of the computation is displayed in Figure 5.8(c). The algorithm used computes the lightest paths between each pair of biomarkers. It is applied on the bipartite graph and avoids cycles within a path. The zoom-in box in Figure 5.8(c) shows that we come to the same

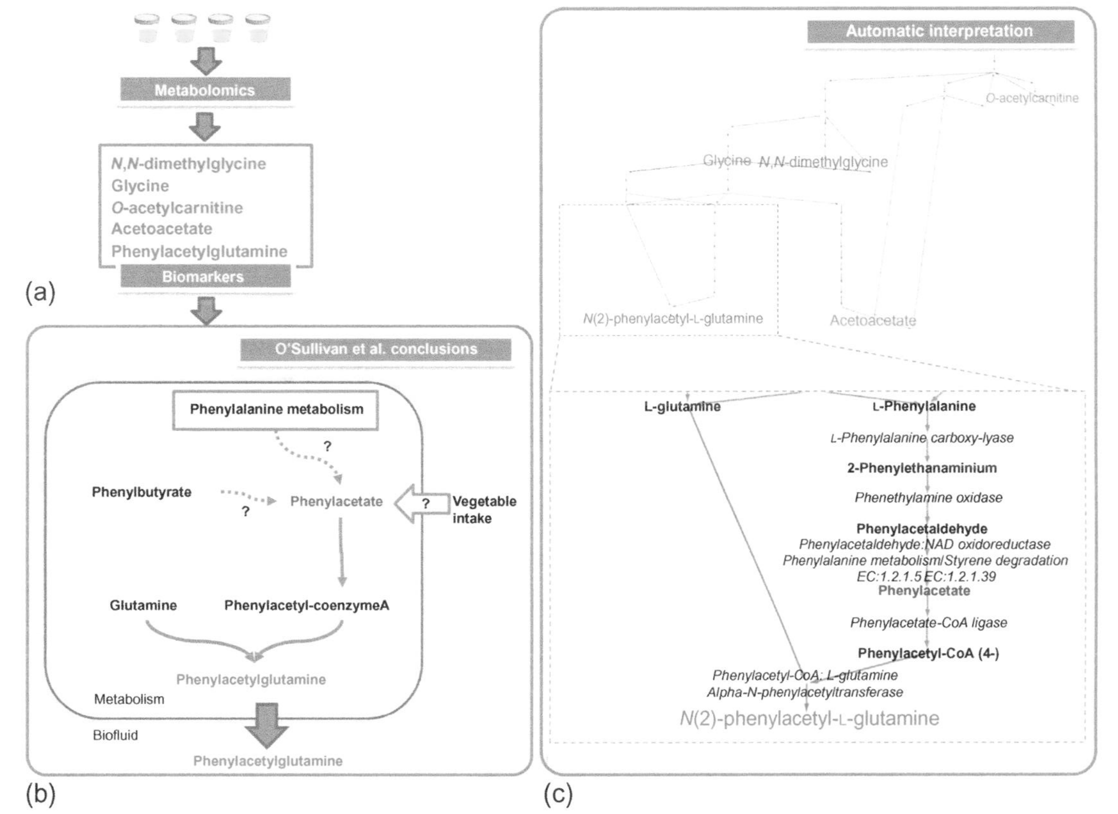

Figure 5.8 Comparison between manual and automatic network analysis of metabolomics data. (a) The list of biomarkers identified in the O'Sullivan et al. (2011) article as discriminated metabolites between identified with either meat or vegetable diets. Red (resp. green; light grey in the print version) metabolites are the ones with lower urinal concentrations (resp. higher) in subjects consuming unhealthy diets compared to subjects with favourable food intake. (b) The interpretation made in the article for the concentration decrease of phenylacetylglutamine in biofluids. Dashed arrows with question marks show the hypothesis made by authors. (c) The automatic output obtained using the MetExplore web server. Note that all biomarkers are connected. The zoom-in box shows that some of the conclusions in the article are supported by this subnetwork extraction.

conclusion as the one raised in the article. But, in addition, potential metabolic connections are retrieved using the algorithm because it connects all the biomarkers into a single subnetwork.

5.6.3 Metabolic stories

Many alternative paths with the same weight may connect two metabolites. Moreover, given two metabolites such as glucose and pyruvate, it may be important to distinguish the subnetwork going from glucose to pyruvate (glycolysis) and the one going from pyruvate to glucose (gluconeogenesis). This notion was recently formalised in the so-called metabolic stories (Milreu et al., 2014) that search for subnetworks without cycles (there is no path traversing a node twice) and with sources and targets that are interesting compounds. A large number of stories are generated from a given set of compounds. These stories must then be classified in order to exhibit biological trends related to the input biomarkers. This part is still an ongoing research topic. Yet, work with a metabolomics dataset extracted from a study by Madalinski et al. (2008) has shown that metabolic stories can help find new insights on metabolite shifts induced by toxicological agents like cadmium metal.

Both path-based subnetwork extraction and metabolic stories only rely on the graph structure of the metabolic network, however. They do not take into account the stoichiometry of reactions between biomarkers along the paths. Stoichiometry and weight optimisation along paths (i.e. based on energy consumption) are two future research directions in this field. Advances in these areas will allow the reduction of the number of possible subnetworks, while finding more biologically relevant ones.

5.6.4 Usage in metabolomics and other multi-omics analysis

No spectrometry solution allows the simultaneous detection of all metabolites in a sample. Moreover, data-processing tools can discard some detected metabolites if their concentrations are too low (i.e. due to a quick turnover). A subnetwork is a way to identify metabolites that may be hidden in the background noise of raw data. In Jourdan et al. (2010), we showed that metabolomics data processing can be improved by using this approach. We applied the subnetwork approach to hepatic cell lines (HepG2) processed using high-resolution mass spectrometry, and this method helped to identify metabolites under the noise-intensity threshold. In a more systematic way, network structure can also be used to identify and classify metabolites with the same molecular weight (Rogers et al., 2009).

Because networks contain the information linking reactions to proteins and then to genes, we can use them for multi-omics data interpretation. In particular, subnetwork extraction based on metabolomics data may point out reactions of interest between biomarkers. Searching omics databases and bibliographies can then enhance the interpretation.

5.7 Conclusion and future directions

Metabolism can now be investigated on a global scale using both experimental and in silico approaches. One of the main remaining challenges is the faithful reconstruction of genome-scale metabolic networks, however. Research groups have formed to create genome-scale networks for humans, and some efforts are currently aimed at extracting subnetworks for different tissues and cell lines. All these improvements in reconstruction will lead to better interpretation of biological experimental data.

Metabolism modelling can range from low-scale dynamic simulation to large-scale descriptive approaches. The large-scale approaches, which employ graph models, are quite useful for handling global metabolomics data. In fact, they allow identification of metabolic shifts between different experimental conditions without any a priori knowledge. Before performing this large-scale interpretation, one must map identified metabolites in the network structure. This is a challenging problem because of the lack of metabolite identifier standards in the modelling community. Moreover, metabolic networks, and consequently metabolic graphs, contain thousands of interconnected elements, so that visual inspection of the data is not directly possible. The main solution proposed here consists in extracting subnetworks that connect the identified biomarkers. In a metabolomics dietary experiment, we have shown that this whole analysis pipeline can be used to automatically interpret data. In the experiment, we were able to retrieve the metabolic processes suggested by other authors and to complete this interpretation by adding other potentially involved reactions.

Finally, metabolic networks constitute a relevant framework for the simultaneous interpretation of multi-omics data because they maintain a link between genes, proteins, reactions, and metabolites. While graph modelling is mainly a descriptive approach, human genome-scale network modelling is now evolving towards more predictive methods based on constraint-based modelling. These approaches will be particularly useful in the field of nutrition because they will allow the association of genetic trends or perturbations with biomarkers in biofluids. Nevertheless, researchers will still need to adequately define the constraints on the network. Metabolic networks have now been built for many microorganisms, and they can also be reconstructed based on the metagenome. One potential future direction will be to model the interplay between gut microflora and human metabolism. This research could provide a relevant framework to interpret diet impacts and metabolism.

Acknowledgements

The authors would like to thank Ludovic Cottret, Florence Vinson, Yoann Gloaguen, and Benjamin Merlet for the development of MetExplore, as well as the INRA Nutrition, Chemical Food Safety, and Consumer Behaviour division for funding the authors' research on genome-scale network modelling. This work is supported by France's metabolomics and fluxomics infrastructure, MetaboHub (project ANR-11-INBS-0010).

References

Agren, R., Bordel, S., Mardinoglu, A., Pornputtapong, N., Nookaew, I., Nielsen, J., 2012. Reconstruction of genome-scale active metabolic networks for 69 human cell types and 16 cancer types using INIT. PLoS Comput. Biol. 8, e1002518.

Albert, R., Jeong, H., Barabasi, A., 2000. Error and attack tolerance of complex networks. Nature 406, 378–382.

Antonov, A.V., Dietmann, S., Wong, P., Mewes, H.W., 2009. TICL—a web tool for network-based interpretation of compound lists inferred by high-throughput metabolomics. FEBS J. 276, 2084–2094.

Arakawa, K., Kono, N., Yamada, Y., Mori, H., Tomita, M., 2005. KEGG-based pathway visualization tool for complex omics data. In Silico Biol. 5, 419–423.

Bairoch, A., 2000. The ENZYME database in 2000. Nucleic Acids Res. 28, 304–305.

Bordbar, A., Feist, A.M., Usaite-Black, R., Woodcock, J., Palsson, B.O., Famili, I., 2011a. A multi-tissue type genome-scale metabolic network for analysis of whole-body systems physiology. BMC Syst. Biol. 5, 180.

Bordbar, A., Jamshidi, N., Palsson, B.Ø., 2011b. iAB-RBC-283: a proteomically derived knowledge-base of erythrocyte metabolism that can be used to simulate its physiological and patho-physiological states. BMC Syst. Biol. 5, 110.

Breitling, R., Pitt, A.R., Barrett, M.P., 2006a. Precision mapping of the metabolome. Trends Biotechnol. 24, 543–548.

Breitling, R., Ritchie, S., Goodenowe, D., Stewart, M.L., Barrett, M.P., 2006b. Ab initio prediction of metabolic networks using Fourier transform mass spectrometry data. Metabolomics 2, 155–164.

Carbonell, P., Planson, A.-G., Fichera, D., Faulon, J.-L., 2011. A retrosynthetic biology approach to metabolic pathway design for therapeutic production. BMC Syst. Biol. 5, 122.

Caspi, R., Altman, T., Dreher, K., Fulcher, C.A., Subhraveti, P., Keseler, I.M., Kothari, A., Krummenacker, M., Latendresse, M., Mueller, L.A., Ong, Q., Paley, S., Pujar, A., Shearer, A.G., Travers, M., Weerasinghe, D., Zhang, P., Karp, P.D., 2012. The MetaCyc database of metabolic pathways and enzymes and the BioCyc collection of pathway/genome databases. Nucleic Acids Res. 40, D742–D753.

Chang, R.L., Xie, Li, Xie, Lei, Bourne, P.E., Palsson, B.Ø., 2010. Drug off-target effects predicted using structural analysis in the context of a metabolic network model. PLoS Comput. Biol. 6, e1000938.

Chavali, A.K., Whittemore, J.D., Eddy, J.A., Williams, K.T., Papin, J.A., 2008. Systems analysis of metabolism in the pathogenic trypanosomatid Leishmania major. Mol. Syst. Biol. 4, 177.

Cottret, L., Jourdan, F., 2010. Graph methods for the investigation of metabolic networks in parasitology. Parasitology 137, 1393–1407.

Cottret, L., Wildridge, D., Vinson, F., Barrett, M.P., Charles, H., Sagot, M.-F., Jourdan, F., 2010. MetExplore: a web server to link metabolomic experiments and genome-scale metabolic networks. Nucleic Acids Res. 38, W132–W137.

Croes, D., Couche, F., Wodak, S.J., Van Helden, J., 2005. Metabolic PathFinding: inferring relevant pathways in biochemical networks. Nucleic Acids Res. 33, W326–W330.

Croft, D., Mundo, A.F., Haw, R., Milacic, M., Weiser, J., Wu, G., Caudy, M., Garapati, P., Gillespie, Marc, Kamdar, M.R., Jassal, B., Jupe, S., Matthews, L., May, B., Palatnik, S., Rothfels, K., Shamovsky, V., Song, H., Williams, M., Birney, E., Hermjakob, H., Stein, L., D'Eustachio, P., 2013. The Reactome pathway knowledgebase. Nucleic Acids Res. 42, D472–D477.

DeJongh, M., Formsma, K., Boillot, P., Gould, J., Rycenga, M., Best, A., 2007. Toward the automated generation of genome-scale metabolic networks in the SEED. BMC Bioinformatics 8, 139.

Deo, R.C., Hunter, L., Lewis, G.D., Pare, G., Vasan, R.S., Chasman, D., Wang, T.J., Gerszten, R.E., Roth, F.P., 2010. Interpreting metabolomic profiles using unbiased pathway models. PLoS Comput. Biol. 6, e1000692.

Duarte, N.C., Becker, S.A., Jamshidi, N., Thiele, I., Mo, M.L., Vo, T.D., Srivas, R., Palsson, B.Ø., 2007. Global reconstruction of the human metabolic network based on genomic and bibliomic data. Proc. Natl. Acad. Sci. U. S. A. 104, 1777–1782.

Euler, L., 1741. Solutio problematis ad geometriam situs pertinentis. Academiae Scientiarum Imperialis Petropolitanae 8, 128–140.

Faust, K., Van Helden, J., 2012. Predicting metabolic pathways by sub-network extraction. Methods Mol. Biol. 804, 107–130.

Faust, K., Croes, D., Van Helden, J., 2009. Metabolic pathfinding using RPAIR annotation. J. Mol. Biol. 388, 390–414.

Folger, O., Jerby, L., Frezza, C., Gottlieb, E., Ruppin, E., Shlomi, T., 2011. Predicting selective drug targets in cancer through metabolic networks. Mol. Syst. Biol. 7, 501.

Forth, T., McConkey, G.A., Westhead, D.R., 2010. MetNetMaker: a free and open-source tool for the creation of novel metabolic networks in SBML format. Bioinformatics 26, 2352–2353.

Frezza, C., Zheng, L., Folger, O., Rajagopalan, K.N., MacKenzie, E.D., Jerby, L., Micaroni, M., Chaneton, B., Adam, J., Hedley, A., Kalna, G., Tomlinson, I.P.M., Pollard, P.J., Watson, D. G., Deberardinis, R.J., Shlomi, T., Ruppin, E., Gottlieb, E., 2011. Haem oxygenase is synthetically lethal with the tumour suppressor fumarate hydratase. Nature 477, 225–228.

Ganter, M., Bernard, T., Moretti, S., Stelling, J., Pagni, M., 2013. MetaNetX.org: a website and repository for accessing, analysing and manipulating metabolic networks. Bioinformatics 29, 815–816.

Gille, C., Bölling, C., Hoppe, A., Bulik, S., Hoffmann, S., Hübner, K., Karlstädt, A., Ganeshan, R., König, M., Rother, K., Weidlich, M., Behre, J., Holzhütter, H.-G., 2010. HepatoNet1: a comprehensive metabolic reconstruction of the human hepatocyte for the analysis of liver physiology. Mol. Syst. Biol. 6, 411.

Ginsburg, H., 2006. Progress in in silico functional genomics: the malaria Metabolic Pathways database. Trends Parasitol. 22, 238–240.

Hao, T., Ma, H., Zhao, X.-M., Goryanin, I., 2010. Compartmentalization of the Edinburgh Human Metabolic Network. BMC bioinformatics 11, 393.

Hucka, M., Finney, A., Sauro, H.M., Bolouri, H., Doyle, J.C., Kitano, H., Arkin, A.P., Bornstein, B.J., Bray, D., Cornish-Bowden, A., Cuellar, A.A., Dronov, S., Gilles, E.D., Ginkel, M., Gor, V., Goryanin, I.I., Hedley, W.J., Hodgman, T.C., Hofmeyr, J.-H., Hunter, P.J., Juty, N.S., Kasberger, J.L., Kremling, A., Kummer, U., Le Novère, N., Loew, L.M., Lucio, D., Mendes, P., Minch, E., Mjolsness, E.D., Nakayama, Y., Nelson, M.R., Nielsen, P.F., Sakurada, T., Schaff, J.C., Shapiro, B.E., Shimizu, T.S., Spence, H.D., Stelling, J., Takahashi, K., Tomita, M., Wagner, J., Wang, J., 2003. The systems biology markup language (SBML): a medium for representation and exchange of biochemical network models. Bioinformatics 19, 524–531.

Joshi-Tope, G., Gillespie, M., Vastrik, I., D'Eustachio, P., Schmidt, E., De Bono, B., Jassal, B., Gopinath, G.R., Wu, G.R., Matthews, L., Lewis, S., Birney, E., Stein, L., 2005. Reactome: a knowledgebase of biological pathways. Nucleic Acids Res. 33, D428–D432.

Jourdan, F., Breitling, R., Barrett, M.P., Gilbert, D., 2008. MetaNetter: inference and visualization of high-resolution metabolomic networks. Bioinformatics 24, 143–145.

Jourdan, F., Cottret, L., Huc, L., Wildridge, D., Scheltema, R., Hillenweck, A., Barrett, M.P., Zalko, D., Watson, D.G., Debrauwer, L., 2010. Use of reconstituted metabolic networks to assist in metabolomic data visualization and mining. Metabolomics 6, 312–321.

Kanehisa, M., Araki, M., Goto, S., Hattori, M., Hirakawa, M., Itoh, M., Katayama, T., Kawashima, S., Okuda, S., Tokimatsu, T., Yamanishi, Y., 2008. KEGG for linking genomes to life and the environment. Nucleic Acids Res. 36, D480–D484.

Kanehisa, M., Goto, S., Sato, Y., Furumichi, M., Tanabe, M., 2012. KEGG for integration and interpretation of large-scale molecular data sets. Nucleic Acids Res. 40, D109–D114.

Karp, P.D., Latendresse, M., Caspi, R., 2011. The pathway tools pathway prediction algorithm. Stand. Genomic Sci. 5, 424–429.

Khatri, P., Sirota, M., Butte, A.J., 2012. Ten years of pathway analysis: current approaches and outstanding challenges. PLoS Comput. Biol. 8, e1002375.

Lacroix, V., Fernandes, C.G., Sagot, M.-F., 2006. Motif search in graphs: application to metabolic networks. IEEE/ACM Trans. Comput. Biol. Bioinform. 3, 360–368.

Lacroix, V., Cottret, L., Thébault, P., Sagot, M.-F., 2008. An introduction to metabolic networks and their structural analysis. IEEE/ACM Trans. Comput. Biol. Bioinform. 5, 594–617.

Lander, E.S., Linton, L.M., Birren, B., Nusbaum, C., Zody, M.C., Baldwin, J., et al., 2004. Finishing the euchromatic sequence of the human genome. Nature 431, 931–945.

Lespinet, O., Labedan, B., 2005. Orphan enzymes? Science 307, 42.

Lewis, N.E., Schramm, G., Bordbar, A., Schellenberger, J., Andersen, M.P., Cheng, J.K., Patel, N., Yee, A., Lewis, R.A., Eils, R., König, R., Palsson, B.Ø., 2010. Large-scale in silico modeling of metabolic interactions between cell types in the human brain. Nat. Biotechnol. 28, 1279–1285.

Ma, H., Sorokin, A., Mazein, A., Selkov, A., Selkov, E., Demin, O., Goryanin, I., 2007. The Edinburgh human metabolic network reconstruction and its functional analysis. Mol. Syst. Biol. 3, 135.

Madalinski, G., Godat, E., Alves, S., Lesage, D., Genin, E., Levi, P., Labarre, J., Tabet, J.-C., Ezan, E., Junot, C., 2008. Direct introduction of biological samples into a LTQ-Orbitrap hybrid mass spectrometer as a tool for fast metabolome analysis. Anal. Chem. 80, 3291–3303.

Maglott, D., Ostell, J., Pruitt, K.D., Tatusova, T., 2005. Entrez Gene: gene-centered information at NCBI. Nucleic Acids Res. 33, D54–D58.

Mardinoglu, A., Agren, R., Kampf, C., Asplund, A., Nookaew, I., Jacobson, P., Walley, A.J., Froguel, P., Carlsson, L.M., Uhlen, M., Nielsen, J., 2013. Integration of clinical data with a genome-scale metabolic model of the human adipocyte. Mol. Syst. Biol. 9, 649.

May, J.W., James, A.G., Steinbeck, C., 2013. Metingear: a development environment for annotating genome-scale metabolic models. Bioinformatics 29, 2213–2215.

Milreu, P.V., Klein, C.C., Cottret, L., Acuña, V., Birmelé, E., Borassi, M., Junot, C., Marchetti-Spaccamela, A., Marino, A., Stougie, L., Jourdan, F., Crescenzi, P., Lacroix, V., Sagot, M.-F., 2014. Telling metabolic stories to explore metabolomics data: a case study on the yeast response to cadmium exposure. Bioinformatics 30, 61–70.

Mintz-Oron, S., Aharoni, A., Ruppin, E., Shlomi, T., 2009. Network-based prediction of metabolic enzymes' subcellular localization. Bioinformatics 25, i247–i252.

Mo, M.L., Palsson, B.Ø., 2009. Understanding human metabolic physiology: a genome-to-systems approach. Trends Biotechnol. 27, 37–44.

O'Sullivan, A., Gibney, M.J., Brennan, L., 2011. Dietary intake patterns are reflected in metabolomic profiles: potential role in dietary assessment studies. Am. J. Clin. Nutr. 93, 314–321.

Orth, J.D., Conrad, T.M., Na, J., Lerman, J.A., Nam, H., Feist, A.M., Palsson, B.Ø., 2011. A comprehensive genome-scale reconstruction of Escherichia coli metabolism–2011. Mol. Syst. Biol. 7, 535.

Paley, S.M., Karp, P.D., 2006. The Pathway Tools cellular overview diagram and Omics Viewer. Nucleic Acids Res. 34, 3771–3778.

Price, N.D., Reed, J.L., Palsson, B.Ø., 2004. Genome-scale models of microbial cells: evaluating the consequences of constraints. Nat. Rev. Microbiol. 2, 886–897.

Rahman, S.A., Schomburg, D., 2006. Systems biology observing local and global properties of metabolic pathways: "load points" and "choke points" in the metabolic networks. Bioinformatics 22, 1767–1774.

Raman, K., Chandra, N., 2009. Flux balance analysis of biological systems: applications and challenges. Brief. Bioinform. 10, 435–449.

Rogers, S., Scheltema, R.A., Girolami, M., Breitling, R., 2009. Probabilistic assignment of formulas to mass peaks in metabolomics experiments. Bioinformatics 25, 512–518.

Romero, P., Wagg, J., Green, M.L., Kaiser, D., Krummenacker, M., Karp, P.D., 2005. Computational prediction of human metabolic pathways from the complete human genome. Genome Biol. 6, R2.

Sahoo, S., Thiele, I., 2013. Predicting the impact of diet and enzymopathies on human small intestinal epithelial cells. Hum. Mol. Genet. 22, 2705–2722.

Schellenberger, J., Park, J.O., Conrad, T.M., Palsson, B.Ø., 2010. BiGG: a biochemical genetic and genomic knowledgebase of large scale metabolic reconstructions. BMC bioinformatics 11, 213.

Schellenberger, J., Que, R., Fleming, R.M.T., Thiele, I., Orth, J.D., Feist, A.M., Zielinski, D.C., Bordbar, A., Lewis, N.E., Rahmanian, S., Kang, J., Hyduke, D.R., Palsson, B.Ø., 2011. Quantitative prediction of cellular metabolism with constraint-based models: the COBRA Toolbox v2.0. Nat. Protoc. 6, 1290–1307.

Schomburg, I., Chang, A., Ebeling, C., Gremse, M., Heldt, C., Huhn, G., Schomburg, D., 2004. BRENDA, the enzyme database: updates and major new developments. Nucleic Acids Res. 32, D431–D433.

Schomburg, I., Chang, A., Placzek, S., Söhngen, C., Rother, M., Lang, M., Munaretto, C., Ulas, S., Stelzer, M., Grote, A., Scheer, M., Schomburg, D., 2013. BRENDA in 2013: integrated reactions, kinetic data, enzyme function data, improved disease classification: new options and contents in BRENDA. Nucleic Acids Res. 41, D764–D772.

Schuster, S., Hilgetag, C., 1994. On elementary flux modes in biochemical reaction systems at steady state. J. Biol. Syst. 2, 165–182.

Schuster, R., Schuster, S., 1993. Refined algorithm and computer program for calculating all non-negative fluxes admissible in steady states of biochemical reaction systems with or without some flux rates fixed. Comput. Appl. Biosci. 9, 79–85.

Schuster, S., Fell, D.A., Dandekar, T., 2000. A general definition of metabolic pathways useful for systematic organization and analysis of complex metabolic networks. Nat. Biotechnol. 18, 326–332.

Shannon, P., Markiel, A., Ozier, O., Baliga, N.S., Wang, J.T., Ramage, D., Amin, N., Schwikowski, B., Ideker, T., 2003. Cytoscape: a software environment for integrated models of biomolecular interaction networks. Genome Res. 13, 2498–2504.

Shatkay, H., Höglund, A., Brady, S., Blum, T., Dönnes, P., Kohlbacher, O., 2007. SherLoc: high-accuracy prediction of protein subcellular localization by integrating text and protein sequence data. Bioinformatics 23, 1410–1417.

Shlomi, T., Cabili, M.N., Herrgård, M.J., Palsson, B.Ø., Ruppin, E., 2008. Network-based prediction of human tissue-specific metabolism. Nat. Biotechnol. 26, 1003–1010.

Shlomi, T., Cabili, M.N., Ruppin, E., 2009. Predicting metabolic biomarkers of human inborn errors of metabolism. Mol. Syst. Biol. 5, 263.

Terzer, M., Stelling, J., 2008. Large-scale computation of elementary flux modes with bit pattern trees. Bioinformatics 24, 2229–2235.

The UniProt Consortium, 2013. Update on activities at the Universal Protein Resource (UniProt) in 2013. Nucleic Acids Res. 41, D43–D47.

Thiele, I., Palsson, B.Ø., 2010a. A protocol for generating a high-quality genome-scale metabolic reconstruction. Nat. Protoc. 5, 93–121.

Thiele, I., Palsson, B.Ø., 2010b. Reconstruction annotation jamborees: a community approach to systems biology. Mol. Syst. Biol. 6, 361.

Thiele, I., Swainston, N., Fleming, R.M.T., Hoppe, A., Sahoo, S., Aurich, M.K., Haraldsdottir, H., Mo, M.L., Rolfsson, O., Stobbe, M.D., Thorleifsson, S.G., Agren, R., Bölling, C., Bordel, S., Chavali, A.K., Dobson, P., Dunn, W.B., Endler, L., Hala, D., Hucka, M., Hull, D., Jameson, D., Jamshidi, N., Jonsson, J.J., Juty, N., Keating, S., Nookaew, I., Le Novère, N., Malys, N., Mazein, A., Papin, J.A., Price, N.D., Selkov, E., Sigurdsson, M.I., Simeonidis, E., Sonnenschein, N., Smallbone, K., Sorokin, A., Van Beek, J.H.G.M., Weichart, D., Goryanin, I., Nielsen, J., Westerhoff, H.V., Kell, D.B., Mendes, P., Palsson, B.Ø., 2013. A community-driven global reconstruction of human metabolism. Nat. Biotechnol. 31, 419–425.

Vlassis, N., Pacheco, M.P., Sauter, T., 2014. Fast reconstruction of compact context-specific metabolic network models. PLoS Comput. Biol. 10, e1003424.

Vo, T.D., Paul Lee, W.N., Palsson, B.Ø., 2007. Systems analysis of energy metabolism elucidates the affected respiratory chain complex in Leigh's syndrome. Mol. Genet. Metab. 91, 15–22.

Wägele, B., Witting, M., Schmitt-Kopplin, P., Suhre, K., 2012. MassTRIX reloaded: combined analysis and visualization of transcriptome and metabolome data. PLoS One 7, e39860.

Wishart, D.S., Jewison, T., Guo, A.C., Wilson, M., Knox, C., Liu, Y., Djoumbou, Y., Mandal, R., Aziat, F., Dong, E., Bouatra, S., Sinelnikov, I., Arndt, D., Xia, J., Liu, P., Yallou, F., Bjorndahl, T., Perez-Pineiro, R., Eisner, R., Allen, F., Neveu, V., Greiner, R., Scalbert, A., 2013. HMDB 3.0—the human metabolome database in 2013. Nucleic Acids Res. 41, D801–D807.

Yamada, T., Waller, A.S., Raes, J., Zelezniak, A., Perchat, N., Perret, A., Salanoubat, M., Patil, K.R., Weissenbach, J., Bork, P., 2012. Prediction and identification of sequences coding for orphan enzymes using genomic and metagenomic neighbours. Mol. Syst. Biol. 8, 581.

Zelezniak, A., Pers, T.H., Soares, S., Patti, M.E., Patil, K.R., 2010. Metabolic network topology reveals transcriptional regulatory signatures of type 2 diabetes. PLoS Comput. Biol. 6, e1000729.

Using metabolomics to analyse the role of gut microbiota in nutrition and disease

G. Xie, W. Jia
University of Hawaii Cancer Center, Honolulu, HI, USA

6.1 Introduction: gut microbiota and human health

6.1.1 Gut microbiota: an extragenome organ in the human host

Evidence has increasingly revealed that the gut microbiota is involved in the regulation of multiple mammalian metabolic pathways through a series of interactive gut microbiota–host metabolic, signalling, and immune–inflammatory axes that physiologically connect the gut, liver, brain, and other organs. The human microbiota contains as many as 10^{14} bacterial cells, a number that is 10 times greater than all of the eukaryotic cells of the host combined (Musso et al., 2011). The microbiome exceeds the size of the human nuclear genome by two orders of magnitude and contributes to a broad range of biochemical and metabolic functions that the host could not otherwise perform (Ley et al., 2008). Therefore, humans are considered to be a "superorganism" (Wilson and Sober, 1989), and the gut microbiota can be regarded as an extragenome organ in the human host. The microbiota colonises virtually every surface of the human body that is exposed to the external environment, including the skin, oral cavity, and genitourinary, gastrointestinal, and respiratory tracts (Chiller et al., 2001; Hull and Chow, 2007; Neish, 2009; Verstraelen, 2008). By far, the most densely colonised organ is the gastrointestinal (GI) tract, particularly the colon, with an estimated percentage of over 70% of all the microbes in the human body (Ley et al., 2006a; Verstraelen, 2008).

The GI tract is a complex and dynamic ecosystem containing a diverse collection of microorganisms. These microorganisms are either resident members of the intestinal microbiota or transient passengers introduced from the environment, for example, by the regular influx of microorganisms by the intake of food (Gerritsen et al., 2011). The majority of the gut microbiota is composed of strict anaerobes, which dominate the facultative anaerobes and aerobes by two to three orders of magnitude (Gordon and Dubos, 1970; Harris et al., 1976; Savage, 1970). Although there have been over 70 bacterial phyla described to date (Marchesi, 2010), both culture-dependent and culture-independent studies have demonstrated that the majority of the intestinal bacteria belong to two phyla, the Bacteroidetes and the Firmicutes, whereas Proteobacteria, Verrucomicrobia, Actinobacteria, Fusobacteria, and Cyanobacteria are present in minor proportions (Eckburg et al., 2005). The generally accepted number of

Metabolomics as a Tool in Nutrition Research. http://dx.doi.org/10.1016/B978-1-78242-084-2.00006-X

bacterial species present in the human gut is ~500–1000 (Xu and Gordon, 2003), although the number varies widely between different studies. However, a recent analysis involving multiple subjects suggested that the collective human gut microbiota is composed of over 35,000 bacterial species (Frank et al., 2007).

Host physiology and gut microbiota are intimately connected, which is evident from the fact that each distinct anatomical region along the GI tract is characterised by its own physicochemical conditions, and these changing conditions exert a selective pressure on the microbiota. The composition of gut microbiota is influenced by several physicochemical conditions including intestinal motility, pH, redox potential, nutrient supplies, host secretions (e.g. hydrochloric acid, digestive enzymes, bile, and mucus), and the presence of an intact ileocaecal valve (Booijink et al., 2007). Thus, the GI tract harbours many distinct regions, each containing a different microbial ecosystem that varies according to the location within the GI tract. The number of bacterial cells present in the mammalian gut shows a continuum that goes from 10^1 to 10^3 bacteria per gram of contents in the stomach and duodenum, progressing to 10^4 to 10^7 bacteria per gram in the jejunum and ileum and culminating in 10^{11} to 10^{12} cells per gram in the colon and faces (Booijink et al., 2007; Dethlefsen et al., 2006; O'Hara and Shanahan, 2006). Despite the fact that it is well known that the intestinal microbiota is not homogeneously distributed within the GI tract, it is still largely unknown how the diversity varies in the different regions along the GI tract.

6.1.2 The relationships between changes in gut microbiota composition and diversity and disease

GI homeostasis relies on a stable immune system, good intestinal mucosal barrier function, and a balanced gut microbial ecosystem. Alteration or instability of the gut microbiota and changes in its biodiversity are characteristic of a number of GI disorders and metabolic diseases (Aziz et al., 2013). The consortium of symbiotic gut microbes can be viewed as a metabolically adaptable, rapidly renewable, and compositionally flexible ecosystem varying with the host's age, diet, and health status (Gordon, 2012; Nicholson et al., 2005a). Unlike its host's genome, the collective genome of the microbiota can dynamically change the configuration of its components to adapt to the needs of its individual constituents, of the community as a whole, and of the host, whose environment varies widely in response to factors such as dietary nutrients, illness, and antibiotic use. The lifelong metabolic communication between the gut microbiota and the mammalian host is accompanied with many channels of chemical information exchange operating between various microbial players and pathways in multiple host tissue compartments (Nicholson et al., 2012). Both system-wide and organ-specific changes in metabolic profiles may have components driven by gut microbial activities (Nicholson et al., 2005a; Zheng et al., 2011). As a result, the metabolic processes encompass not only the indigenous metabolic processes encoded by the human genome but also those of the gut microbiome.

Humans cannot survive without these commensal microorganisms, as they interact extensively with the hosts by modulating the metabolism (Nicholson et al., 2005b), immunity (Kelly et al., 2007), energy harvest (Turnbaugh et al., 2006) and fat storage (Backhed et al., 2004). Perturbation of the microbiota composition, also known as dysbiosis, has been recognised in various diseases such as obesity (Ley, 2010; Ley et al., 2006b), diabetes (Brugman et al., 2006; Turnbaugh et al., 2006), inflammatory bowel disease (IBD) (Mahida and Rolfe, 2004; Peterson et al., 2008), gastrointestinal cancers (Huycke and Gaskins, 2004; Mahida and Rolfe, 2004), and infectious diseases (Lupp et al., 2007; Sekirov et al., 2008), of which many are associated with the GI tract. However, before dysbiosis can be established, the composition of a healthy normal microbiota has to be defined. From an operational point of view, it could be stated that a healthy gut microbiota is the microbiota composition as it can be found in healthy individuals. For practical reasons, the phylogenetic characterisation of the microbiota of diseased individuals in comparison with apparently healthy individuals is, at this moment, the main approach to study changes in composition of the gut microbiota in relation to disease. However, since there are substantial inter-individual and intra-individual variations in the composition of the gut microbiota, it is difficult to establish the precise relations between human health and the presence and relative abundance of specific microbial communities. In the future, specific changes in compositional diversity, or even functional diversity, may be applied as biomarkers for health or specific diseases. It must be noted, however, that it is questionable whether changes in phylogenetic composition are really cause or consequence of a given disease. Intensively studied examples for which dysbiosis of the intestinal microbiota has been described include IBD, irritable bowel syndrome (IBS), obesity, and several other (chronic) diseases and disorders such as coeliac disease, colorectal cancer (CRC), pouchitis, and necrotising enterocolitis (Table 6.1).

6.2 Metagenomics of gut microbiota

The extent of diversity of the microbiota is a fundamental question in intestinal microbial ecology. The 10-metre long human intestinal tract was like a dark tunnel. Some light had been shed on it by culturing bacteria from the faeces, but the darkness was overwhelming. Cultivation-based techniques traditionally were used to study GI bacteria. However, cultivation-based approaches have several limitations (Pandeya et al., 2012) because metagenomic studies demonstrated that about 65% of the bacteria identified in the intestinal microbiota were previously unknown, and among them, 80% were unculturable (Turnbaugh et al., 2009). The molecular basis underlying the mutual relationships remains poorly understood partly due to the fact that 70–90% of the bacteria are difficult, or sometimes impossible, to cultivate in the laboratory, although the crucial roles of commensal microbes in human health and disease are being increasingly recognised. Even if the mammalian gut microbiota is one of the most densely populated microbial ecosystems in nature, sequence-based analysis demonstrated that it is characterised by a peculiarly low phylogenetic diversity. Metagenomics, the culture-independent and sequencing-based studies of the collective set of genomes of mixed microbial communities (metagenomes), aimed to explore their compositional and functional characteristics (Petrosino et al., 2009)

Table 6.1 Overview of human studies that demonstrate changes in the gut microbiota associated with diseases

Study material	Key findings	Changes in microbiota presence/function	References
Allergies			
Colon tissue	*Lactobacillus* spp. ↓	Early colonisation with *Lactobacillus* associated with decreased allergies	Round et al. (2011)
Faeces	*Bifidobacterium adolescentis* ↓ *Clostridium difficile* ↓	Early colonisation with more diverse microbiota, might prevent allergies	Round and Mazmanian (2009)
Cell	*Helicobacter pylori* ↓	*H. pylori* tolerance mediated by Tregs (regulatory T cells) that suppress asthma	Arnold et al. (2011)
Coeliac disease			
Faeces	*Bacteroides vulgatus* ↑ *Escherichia coli* ↓ *Clostridium coccoides* ↓	Higher diversity (Shannon-Wiener index) in Coeliac disease patients versus controls	Elinav et al. (2011)
Faeces	*Bacteroides–Prevotella* ↑		De Palma et al. (2010), Schippa et al. (2010)
Faeces	*Bifidobacterium* ↓ *Clostridium histolyticum* ↓ *C. lituseburense* ↓ *F. prausnitzii* ↓		De Palma et al. (2010)
Gastric cancer			
T cells	*H. pylori* ↑	Important element in carcinogenic pathway for developing gastric adenocarcinomas	Lathrop et al. (2011)
Autism			
Faeces	Bacteroidetes ↑ Proteobacteria ↑ Actinobacteria ↓ Firmicutes ↓	Increased bacterial diversity in faeces of autistic children compared to controls	Robinson et al. (2010)
Obesity			
Faeces	Bacteriodetes ↓ Firmicutes ↑	Obese individuals compared with lean	Ley et al. (2006b)
Faeces	Roseburia ↓ *Eubacterium rectale* subgroup of cluster XIVa ↓ Bifidobacteria ↓	Obese individuals on diet of decreased carbohydrate intake	Duncan et al. (2007)

Continued

Table 6.1 **Continued**

Study material	Key findings	Changes in microbiota presence/function	References
Faeces	*Bacteroides* ↑ *Clostridium* ↑ *Staphylococcus* ↓	Overweight pregnant women	Collado et al. (2008)
Faeces	Bacteriodetes ↔ Butyrate-producing Firmicutes ↓	During weight-loss diet	Duncan et al. (2008)
Faeces	Bifidobacteria ↓ *Staphylococcus aureus* ↑	Intestinal microbiota during infancy preceding overweight during childhood	Kalliomaki et al. (2008)
Faeces	Bacteriodetes ↑ Firmicutes ↓	Obese individuals compared with lean	Schwiertz et al. (2010)
Faeces	*Bifidobacterium* ↓ *Bacteroides* ↓ *Staphylococcus* ↑ Enterobacteriaceae ↑ *E. coli* ↑	Overweight pregnant women	Santacruz et al. (2010)
Faeces	H2-producing Prevotellaceae ↑ H2-utilising methanogenic Archaea ↑	Obese individuals	Zhang et al. (2009)
Caecum content	Bacteroidetes ↓ *Lactobacillus* ↑	Significant changes in gut microbiota are associated with increasing obesity	Ley et al. (2005), Pflughoeft and Versalovic (2012)
	Firmicutes/Bacteroidetes ratio ↓		Ley et al. (2005)
	Methanobrevibacter smithii ↓		Turnbaugh et al. (2009b)
Anorexia			
Faeces	*M. smithii* ↑	Bacteroidetes, Firmicutes, and *Lactobacillus* similar to lean patients, though *M. smithii* significantly increased	Armougom et al. (2009), Pflughoeft and Versalovic (2012)
IBS			
Duodenal mucosal brush and faecal samples	*P. aeruginosa* ↑	*P. aeruginosa* is detected more frequently and at higher levels in IBS patients than in healthy subjects	Kerckhoffs et al. (2011)

Continued

Table 6.1 **Continued**

Study material	Key findings	Changes in microbiota presence/function	References
Faeces	*Veillonella* ↑ *Lactobacillus* ↑	Altered profiles of intestinal microbiota may be the origin of symptoms in irritable bowel syndrome	Tana et al. (2010)
Faeces	Aerobic bacteria ↓ *Lactobacillus* species ↑	Quantitative differences exist in specific bacterial groups in the microbiota between D-IBS and healthy subjects	Carroll et al. (2010)
Faeces	*Lactobacillus* spp. ↓ *Veillonella* spp. ↑	Suggested differences in the *C. coccoides* subgroup and *Bifidobacterium* catenulatum group between IBS patients ($n=21$) and controls ($n=15$)	Malinen et al. (2005)
IBD—Crohn's disease			
Faeces	*Bacteroides ovatus* ↑ *Bacteroides vulgatus* ↑ *Bacteroides uniformis* ↓	Less diversity in patients with Crohn's disease compared to healthy patients	Dicksved et al. (2008)
Faeces	*Dialister invisus* ↑ *Clostridium* cluster XIVa ↔ *Faecalibacterium prausnitzii* ↔ *B. adolescentis* ↔ *Ruminococcus gnavus* ↓	A set of five bacterial species that characterised the predominant dysbiosis in CD patients compared with unaffected relatives and healthy individuals	Joossens et al. (2011)
IBD (General)			
Serum stool	Bacteroidetes ↓ Lachnospiraceae ↓ Actinobacteria ↑ Proteobacteria ↑ *Clostridium leptum* ↓ *C. coccoides* ↓ *Faecalibacterium prasnitzii* ↓ Firmicutes/Bacteroidetes ratio ↓ Bifidobacteria ↓	IBD associated with overall community dysbiosis rather than single causal bacterial species	Spor et al. (2011), Perry et al. (2006)

Continued

Table 6.1 **Continued**

Study material	Key findings	Changes in microbiota presence/function	References
Type 2 diabetes			
Faeces	Firmicutes ↓ Clostridia ↓ *Bacteroides–Prevotella* ↑ versus *C. coccoides–E. rectale* ↓ Betaproteobacteria ↑ Bacteroidetes/Firmicutes ratio ↑	Shifts in gut microbiota associated with increases in plasma glucose concentrations	Brown (2000)
Colorectal cancer			
Colonic mucosa	Proteobacteria ↑ Bacteroidetes ↓ *Dorea* spp. ↑ *Faecalibacterium* spp. ↑ *Bacteroides* spp. ↓ *Coprococcus* spp. ↓	Cases had higher bacterial diversity and richness than controls	Shen et al. (2010)
Ulcerative colitis pouchitis			
Mucocal and faecal	*Clostridium* ↑ *Eubacterium* ↑ *Lactobacillus* ↓ *Streptococcus* ↓	Compared with the microbiota of healthy pouches from familial adenomatous polyposis (FAP) patients	Lim et al. (2009), Zella et al. (2011)
Rheumatoid arthritis			
Colonic mucosa	Bifidobacteria ↓ Bacteria of the *Bacteroides–Prevotella* group ↓ Bacteria of the *Bacteroides fragilis* subgroup ↓ Bacteria of the *E. rectale–C. coccoides* group ↓	Comparison to patients with fibromyalgia	Vaahtovuo et al. (2008)

Source: Clemente *et al.* (2012).

without the need of cultivation. While in the last decade Sanger sequencing was used to generate data in most microbial genomics and metagenomics sequencing projects, next-generation sequencing technologies have been widely used to study the complex microbial ecosystem populating the GI tract. Next-generation sequencing phylogenetic analysis of the gut microbiota is based on the amplification of selected target regions of the 16S rRNA genes and two main platforms have been developed for next-generation sequencing studies: the Genome Sequencer FLX+ System (454 Life Sciences) and the Genome Analyzer system (Illumina). It was reported that culture-independent 18S rRNA gene-based methods have been used, demonstrating that the genera *Blastocystis* and *Ascomycota* were the predominant microeukaryotes populating the intestinal ecosystem (Marchesi, 2010). A study on the virome with next-generation sequencing approach (Reyes et al., 2010) was performed on the collective metagenome of virus-like particles isolated from human faecal samples, which demonstrated that 81% of reads generated in this study did not match any known viruses, and that the human virome consists of prophages or phages generally classified as temperate (i.e. coliphage P22-like), commonly hosted by Firmicutes and Bacteroidetes members.

Bacterial small-subunit rRNA (16S rRNA) gene sequencing, quantitative PCR coupled to denaturing gradient gel electrophoresis (DGGE) (Muyzer et al., 1993), and fluorescent *in situ* hybridisation (FISH) (Amann et al., 1991) have proven to be robust techniques for characterising the gut microbial community, with regards to bacterial population and species diversity in their native environment of growth and development. Out of the 70 phyla described to date, next-generation sequencing-based survey indicated that 6–10 is the number of bacterial phyla per individual represented in the gut microbiota: Acidobacteria, Actinobacteria, Bacteroidetes, Firmicutes, Fusobacteria, Lentisphaerae, Proteobacteria, candidate division TM7, Verrucomicrobia, and Deinococcus–Thermus (Figure 6.1a) (Candela et al., 2010; Marchesi, 2010). Among these, Firmicutes and Bacteroidetes represent up to 90% of the intestinal microbiota, with a relative abundance of approximately 65% and 25%, respectively. One single archaeal phylotype, *Methanobrevibacter smithii*, has been observed in the GI tract. On the other hand, a great diversity at lower taxonomic levels and a considerable inter-individual variability in the bacterial species and strains have been described, with at least 1800 genera and 16,000 phylotypes (Peterson et al., 2008).

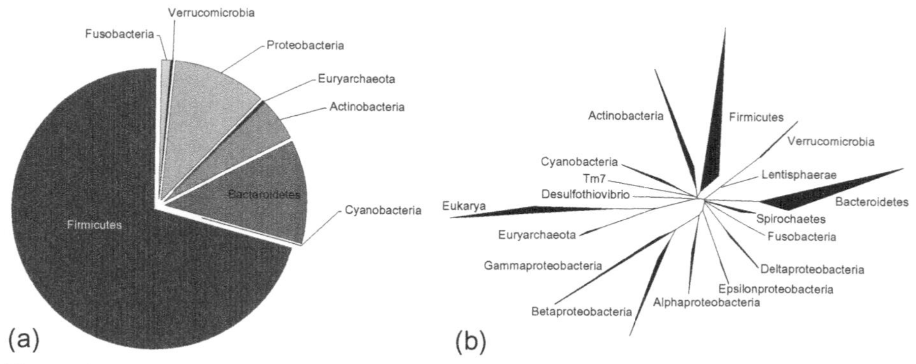

Figure 6.1 (a) Relative proportion of the phylotypes belonging to the eight main bacterial divisions which have been found in the human gut microbiota, out of the over 70 globally known (Candela et al., 2010). (b) Phylogenetic tree representing the groups of bacteria most frequently detected in human faces using 16S rRNA gene sequencing. The extent of the bold areas indicates diversity and abundance of the bacterial groups. The phylogenetic tree is reported by Vrieze et al. (2010).

Interestingly, 70% of these phylotypes are subject specific, none of which is present at more than about 0.5% abundance in all subjects (Figure 6.1b).

Metabolic profiling approach has been proved to be a powerful tool for detecting various metabolites originating from microorganisms that are commonly found in mammals. Microbial community structure can also be analysed by fingerprinting techniques, whereas dot-blot hybridisation, FISH, or quantitative PCR that targets known taxa can measure the abundance of particular microbes (Pandeya et al., 2012). Emerging approaches, such as those based on functional genes and their expression and the combined use of stable isotopes and biomarkers, are also being developed and optimised to study metabolic activities of groups or individual organisms *in situ*. Functional metagenomics, the studies of gut microbiota interactions with metabolic phenotypes, are now possible through the use of ^{1}H-nuclear magnetic resonance (NMR) spectroscopy and mass spectrometry (MS)-based profiling of faecal, urine, or other extracts.

Besides for generating the composition data, the metagenomics approach also provides a powerful tool for measuring the metabolic potential of the gut microbiota. The gut microbiome enlarges the genome of the host and enhances the host's metabolic potential (Possemiers et al., 2009). Indeed, it is estimated that the collection of all microbial genomes in the gut comprises between 2 and 4 million genes, which is 70–140 times more than that of their host (Qin et al., 2010). This microbiome encompasses all genes that are responsible for numerous processes such as substrate breakdown, protein synthesis, biomass production, and signalling molecule and antimicrobial compound production, and it encodes biochemical pathways that humans have not evolved (Egert et al., 2006).

The intestinal microbiota can therefore be regarded as a separate organ within the human host that is capable of even more conversions than the human liver, and we can view ourselves as a composite of human cells and bacteria and our genetic landscape as a "metagenome", an amalgam of genes embedded in our genome and in the genomes of all our microbial partners (Turnbaugh et al., 2007). Through its immense metabolic capabilities, the gut microbiota contributes to human physiology by transforming complex nutrients, such as dietary fibre or intestinal mucins that otherwise would be lost to the human host, into simple sugars, short-chain fatty acids (SCFAs), and other nutrients that can be absorbed (Mai et al., 2010). Over the past few years, studies have demonstrated that the gut microbes are required for many of the host's important metabolic processes, including lipid (Fava et al., 2006), choline (Spencer et al., 2011), and bile acid (Jones et al., 2008) metabolism. Gut microbiota–host co-metabolism also produces SCFAs as an energy source for the host, as well as substrates needed for *de novo* lipogenesis (Han et al., 2010). Therefore, the microbiome has become a nutritional target that may also become the foundation of future drug targeting and interventions (Jia et al., 2008; Nicholson et al., 2012).

In contrast to the oxidative and conjugative nature of liver metabolism, which generates hydrophilic high-molecular-weight biotransformation products, the metabolic nature of the gut microbial community in an anaerobic environment is mainly reductive and hydrolytic, generating non-polar low-molecular-weight by-products (Sousa et al., 2008). Additionally, the intestinal microbiota also interferes with the human biotransformation process through the enterohepatic circulation of xenobiotic compounds.

Compounds that have been absorbed in the intestine and subsequently detoxified are usually conjugated with polar groups (glucuronic acid, glycine, sulphate, glutathione, and taurine) in the epithelium or liver. Such metabolites may enter the blood stream prior to excretion in the urine, but depending on the compound, a considerable fraction may also enter again into the intestine via secretion with the bile (Ilett et al., 1990). Once released in the intestinal lumen, these conjugates may be hydrolysed again by bacterial enzymes such as β-glucuronidases, sulphatases, and glucosidases.

6.3 Metabolomics: uncovering complex host–microbe interactions

Recent research has disclosed tight and coordinated interactions between gut microbes and host metabolism (Holmes et al., 2012; Nicholson et al., 2012), and it is well known that there is great symbiosis between the human host and its gut microbiota. Modulation of the gut microbiota composition has potential effects on health improvement or even disease prevention (Moco et al., 2012). Therefore, it is of utmost importance to obtain a greater understanding and characterisation of the interactive processes between the host and its microbiome. Diversity in gut microbial communities and functions creates differences in nutrient milieu, digesta retention times, and temperatures that create diverse microbial niches and inhabitants. With the recent advances in the new profiling technologies such as metagenomics and metabolomics (Metges et al., 2006; Pang et al., 2007), the direct correlation of global metabolic changes with gut microbiome becomes increasingly important to decipher the host–microbe relationships and to gain mechanistic understanding of nutritional and drug intervention in the "gateway" of host–microbe co-metabolism. Scientists from different disciplines are working together and beginning to determine the details of gut microbial diversity and manipulate the complex interactions between the host metabolism and its symbionts for improved nutrition and disease treatment (Li et al., 2008b; Pang et al., 2007; Wei et al., 2010). A recent review (Nicholson et al., 2012) on host–gut microbiota metabolic interactions describes in detail the symbiotic signalling interactions of necessity changes during human development, which are in line with changes in the developing microbial ecology and diverse gut microbiome structure. Some of the main chemical classes involved in the host microbiome are provided (Nicholson et al., 2012) including SCFAs, bile acids, choline metabolites, indole derivatives, phenolic derivatives, benzoyl derivatives, and phenyl derivatives. However, it is likely that there are many more classes of compounds and interactions still to be discovered given the vast numbers of gut microbial genes of unknown function. Metabolomics (Fiehn, 2002), or metabonomics (Nicholson et al., 2002), which is the quantitative measurement of dynamic metabolic changes of living systems in response to genetic modifications or physiological stimuli mainly based on ^{1}H-NMR spectroscopy and MS, offers new opportunities to explore individual needs, foods, and nutrient functionalities and formulate tangible biological hypotheses that can be followed-up and tested at the individual and population scales. Monitoring the metabolic variations provides a unique insight into intra- and extracellular regulatory processes involved in our metabolic homeostasis. By analysing low-molecular-weight metabolites in biofluids (blood and urine), intestinal contents, and tissues, metabolomics provides the characterisation of metabolic fingerprints that can be associated with individual phenotypes encompassing dietary or disease statuses (Martin et al., 2012).

The gut microbiome tremendously increases the diversity of metabolic pathways accessible to mammalian hosts, enabling them to metabolise many things that they otherwise could not. As a result, gut microbes have been associated with various essential biological functions in humans through a "network" of gut microbiot–host co-metabolism to process nutrients and drugs and modulate the activities of multiple pathways in a variety of organ systems (Claus et al., 2008; Martin et al., 2007a, 2009). Gut microbes enable us to digest cellulose, the single largest nutritional energy source on the planet, and to survive on diets with low levels of particular nutrients and high levels of particular toxins. For example, gut microbes metabolise unabsorbed carbohydrates to SCFAs, the monocarboxylic acids with a chain-length up to six carbon atoms, that is, acetic, propionic, butyric, isovaleric, valeric, isocaproic, and caproic acids in the colon. SCFAs function both as an energy source and as a signalling molecule, and their abundance and type (e.g. butyric, propionic, and acetic acids) are directly related to the speciation of the microbiota and their syntrophic interactions.

An interesting study (Zheng et al., 2011) was performed to profile the urinary and faecal metabolites in Wistar rats exposed to an antibiotic, imipenem/cilastatin sodium, at 50 mg/kg/daily for 4 days followed by a 14-day recovery period in a specific pathogen-free (SPF) environment using GC-MS- and LC-MS-based metabolomics approach. The time-dependent metabolic 'footprints' in urine and faeces of experimental rats resulting from antibiotic exposure were visualised. A 4-day antibiotic intervention resulted in significantly altered human metabolic profile, and a panel of 202 urinary and 223 faecal metabolites significantly related to end points of a "functional metagenome" was characterised. This study shows extensive gut microbiota modulation of host systemic metabolism involving SCFAs, tryptophan, tyrosine metabolism, and possibly a compensatory mechanism of indole-melatonin production and also provides important baseline information of a complete spectrum of metabolites produced from the gut microbiota–host co-metabolism, which will improve our understanding of the "functional metagenome" as well as the molecular mechanisms underlying multilevel host–microbe interactions. The microbiome has a strong impact on the metabolic phenotypes of the host, and hence, metabolic readouts can provide insight into functional metagenomic activity.

The impact of gut microbiota on bacterial SCFAs has been widely studied (Martin et al., 2007a, 2008b, 2010). They found that the production of SCFAs by the gut microbiota of re-conventionalised mice was similar to that of conventional mice, except the latter had higher levels of acetate. Compared to the conventional group, mice colonised with human baby flora were associated with lower concentrations and different proportions of SCFAs. In particular, a higher proportion of propionate and a lower proportion of *n*-butyrate were observed in colonised mice. Another study by the same group (Martin et al., 2008b) demonstrated a significant association between the probiotic modulation of the gut microbiome and the metabolism of SCFAs. The production of acetate and butyrate by the human baby flora mice supplemented with *Lactobacillus paracasei* or *Lactobacillus rhamnosus* probiotics was also reduced. The concentrations of isobutyrate and isovalerate were increased in mice fed with *L. paracasei*. Interestingly, a faecal metabonomics study revealed that the synbiotic combination of *L. paracasei* (probiotic) and galactosyl-oligosaccharides (prebiotics) in mice was directly related to enhanced growth of bifidobacteria and lactobacilli compared to mice colonised to other human baby microbiota. These bacterial variations were associated with a modulation of bacterial metabolism of carbohydrates and SCFAs, which was marked by a lower level of unassigned fatty acids and a larger increase in acetate levels (Martin et al., 2010).

Recently, two studies of MS-based metabolomics study revealed distinct alterations of the intestinal content metabolites in the whole gastrointestinal tract (the stomach, duodenum, jejunum, ileum, caecum, colon, and rectum) in male Sprague-Dawley rats following 8 weeks' ethanol exposure, which were characterised by increased fatty acids and steroids (bile acids), a significant decrease of all amino acids and branched chain amino acids, and significantly decreased SCFAs except for acetic acid (Xie et al., 2013a; Zheng et al., 2013). The findings have shown that the metabolomics approach would be an effective tool to characterise the host–gut microbiota interactions.

Martin et al. also used a targeted UPLC-MS profiling approach to assess the impact of gut microbiota perturbations on the bile acid enterohepatic cycle and host tissue-specific metabolic profiles (Martin et al., 2007b). Interestingly, when compared with conventional gut microbiota, mice colonised with human baby intestinal microbiota presented higher ileal concentrations of tauroconjugated bile acids, which were mainly tauro-β-muricholic acid and taurocholic acid, owing to lower deconjugation activity from the human baby microbiota. These changes had a direct impact on emulsification and absorption of bile acids and indirectly affected hepatic fatty acid storage and lipoperoxidation, resulting in higher triglyceride and lower glutathione content in the liver of mice harbouring the human flora. They further found that supplementation with probiotic *Lactobacillus* spp. significantly impacted the tauroconjugated/unconjugated ratio of bile acids and the metabolism of SCFAs, amino acids, and methylamines (Martin et al., 2008a). Xie et al. also used a targeted metabolomics approach to characterise the bile acid profiles of the serum, GI tract (duodenum, jejunum, ileum, caecum, colon, and rectum) content, and liver in male Sprague-Dawley rats consuming ethanol chronically for 8 weeks. They found that ethanol consumption substantially impacted the bile acid profiles of different tissues. Tauroconjugated bile acids were significantly decreased in the liver and gastrointestinal tract of ethanol-treated rats, while unconjugated and glycine-conjugated species increased. The authors proposed that altered bile acid profile may be due to ethanol-induced changes in the gut microbiota and may indicate another mechanism by which the gut microbiota influence host metabolism (Xie et al., 2013b).

Another excellent example by Nicholson's group (Swann et al., 2011) to study the impact of gut microbiota on bile acid metabolism also demonstrated the effect of metabolomics in the host–gut microbiota interaction study. They found that conjugated bile acids dominated the hepatic profile of conventional animals and unconjugated bile acids comprised the largest proportion of the total measured bile acid profile in the kidney and heart tissues. In the germ-free animal, tauroconjugated bile acids (especially taurocholic acid and tauro-β-muricholic acid) dominated the bile acid profiles in all of the tissue compartments, with unconjugated and glycine-conjugated species representing a small proportion of the profile.

IBD is another chronic inflammatory disorder of the GI tract, with both genetic and environmental contributions. Crohn's disease (CD) and ulcerative colitis are two principal forms of IBD (Bonen and Cho, 2003; Katz et al., 1999; Young and Abreu, 2006), but their aetiologies are not well realised. Metabolic profiling by non-invasive ^{1}H-NMR spectroscopy of faecal extracts from CD and ulcerative colitis patients showed reduced levels of microbial co-metabolites, such as acetate, butyrate, methylamine, and trimethylamine (Marchesi et al., 2007b).

Such broad metabolomics profiling studies combined with microbial profiles in mammals have revealed the existence of multilevel host–microbe interactions, and therefore, this approach promises to be a powerful tool for the deconvolution of the complex interplay between mammalian and bacterial metabolic processes.

6.4 The marriage of metagenomics and metabolomics: microbiome–metabolome interactions

Metagenomics seeks to characterise the composition of microbial communities, their operations, and their dynamically coevolving relationships with the habitats they occupy without having to culture community members. Uniting metagenomics with the analyses of the products of microbial community metabolism (metabolomics) will shed light on how microbial communities function in a variety of environments, including the human body. The gut microbiota acts in a concerted manner to achieve metabolic communication with the host, and many different bacterial genera and species are involved in metabolite production (Nicholson et al., 2012). The microbiome represents a first step in exploring the largely mysterious bio-transformations that are supported by its constituents. The metabolome, the set of metabolites generated by one or more organisms under a particular set of physiological/environmental conditions, holds the key to moving beyond descriptions of the composition of our indigenous microbial communities. The metabolome will enable a better understanding of the dynamic operations of our indigenous microbial communities and their functional contributions to the various body habitats that they occupy (Turnbaugh and Gordon, 2008). These contributions include metabolic activities that are not encoded in our human genome, for example, the breakdown of otherwise difficult to digest plant glycans, synthesis of vitamins, and the processing of various xenobiotics that we consume. For example, hippurate is the most widely detected urinary metabolite of host–microbe origin in humans, dogs, ruminants, and rodents, and its urinary concentrations are modulated by diet, stress, disease, and microbial presence or activity (Holmes et al., 2008).

Given the integral nature of a specific gut microbiome and metabolome, any differences in the microbial communities could result in significant alterations in the extracellular metabolome that may account for important findings commonly encountered in pathology, toxicology, or drug metabolism studies. Global systems biology (Nicholson, 2006), which examines the complex interactions between genes, proteins, metabolites, and other cellular components at the whole-organism or community levels, provides new opportunities to deepen and model the complex interactions between the gut microbiome and host. Integration of gut microbial profiling with high-throughput metabolic phenotyping promises to delineate the microbiome and the host metabolic phenotypes at a global level to uncover their inherent associations. These studies represent an exciting frontier in human biology and are improving our understanding of the mechanisms underlying complex host–microbe interactions.

There are various methods for establishing biological or statistical links between the microbes and the metabolites that they may produce. Next-generation sequencing methods can provide a reconstruction of DNA sequences and insight into the capability of organisms to perform metabolic functions. Metabolic profiling of biofluids (such as urine, plasma, or faecal water) that uses high-resolution spectroscopy offers an alternative strategy for characterising metabolites of microbial origin, and the profiles can subsequently be statistically integrated with metagenomics data by using multivariate computational modelling. Evidence is accumulating that gut microbes influence the metabolite profiles of human blood (Wikoff et al., 2009), urine (Li et al., 2008a) and faecal extracts (Marchesi et al., 2007a; Saric et al., 2008). Metabolic profiling of urine samples in a Chinese family and co-variation of 16S rRNA PCR–DGGE profiles of the inter- and intra-individual variations in gut microbiota within this single family demonstrated that symbiotic gut microbes have a strong correlation with the human metabolic phenotypes (metabotypes) (Li et al., 2008a).

Co-metabolism and metabolic exchange between the host and the gut microbial consortia significantly contribute to host metabotypes (Nicholson et al., 2005a). The ^{1}H-NMR metabolic profiling of human faecal water from CRC patients and healthy controls demonstrated decreased levels of health-promoting acetate and butyrate and some correlation of proline and cysteine concentrations with disease (Monleon et al., 2009). Subsequently, metagenomic analysis using 16S rRNA PCR–DGGE, ribosomal intergenic spacer analysis, and in-parallel ^{1}H-NMR metabonomic analysis of the faecal extracts from colon cancer and polyposis patients compared to healthy controls (Monleon et al., 2009; Scanlan et al., 2008) demonstrated that the gut microbes and the detected metabolites were significantly altered in both the CRC and the polyposis subjects, with reduced temporal stability and increased diversity of the *Clostridium leptum* and *Clostridium coccoides* subgroups in both disease groups.

6.5 Future perspectives: personalised nutrition

The goal of nutrition has extended beyond just ameliorating or curing diseases and now aims to achieve an overall objective in preventing diseases and improving health. Therefore, the pivotal scientific objective has become understanding the relationship between diet and health/diseases. Together these developments indicate that the future goal of nutritional research will be to predict the likelihood of future diseases within the context of an individual's overall heath and identify causal risk factors, leading to recommendations for appropriate intervention, such as dietary habit changes, to avoid homeostasis loss and maintain healthy status.

Personalised nutrition is the outcome for individuals who will adapt their diet and lifestyle according to knowledge about their current or future healthy status (Rezzi et al., 2007). The concept of personalised medicine, first noted in the 1970s, began to emerge and with it the concept of personalised nutrition (Kaput, 2008). Generally speaking, personalised nutrition has, alongside personalised medicine, had a gene-centric approach. However, the delivery of personalised nutrition is increasingly seen as existing at three levels: personalised nutrition advice based on personalised dietary data, personalised nutrition advice based on personalised phenotypic data, and personalised nutrition advice based on personalised genomic data (Gibney and Walsh, 2013). Clayton and his colleagues have described a novel "pharmacometabolomics" concept of personalised drug treatment (Clayton et al., 2006), which applies a combination of predose metabolic profiling and bio-informatic tools to model and predict the response of individual subjects. The concept of "pharmacometabolomics" is sensitive to both genetic and environmental influences and addresses the metabolic response at the individual level. This concept could be alternatively applied to nutritional research as a means of assessing individual response to diets. In the future, researchers could use such metabolic profiling to measure, predict, and optimise the metabolic response of individual response to dietary interventions or modulations. Likely, in cases of impairment of human homeostasis, the patients would thus develop a coordinated approach to re-establish a metabolic trajectory for the individual consistent with their metabotypes.

Combining metabolomics with metagenomics provides a new "top-down" systems biology approach to uncover the molecular mechanisms underlying multilevel host–gut microbe interactions and their interdependencies. This approach will also be important in determining the effects of these interactions on the aetiology of human diseases as a function of unfavourable host–gut microbiota interactions. Metabolomic profiling of the microbial metabolites or co-metabolites resulting from crosstalk between the host and commensal microbes will assist in understanding the extent to which the gut microbiota affects the responses of the human host to dietary modulation or intervention. As the gut microbiota is involved in the predisposition to, or the onset of, many human diseases, quantitative profiling of the gut microbiota can help predict what types of metabolites and metabolic processes can be affected. These metabolites may be potential biomarkers for the evaluation of disease progression and human responses to specific therapeutic regimens at the metabolome level.

Although many efforts on metagenomics and metabolomics for personalised nutrition have been made, most of the published work in this area demonstrates only statistical associations between the metabolic phenotypes and the compositional changes of gut microbiota, with the exception of some well-known pathways, such as those of SCFAs, bile acids, and amino acids. To further discover connections between our supraorganismal metabolism and our microbial ecology, several advances should be made. We need to improve the knowledge about the mechanisms of those metabolic processes impacted by each individual microbial species regarding which of the many microbial species are vital for modulation of the "transgenomic" metabolism between the human host and gut microbes. We need to improve our current metabolomics technology to get more detected metabolites identified and get more low-abundance metabolites detected. These difficulties have limited our ability to retrieve all of the biological information contained in these studies on host–microbe associations. A clear understanding of the important host–gut microbiota interactions within our bodies will depend on future advancements in metabolomics, metagenomics, systems biology, and other related technologies.

References

Amann, R., Springer, N., Ludwig, W., Gortz, H.D., Schleifer, K.H., 1991. Identification in situ and phylogeny of uncultured bacterial endosymbionts. Nature 351, 161–164.

Armougom, F., Henry, M., Vialettes, B., Raccah, D., Raoult, D., 2009. Monitoring bacterial community of human gut microbiota reveals an increase in Lactobacillus in obese patients and Methanogens in anorexic patients. PLoS One 4, e7125.

Arnold, I.C., Dehzad, N., Reuter, S., Martin, H., Becher, B., Taube, C., Muller, A., 2011. Helicobacter pylori infection prevents allergic asthma in mouse models through the induction of regulatory T cells. J. Clin. Invest. 121, 3088–3093.

Aziz, Q., Dore, J., Emmanuel, A., Guarner, F., Quigley, E.M., 2013. Gut microbiota and gastrointestinal health: current concepts and future directions. Neurogastroenterol. Motil. 25, 4–15.

Backhed, F., Ding, H., Wang, T., Hooper, L.V., Koh, G.Y., Nagy, A., Semenkovich, C.F., Gordon, J.I., 2004. The gut microbiota as an environmental factor that regulates fat storage. Proc. Natl. Acad. Sci. U. S. A. 101, 15718–15723.

Bonen, D.K., Cho, J.H., 2003. The genetics of inflammatory bowel disease. Gastroenterology 124, 521–536.

Booijink, C.C., Zoetendal, E.G., Kleerebezem, M., de Vos, W.M., 2007. Microbial communities in the human small intestine: coupling diversity to metagenomics. Future Microbiol 2, 285–295.

Brown, L.M., 2000. Helicobacter pylori: epidemiology and routes of transmission. Epidemiol. Rev. 22, 283–297.

Brugman, S., Klatter, F.A., Visser, J.T., Wildeboer-Veloo, A.C., Harmsen, H.J., Rozing, J., Bos, N.A., 2006. Antibiotic treatment partially protects against type 1 diabetes in the Bio-Breeding diabetes-prone rat. Is the gut flora involved in the development of type 1 diabetes? Diabetologia 49, 2105–2108.

Candela, M., Consolandi, C., Severgnini, M., Biagi, E., Castiglioni, B., Vitali, B., DeBellis, G., Brigidi, P., 2010. High taxonomic level fingerprint of the human intestinal microbiota by ligase detection reaction—universal array approach. BMC Microbiol. 10, 116.

Carroll, I.M., Chang, Y.H., Park, J., Sartor, R.B., Ringel, Y., 2010. Luminal and mucosal-associated intestinal microbiota in patients with diarrhea-predominant irritable bowel syndrome. Gut. Pathog. 2.

Chiller, K., Selkin, B.A., Murakawa, G.J., 2001. Skin microflora and bacterial infections of the skin. J. Investig. Dermatol. Symp. Proc. 6, 170–174.

Claus, S.P., Tsang, T.M., Wang, Y., Cloarec, O., Skordi, E., Martin, F.P., Rezzi, S., Ross, A., Kochhar, S., Holmes, E., Nicholson, J.K., 2008. Systemic multicompartmental effects of the gut microbiome on mouse metabolic phenotypes. Mol. Syst. Biol. 4, 219.

Clayton, T.A., Lindon, J.C., Cloarec, O., Antti, H., Charuel, C., Hanton, G., Provost, J.P., Le Net, J.L., Baker, D., Walley, R.J., Everett, J.R., Nicholson, J.K., 2006. Pharmaco-metabonomic phenotyping and personalized drug treatment. Nature 440, 1073–1077.

Clemente, J.C., Ursell, L.K., Parfrey, L.W., Knight, R., 2012. The impact of the gut microbiota on human health: an integrative view. Cell 148, 1258–1270.

Collado, M.C., Isolauri, E., Laitinen, K., Salminen, S., 2008. Distinct composition of gut microbiota during pregnancy in overweight and normal-weight women. Am. J. Clin. Nutr. 88, 894–899.

De Palma, G., Nadal, I., Medina, M., Donat, E., Ribes-Koninckx, C., Calabuig, M., Sanz, Y., 2010. Intestinal dysbiosis and reduced immunoglobulin-coated bacteria associated with coeliac disease in children. BMC Microbiol. 10, 63.

Dethlefsen, L., Eckburg, P.B., Bik, E.M., Relman, D.A., 2006. Assembly of the human intestinal microbiota. Trends Ecol. Evol. 21, 517–523.

Dicksved, J., Halfvarson, J., Rosenquist, M., Jarnerot, G., Tysk, C., Apajalahti, J., Engstrand, L., Jansson, J.K., 2008. Molecular analysis of the gut microbiota of identical twins with Crohn's disease. Isme. J. 2, 716–727.

Duncan, S.H., Belenguer, A., Holtrop, G., Johnstone, A.M., Flint, H.J., Lobley, G.E., 2007. Reduced dietary intake of carbohydrates by obese subjects results in decreased concentrations of butyrate and butyrate-producing bacteria in feces. Appl. Environ. Microbiol. 73, 1073–1078.

Duncan, S.H., Lobley, G.E., Holtrop, G., Ince, J., Johnstone, A.M., Louis, P., Flint, H.J., 2008. Human colonic microbiota associated with diet, obesity and weight loss. Int. J. Obes. (Lond) 32, 1720–1724.

Eckburg, P.B., Bik, E.M., Bernstein, C.N., Purdom, E., Dethlefsen, L., Sargent, M., Gill, S.R., Nelson, K.E., Relman, D.A., 2005. Diversity of the human intestinal microbial flora. Science 308, 1635–1638.

Egert, M., de Graaf, A.A., Smidt, H., de Vos, W.M., Venema, K., 2006. Beyond diversity: functional microbiomics of the human colon. Trends Microbiol. 14, 86–91.

Elinav, E., Strowig, T., Kau, A.L., Henao-Mejia, J., Thaiss, C.A., Booth, C.J., Peaper, D.R., Bertin, J., Eisenbarth, S.C., Gordon, J.I., Flavell, R.A., 2011. NLRP6 inflammasome regulates colonic microbial ecology and risk for colitis. Cell 145, 745–757.

Fava, F., Lovegrove, J.A., Gitau, R., Jackson, K.G., Tuohy, K.M., 2006. The gut microbiota and lipid metabolism: implications for human health and coronary heart disease. Curr. Med. Chem. 13, 3005–3021.

Fiehn, O., 2002. Metabolomics—the link between genotypes and phenotypes. Plant Mol. Biol. 48, 155–171.

Frank, D.N., St Amand, A.L., Feldman, R.A., Boedeker, E.C., Harpaz, N., Pace, N.R., 2007. Molecular-phylogenetic characterization of microbial community imbalances in human inflammatory bowel diseases. Proc. Natl. Acad. Sci. U. S. A. 104, 13780–13785.

Gerritsen, J., Smidt, H., Rijkers, G.T., de Vos, W.M., 2011. Intestinal microbiota in human health and disease: the impact of probiotics. Genes Nutr. 6, 209–240.

Gibney, M.J., Walsh, M.C., 2013. The future direction of personalised nutrition: my diet, my phenotype, my genes. Proc. Nutr. Soc. 72, 219–225.

Gordon, J.I., 2012. Honor thy gut symbionts redux. Science 336, 1251–1253.

Gordon, J.H., Dubos, R., 1970. The anaerobic bacterial flora of the mouse cecum. J. Exp. Med. 132, 251–260.

Han, J., Antunes, L.C., Finlay, B.B., Borchers, C.H., 2010. Metabolomics: towards understanding host-microbe interactions. Future Microbiol 5, 153–161.

Harris, M.A., Reddy, C.A., Carter, G.R., 1976. Anaerobic bacteria from the large intestine of mice. Appl. Environ. Microbiol. 31, 907–912.

Holmes, E., Loo, R.L., Stamler, J., Bictash, M., Yap, I.K., Chan, Q., Ebbels, T., De Iorio, M., Brown, I.J., Veselkov, K.A., Daviglus, M.L., Kesteloot, H., Ueshima, H., Zhao, L., Nicholson, J.K., Elliott, P., 2008. Human metabolic phenotype diversity and its association with diet and blood pressure. Nature 453, 396–400.

Holmes, E., Kinross, J., Gibson, G.R., Burcelin, R., Jia, W., Pettersson, S., Nicholson, J.K., 2012. Therapeutic modulation of microbiota-host metabolic interactions. Sci. Transl. Med. 4 (137rv6), 137.

Hull, M.W., Chow, A.W., 2007. Indigenous microflora and innate immunity of the head and neck. Infect. Dis. Clin. North Am. 21, 265–282.

Huycke, M.M., Gaskins, H.R., 2004. Commensal bacteria, redox stress, and colorectal cancer: mechanisms and models. Exp. Biol. Med. (Maywood) 229, 586–597.

Ilett, K.F., Tee, L.B., Reeves, P.T., Minchin, R.F., 1990. Metabolism of drugs and other xenobiotics in the gut lumen and wall. Pharmacol. Ther. 46, 67–93.

Jia, W., Li, H., Zhao, L., Nicholson, J.K., 2008. Gut microbiota: a potential new territory for drug targeting. Nat. Rev. Drug Discov. 7, 123–129.

Jones, B.V., Begley, M., Hill, C., Gahan, C.G., Marchesi, J.R., 2008. Functional and comparative metagenomic analysis of bile salt hydrolase activity in the human gut microbiome. Proc. Natl. Acad. Sci. U. S. A. 105, 13580–13585.

Joossens, M., Huys, G., Cnockaert, M., De Preter, V., Verbeke, K., Rutgeerts, P., Vandamme, P., Vermeire, S., 2011. Dysbiosis of the faecal microbiota in patients with Crohn's disease and their unaffected relatives. Gut 60, 631–637.

Kalliomaki, M., Collado, M.C., Salminen, S., Isolauri, E., 2008. Early differences in fecal microbiota composition in children may predict overweight. Am. J. Clin. Nutr. 87, 534–538.

Kaput, J., 2008. Nutrigenomics research for personalized nutrition and medicine. Curr. Opin. Biotechnol. 19, 110–120.

Katz, J.A., Itoh, J., Fiocchi, C., 1999. Pathogenesis of inflammatory bowel disease. Curr. Opin. Gastroenterol. 15, 291–297.

Kelly, D., King, T., Aminov, R., 2007. Importance of microbial colonization of the gut in early life to the development of immunity. Mutat. Res. 622, 58–69.

Kerckhoffs, A.P.M., Ben-Amor, K., Samsom, M., van der Rest, M.E., de Vogel, J., Knol, J., Akkermans, L.M.A., 2011. Molecular analysis of faecal and duodenal samples reveals significantly higher prevalence and numbers of Pseudomonas aeruginosa in irritable bowel syndrome. J. Med. Microbiol. 60, 236–245.

Lathrop, S.K., Bloom, S.M., Rao, S.M., Nutsch, K., Lio, C.W., Santacruz, N., Peterson, D.A., Stappenbeck, T.S., Hsieh, C.S., 2011. Peripheral education of the immune system by colonic commensal microbiota. Nature 478, 250–254.

Ley, R.E., 2010. Obesity and the human microbiome. Curr. Opin. Gastroenterol. 26, 5–11.

Ley, R.E., Backhed, F., Turnbaugh, P., Lozupone, C.A., Knight, R.D., Gordon, J.I., 2005. Obesity alters gut microbial ecology. Proc. Natl. Acad. Sci. U. S. A. 102, 11070–11075.

Ley, R.E., Peterson, D.A., Gordon, J.I., 2006a. Ecological and evolutionary forces shaping microbial diversity in the human intestine. Cell 124, 837–848.

Ley, R.E., Turnbaugh, P.J., Klein, S., Gordon, J.I., 2006b. Microbial ecology: human gut microbes associated with obesity. Nature 444, 1022–1023.

Ley, R.E., Lozupone, C.A., Hamady, M., Knight, R., Gordon, J.I., 2008. Worlds within worlds: evolution of the vertebrate gut microbiota. Nat. Rev. Microbiol. 6, 776–788.

Li, M., Wang, B., Zhang, M., Rantalainen, M., Wang, S., Zhou, H., Zhang, Y., Shen, J., Pang, X., Wei, H., Chen, Y., Lu, H., Zuo, J., Su, M., Qiu, Y., Jia, W., Xiao, C., Smith, L.M., Yang, S., Holmes, E., Tang, H., Zhao, G., Nicholson, J.K., Li, L., Zhao, L., 2008. Symbiotic gut microbes modulate human metabolic phenotypes. Proc. Natl. Acad. Sci. U. S. A. 105, 2117–2122.

Lim, M., Adams, J.D.W., Wilcox, M., Finan, P., Sagar, P., Burke, D., 2009. An assessment of bacterial dysbiosis in pouchitis using terminal restriction fragment length polymorphisms of 16S ribosomal DNA from pouch effluent microbiota. Dis. Colon Rectum 52, 1492–1500.

Lupp, C., Robertson, M.L., Wickham, M.E., Sekirov, I., Champion, O.L., Gaynor, E.C., Finlay, B.B., 2007. Host-mediated inflammation disrupts the intestinal microbiota and promotes the overgrowth of Enterobacteriaceae. Cell Host Microbe 2, 204.

Mahida, Y.R., Rolfe, V.E., 2004. Host-bacterial interactions in inflammatory bowel disease. Clin. Sci. (Lond.) 107, 331–341.

Mai, V., Ukhanova, M., Baer, D.J., 2010. Understanding the Extent and Sources of Variation in Gut Microbiota Studies; a Prerequisite for Establishing Associations with Disease. Diversity 2, 1085–1096.

Malinen, E., Rinttila, T., Kajander, K., Matto, J., Kassinen, A., Krogius, L., Saarela, M., Korpela, R., Palva, A., 2005. Analysis of the fecal microbiota of irritable bowel syndrome patients and healthy controls with real-time PCR. Am. J. Gastroenterol. 100, 373–382.

Marchesi, J.R., 2010. Prokaryotic and eukaryotic diversity of the human gut. Adv. Appl. Microbiol. 72, 43–62.

Marchesi, J.R., Holmes, E., Khan, F., Kochhar, S., Scanlan, P., Shanahan, F., Wilson, I.D., Wang, Y., 2007. Rapid and noninvasive metabonomic characterization of inflammatory bowel disease. J. Proteome Res. 6, 546–551.

Martin, F.P., Dumas, M.E., Wang, Y., Legido-Quigley, C., Yap, I.K., Tang, H., Zirah, S., Murphy, G.M., Cloarec, O., Lindon, J.C., Sprenger, N., Fay, L.B., Kochhar, S., van Bladeren, P., Holmes, E., Nicholson, J.K., 2007. A top-down systems biology view of microbiome-mammalian metabolic interactions in a mouse model. Mol. Syst. Biol. 3, 112.

Martin, F.P., Wang, Y., Sprenger, N., Yap, I.K., Lundstedt, T., Lek, P., Rezzi, S., Ramadan, Z., van Bladeren, P., Fay, L.B., Kochhar, S., Lindon, J.C., Holmes, E., Nicholson, J.K., 2008. Probiotic modulation of symbiotic gut microbial-host metabolic interactions in a humanized microbiome mouse model. Mol. Syst. Biol. 4, 157.

Martin, F.P., Wang, Y., Yap, I.K., Sprenger, N., Lindon, J.C., Rezzi, S., Kochhar, S., Holmes, E., Nicholson, J.K., 2009. Topographical variation in murine intestinal metabolic profiles in relation to microbiome speciation and functional ecological activity. J. Proteome Res. 8, 3464–3474.

Martin, F.P.J., Sprenger, N., Montoliu, I., Rezzi, S., Kochhar, S., Nicholson, J.K., 2010. Dietary modulation of gut functional ecology studied by fecal metabonomics. J. Proteome Res. 9, 5284–5295.

Martin, F.P., Collino, S., Rezzi, S., Kochhar, S., 2012. Metabolomic applications to decipher gut microbial metabolic influence in health and disease. Front. Physiol. 3, 113.

Metges, C.C., Eberhard, M., Petzke, K.J., 2006. Synthesis and absorption of intestinal microbial lysine in humans and non-ruminant animals and impact on human estimated average requirement of dietary lysine. Curr. Opin. Clin. Nutr. Metab. Care 9, 37–41.

Moco, S., Martin, F.P., Rezzi, S., 2012. Metabolomics view on gut microbiome modulation by polyphenol-rich foods. J. Proteome Res. 11, 4781–4790.

Monleon, D., Morales, J.M., Barrasa, A., Lopez, J.A., Vazquez, C., Celda, B., 2009. Metabolite profiling of fecal water extracts from human colorectal cancer. NMR Biomed. 22, 342–348.

Musso, G., Gambino, R., Cassader, M., 2011. Interactions between gut microbiota and host metabolism predisposing to obesity and diabetes. In: Caskey, C.T. (Ed.), Annual Review of Medicine, 62.

Muyzer, G., de Waal, E.C., Uitterlinden, A.G., 1993. Profiling of complex microbial populations by denaturing gradient gel electrophoresis analysis of polymerase chain reaction-amplified genes coding for 16S rRNA. Appl. Environ. Microbiol. 59, 695–700.

Neish, A.S., 2009. Microbes in gastrointestinal health and disease. Gastroenterology 136, 65–80.

Nicholson, J.K., 2006. Global systems biology, personalized medicine and molecular epidemiology. Mol. Syst. Biol. 2, 52.

Nicholson, J.K., Connelly, J., Lindon, J.C., Holmes, E., 2002. Metabonomics: a platform for studying drug toxicity and gene function. Nat. Rev. Drug Discov. 1, 153–161.

Nicholson, J.K., Holmes, E., Wilson, I.D., 2005. Gut microorganisms, mammalian metabolism and personalized health care. Nat. Rev. Microbiol. 3, 431–438.

Nicholson, J.K., Holmes, E., Kinross, J., Burcelin, R., Gibson, G., Jia, W., Pettersson, S., 2012. Host-gut microbiota metabolic interactions. Science 336, 1262–1267.

O'Hara, A.M., Shanahan, F., 2006. The gut flora as a forgotten organ. EMBO Rep. 7, 688–693.

Pandeya, D.R., D'Souza, R., Rahman, M.M., Akhter, S., Kim, H.J., Hong, S.T., 2012. Host-microbial interaction in the mammalian intestine and their metabolic role inside. Biomed. Res. India 23, 9–21.

Pang, X., Hua, X., Yang, Q., Ding, D., Che, C., Cui, L., Jia, W., Bucheli, P., Zhao, L., 2007. Inter-species transplantation of gut microbiota from human to pigs. ISME J. 1, 156–162.

Perry, S., de la Luz Sanchez, M., Yang, S., Haggerty, T.D., Hurst, P., Perez-Perez, G., Parsonnet, J., 2006. Gastroenteritis and transmission of Helicobacter pylori infection in households. Emerg. Infect. Dis. 12, 1701–1708.

Peterson, D.A., Frank, D.N., Pace, N.R., Gordon, J.I., 2008. Metagenomic approaches for defining the pathogenesis of inflammatory bowel diseases. Cell Host Microbe 3, 417–427.

Petrosino, J.F., Highlander, S., Luna, R.A., Gibbs, R.A., Versalovic, J., 2009. Metagenomic pyrosequencing and microbial identification. Clin. Chem. 55, 856–866.

Pflughoeft, K.J., Versalovic, J., 2012. Human microbiome in health and disease. Annu. Rev. Pathol. 7, 99–122.

Possemiers, S., Grootaert, C., Vermeiren, J., Gross, G., Marzorati, M., Verstraete, W., Van de Wiele, T., 2009. The intestinal environment in health and disease—recent insights on the potential of intestinal bacteria to influence human health. Curr. Pharm. Des. 15, 2051–2065.

Qin, J., Li, R., Raes, J., Arumugam, M., Burgdorf, K.S., Manichanh, C., Nielsen, T., Pons, N., Levenez, F., Yamada, T., Mende, D.R., Li, J., Xu, J., Li, S., Li, D., Cao, J., Wang, B., Liang, H., Zheng, H., Xie, Y., Tap, J., Lepage, P., Bertalan, M., Batto, J.M., Hansen, T., Le Paslier, D., Linneberg, A., Nielsen, H.B., Pelletier, E., Renault, P., Sicheritz-Ponten, T., Turner, K., Zhu, H., Yu, C., Jian, M., Zhou, Y., Li, Y., Zhang, X., Qin, N., Yang, H., Wang, J., Brunak, S., Dore, J., Guarner, F., Kristiansen, K., Pedersen, O., Parkhill, J., Weissenbach, J., Bork, P., Ehrlich, S.D., 2010. A human gut microbial gene catalogue established by metagenomic sequencing. Nature 464, 59–65.

Reyes, A., Haynes, M., Hanson, N., Angly, F.E., Heath, A.C., Rohwer, F., Gordon, J.I., 2010. Viruses in the faecal microbiota of monozygotic twins and their mothers. Nature 466, 334–338, U81.

Rezzi, S., Ramadan, Z., Fay, L.B., Kochhar, S., 2007. Nutritional metabonomics: applications and perspectives. J. Proteome Res. 6, 513–525.

Robinson, C.J., Bohannan, B.J., Young, V.B., 2010. From structure to function: the ecology of host-associated microbial communities. Microbiol. Mol. Biol. Rev. 74, 453–476.

Round, J.L., Mazmanian, S.K., 2009. The gut microbiota shapes intestinal immune responses during health and disease (vol 9, pg 313, 2009). Nat. Rev. Immunol. 9, 600.

Round, J.L., Lee, S.M., Li, J., Tran, G., Jabri, B., Chatila, T.A., Mazmanian, S.K., 2011. The toll-like receptor 2 pathway establishes colonization by a commensal of the human microbiota. Science 332, 974–977.

Santacruz, A., Collado, M.C., Garcia-Valdes, L., Segura, M.T., Martin-Lagos, J.A., Anjos, T., Marti-Romero, M., Lopez, R.M., Florido, J., Campoy, C., Sanz, Y., 2010. Gut microbiota composition is associated with body weight, weight gain and biochemical parameters in pregnant women. Brit. J. Nutr. 104, 83–92.

Saric, J., Wang, Y., Li, J., Coen, M., Utzinger, J., Marchesi, J.R., Keiser, J., Veselkov, K., Lindon, J.C., Nicholson, J.K., Holmes, E., 2008. Species variation in the fecal metabolome gives insight into differential gastrointestinal function. J. Proteome Res. 7, 352–360.

Savage, D.C., 1970. Associations of indigenous microorganisms with gastrointestinal mucosal epithelia. Am. J. Clin. Nutr. 23, 1495–1501.

Scanlan, P.D., Shanahan, F., Clune, Y., Collins, J.K., O'Sullivan, G.C., O'Riordan, M., Holmes, E., Wang, Y., Marchesi, J.R., 2008. Culture-independent analysis of the gut microbiota in colorectal cancer and polyposis. Environ. Microbiol. 10, 789–798.

Schippa, S., Iebba, V., Barbato, M., Di Nardo, G., Totino, V., Checchi, M.P., Longhi, C., Maiella, G., Cucchiara, S., Conte, M.P., 2010. A distinctive 'microbial signature' in celiac pediatric patients. BMC Microbiol. 10, 175.

Schwiertz, A., Taras, D., Schafer, K., Beijer, S., Bos, N.A., Donus, C., Hardt, P.D., 2010. Microbiota and SCFA in lean and overweight healthy subjects. Obesity (Silver Spring) 18, 190–195.

Sekirov, I., Tam, N.M., Jogova, M., Robertson, M.L., Li, Y., Lupp, C., Finlay, B.B., 2008. Antibiotic-induced perturbations of the intestinal microbiota alter host susceptibility to enteric infection. Infect. Immun. 76, 4726–4736.

Shen, X.J., Rawls, J.F., Randall, T., Burcal, L., Mpande, C.N., Jenkins, N., Jovov, B., Abdo, Z., Sandler, R.S., Keku, T.O., 2010. Molecular characterization of mucosal adherent bacteria and associations with colorectal adenomas. Gut. Microbes 1, 138–147.

Sousa, T., Paterson, R., Moore, V., Carlsson, A., Abrahamsson, B., Basit, A.W., 2008. The gastrointestinal microbiota as a site for the biotransformation of drugs. Int. J. Pharm. 363, 1–25.

Spencer, M.D., Hamp, T.J., Reid, R.W., Fischer, L.M., Zeisel, S.H., Fodor, A.A., 2011. Association between composition of the human gastrointestinal microbiome and development of fatty liver with choline deficiency. Gastroenterology 140, 976–986.

Spor, A., Koren, O., Ley, R., 2011. Unravelling the effects of the environment and host genotype on the gut microbiome. Nat. Rev. Microbiol. 9, 279–290.

Swann, J.R., Want, E.J., Geier, F.M., Spagou, K., Wilson, I.D., Sidaway, J.E., Nicholson, J.K., Holmes, E., 2011. Systemic gut microbial modulation of bile acid metabolism in host tissue compartments. Proc. Natl. Acad. Sci. U. S. A. 108 (Suppl. 1), 4523–4530.

Tana, C., Umesaki, Y., Imaoka, A., Handa, T., Kanazawa, M., Fukudo, S., 2010. Altered profiles of intestinal microbiota and organic acids may be the origin of symptoms in irritable bowel syndrome. Neurogastroent. Motil. 22, 512–519.

Turnbaugh, P.J., Gordon, J.I., 2008. An invitation to the marriage of metagenomics and metabolomics. Cell 134, 708–713.

Turnbaugh, P.J., Ley, R.E., Mahowald, M.A., Magrini, V., Mardis, E.R., Gordon, J.I., 2006. An obesity-associated gut microbiome with increased capacity for energy harvest. Nature 444, 1027–1031.

Turnbaugh, P.J., Ley, R.E., Hamady, M., Fraser-Liggett, C.M., Knight, R., Gordon, J.I., 2007. The human microbiome project. Nature 449, 804–810.
Turnbaugh, P.J., Hamady, M., Yatsunenko, T., Cantarel, B.L., Duncan, A., Ley, R.E., Sogin, M. L., Jones, W.J., Roe, B.A., Affourtit, J.P., Egholm, M., Henrissat, B., Heath, A.C., Knight, R., Gordon, J.I., 2009a. A core gut microbiome in obese and lean twins. Nature 457, 480–484, U7.
Turnbaugh, P.J., Ridaura, V.K., Faith, J.J., Rey, F.E., Knight, R., Gordon, J.I., 2009b. The effect of diet on the human gut microbiome: a metagenomic analysis in humanized gnotobiotic mice. Sci. Transl. Med. 1, 6ra14.
Vaahtovuo, J., Munukka, E., Korkeamaki, M., Luukkainen, R., Toivanen, P., 2008. Fecal microbiota in early rheumatoid arthritis. J. Rheumatol. 35, 1500–1505.
Verstraelen, H., 2008. Cutting edge: the vaginal microflora and bacterial vaginosis. Verh. K. Acad. Geneeskd. Belg. 70, 147–174.
Vrieze, A., Holleman, F., Zoetendal, E.G., de Vos, W.M., Hoekstra, J.B.L., Nieuwdorp, M., 2010. The environment within: how gut microbiota may influence metabolism and body composition. Diabetologia 53, 606–613.
Wei, H., Dong, L., Wang, T.T., Zhang, M.H., Hua, W.Y., Zhang, C.H., Pang, X.Y., Chen, M.J., Su, M.M., Qiu, Y.P., Zhou, M.M., Yang, S.L., Chen, Z., Rantalainen, M., Nicholson, J.K., Jia, W., Wu, D.Z., Zhao, L.P., 2010. Structural shifts of gut microbiota as surrogate endpoints for monitoring host health changes induced by carcinogen exposure. FEMS Microbiol. Ecol. 73, 577–586.
Wikoff, W.R., Anfora, A.T., Liu, J., Schultz, P.G., Lesley, S.A., Peters, E.C., Siuzdak, G., 2009. Metabolomics analysis reveals large effects of gut microflora on mammalian blood metabolites. Proc. Natl. Acad. Sci. U. S. A. 106, 3698–3703.
Wilson, D.S., Sober, E., 1989. Reviving the superorganism. J. Theor. Biol. 136, 337–356.
Xie, G., Zhong, W., Zheng, X., Li, Q., Qiu, Y., Li, H., Chen, H., Zhou, Z., Jia, W., 2013a. Chronic ethanol consumption alters Mammalian gastrointestinal content metabolites. J. Proteome Res. 12, 3297–3306.
Xie, G.X., Zhong, W., Li, H.K., Li, Q., Qiu, Y.P., Zheng, X.J., Chen, H.Y., Zhao, X.Q., Zhang, S.C., Zhou, Z.X., Zeisel, S.H., Jia, W., 2013b. Alteration of bile acid metabolism in the rat induced by chronic ethanol consumption. FASEB J. 27, 3583–3593.
Xu, J., Gordon, J.I., 2003. Honor thy symbionts. Proc. Natl. Acad. Sci. U. S. A. 100, 10452–10459.
Young, Y., Abreu, M.T., 2006. Advances in the pathogenesis of inflammatory bowel disease. Curr. Gastroenterol. Rep. 8, 470–477.
Zella, G.C., Hait, E.J., Glavan, T., Gevers, D., Ward, D.V., Kitts, C.L., Korzenik, J.R., 2011. Distinct microbiome in pouchitis compared to healthy pouches in ulcerative colitis and familial adenomatous polyposis. Inflamm. Bowel Dis. 17, 1092–1100.
Zhang, H., DiBaise, J.K., Zuccolo, A., Kudrna, D., Braidotti, M., Yu, Y., Parameswaran, P., Crowell, M.D., Wing, R., Rittmann, B.E., Krajmalnik-Brown, R., 2009. Human gut microbiota in obesity and after gastric bypass. Proc. Natl. Acad. Sci. U. S. A. 106, 2365–2370.
Zheng, X., Xie, G., Zhao, A., Zhao, L., Yao, C., Chiu, N.H., Zhou, Z., Bao, Y., Jia, W., Nicholson, J.K., 2011. The footprints of gut microbial-mammalian co-metabolism. J. Proteome Res. 10, 5512–5522.
Zheng, X.J., Qiu, Y.P., Zhong, W., Baxter, S., Su, M.M., Li, Q., Xie, G.X., Ore, B.M., Qiao, S. L., Spencer, M.D., Zeisel, S.H., Zhou, Z.X., Zhao, A.H., Jia, W., 2013. A targeted metabolomic protocol for short-chain fatty acids and branched-chain amino acids. Metabolomics 9, 818–827.

Metabotyping: moving towards personalised nutrition

7

L. Brennan[1,2]
[1]University College Dublin, Dublin, Ireland; [2]Newcastle University, Newcastle upon Tyne, United Kingdom

7.1 Introduction

The concept of personalised nutrition emerged in the context that nutritional recommendations need to be refined for specific subgroups of the population, and was originally described in the 1970s (Nizel, 1972). The nutritional needs of individuals vary according to age, gender, and physiological status such as pregnancy. Considering the substantial interindividual response to dietary interventions performed in the last decade, it has become evident that a more personalised approach to dietary recommendations is needed. In more recent years, various definitions of personalised nutrition have emerged. However, the most comprehensive definition describes a three-level approach: Level 1 describes the delivery of dietary advice following assessment of the individual's dietary intake; level 2 refers to the delivery of personalised advice following assessment of the individual's diet and phenotypic measures (such as blood pressure and clinical chemistry parameters) and level 3 refers to the delivery of advice taking into account the individuals diet, phenotypic measures, and genetic profile (Gibney and Walsh, 2013).

Since the sequencing of the human genome, there has been an increasing interest in using genetic data to derive personalised nutrition advice. From a scientific viewpoint, this is difficult as the evidence is not as strong as we as scientists would like. To date, most of the results are from observational studies with a distinct lack of evidence from dietary intervention studies. However, there are a limited number of examples where evidence from intervention studies exists. One such example includes the C677T variant in the gene encoding the enzyme methylenetetrahydrofolate reductase. A riboflavin intervention for 16 weeks reduced blood pressure significantly in subjects with the TT variant but not in subjects with the C allele of the C677T genotype (Horigan et al., 2010). In a follow-up study in subjects with CVD (cardiovascular disease), the TT genotype riboflavin supplementation again reduced blood pressure (Wilson et al., 2012). More recently, in a group of hypertensive subjects without CVD, a decrease in blood pressure was found following supplementation with riboflavin for 16 weeks. Overall, this provides strong evidence for the proof of concept of delivering dietary advice including analysis of genetic data. However, it should also be recognised that this is a field still in its infancy.

Although there is general agreement that nutritional advice needs to move towards personalised advice, it is also evident that we will not reach a truly personalised level

Metabolomics as a Tool in Nutrition Research. http://dx.doi.org/10.1016/B978-1-78242-084-2.00007-1

where specific foods will be created for individuals. A more realistic approach is the development of personalised advice for groups of individuals also referred to as "targeted nutrition". Stratification of individuals could be achieved based on their metabolic/phenotypic profile, and indeed, examples exist of such an approach (Clayton et al., 2006, 2009; Nicholson et al., 2012a; Winnike et al., 2010). The concept of grouping subjects based on their metabolic phenotype has been demonstrated in a number of studies, and the term "metabotype" has been coined. The present chapter will focus on key pertinent examples where metabotyping has been used with a focus on nutrition examples.

7.2 The concept of the metabotype

Metabolomics has emerged as a tool for determining metabotypes: metabolomic profiles or combinations of specific metabolites can be used to class subjects into groups or clusters. One approach of achieving such grouping is cluster analysis such as *k*-means clustering. The basis of this approach is to group *n* individuals into *k* clusters in which each individual belongs to the cluster with the nearest mean. Other clustering approaches exist such as hierarchical clustering, and each has its own merits and drawbacks. In the metabolomic field, one of the most commonly used data analysis tools is principal component analysis (PCA). PCA is particularly useful in analysing trends in the data but is not a clustering technique itself. Recently, we developed an approach based on PCA to allow group identification: the mixture of probabilistic PCA (Nyamundanda et al., 2010) allows the researcher to ascertain the number of inherent groups in metabolomic data.

The metabotype is known to be influenced by a combination of genetic and environmental factors such as diet and the gut microflora (Figure 7.1). Depending on the metabolites chosen to perform the metabotyping, the influence of each of these factors may be less or more important. Suhre and colleagues had demonstrated elegantly that genotype influences the metabolomic profile and had performed a number of genome-wide association studies with metabolic traits (mGWAS) (Gieger et al., 2008; Illig et al., 2010). With regard to the influence of the gut microflora, there have been numerous publications indicating the important influence of the gut flora on the metabolite levels in urine and faecal water extracts (Claesson et al., 2012; Li et al., 2011; Nicholson et al., 2012b; Wijeyesekera et al., 2012). Thus, if metabotyping is performed using these biofluids, then the influence of the gut microflora will be inherent in defining the groups. In an elderly population, dietary patterns were demonstrated to drive changes in the gut microflora, which in turn were seen in metabolic profiles of the faecal samples (Claesson et al., 2012).

7.3 Examples of metabotyping with a focus on nutrition

With respect to nutrition interventions, metabotyping can be used to identify responders and nonresponders to the intervention. In our previous work, we used such an approach with *k*-means cluster analysis to identify responders and nonresponders to

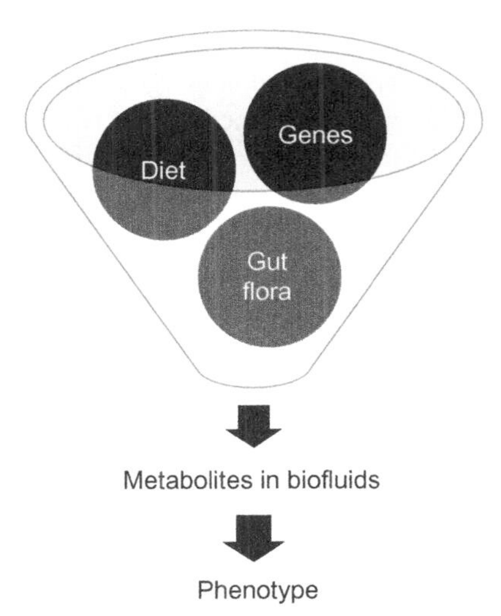

Figure 7.1 Factors that influence the metabolic profile. Metabolite levels in human biofluids are known to be influenced by genetic factors, the diet, and the gut microflora.

a vitamin D intervention (O'Sullivan et al., 2011b). Using the clustering approach, five distinct metabotypes were identified, and analysis of these groups revealed that one was responsive to the dietary intervention. Subjects in this responsive group were characterised by lower serum 25(OH)D and higher levels of adipokines and showed significant responses in insulin, homeostatic model assessment (HOMA)-score, and C-reactive protein (CRP) following supplementation with 15 μg of vitamin D_3 for 4 weeks. Metabolomic analysis revealed further metabolic changes in this group, and the extent of change in 25(OH)D correlated negatively with changes in fasting glucose. This study was an important proof of principle that applying this metabotyping approach could be used for the identification of dietary-responsive phenotypes.

Another example of applying k-means to lipoprotein profiles identified three clusters two of which had a positive response to fenofibrate. The subjects ($n=775$) underwent a 3 week treatment of fenofibrate, and lipoprotein profiling was performed on baseline samples. This approach was more effective in identifying responders compared with traditional approaches based on baseline HDL-c and triglycerides cut-offs (van Bochove et al., 2012).

The above are clear examples where metabolites or metabolic profiles were used to group subjects into distinct groups, which when examined displayed a differential response to the intervention/treatment. Additionally, there are other studies that performed metabotyping on defined groups such as responders and nonresponders. While the approach is different from a statistical viewpoint, the concept of predicting a response to a dietary intervention is the same. In a choline depletion study, analysis of the baseline metabolomic profile could predict which subjects developed liver dysfunction when deprived of dietary choline (Sha et al., 2010). For this study, 53 subjects received a choline-sufficient diet for 10 days (550 mg choline/70 kg/day) followed by a choline-depleted diet (<50 mg choline/70 kg/day) for up to 42 days. Metabolomic analysis was performed using targeted and nontargeted LC–MS approaches. The statistical analysis in this case was performed using two approaches: uncorrelated shrunken centroid was used for selecting markers for predicting which individuals developed liver dysfunction. Partial least squares-discriminant analysis was also used for examining if the profiles could predict class membership defined by whether subjects developed liver disease or not. Interestingly, baseline choline levels alone were not predictive of development of organ dysfunction. This in itself supports the concepts of metabotyping and its use for identifying responders to dietary interventions.

Response to an intervention with calcium and vitamin D also revealed that baseline metabolomic profiles were predictive of response to the intervention (Elnenaei et al., 2011). A 3-month intervention with calcium and vitamin D in 36 females with low bone density identified responders and nonresponders by examination of changes in parathyroid hormone. Distinctive patterns of metabolites separated responders from nonresponders at baseline. The identification of potential "nonresponders" to the vitamin D and calcium therapy could potentially be useful in selection of optimal therapy on an individual basis.

Rezzi et al. investigated whether dietary preferences of individuals were predictive from metabolomic profiles. Twenty-two healthy male volunteers were selected from 75 volunteers based on their chocolate preferences (chocolate loving or hating). Volunteers consumed a standard diet and underwent a 1-week double-crossover intervention where they consumed either chocolate or placebo (bread) on 2 test days. Biofluid samples (blood and 24 h urine) were collected, and metabolomic profiling revealed that the chocolate preference of an individual could be predicted. Prediction of dietary preference could be extremely useful in categorising individuals according to unhealthy dietary habits and developing personalised dietary advice.

All of the above examples clearly demonstrate a potential role of metabotyping in the delivery of personalised nutrition. However, none of the above examples have actually delivered personalised dietary advice. Further work is needed to develop dietary advice based on these metabotypes, thus delivering personalised nutrition at the group rather than individual level (Figure 7.2).

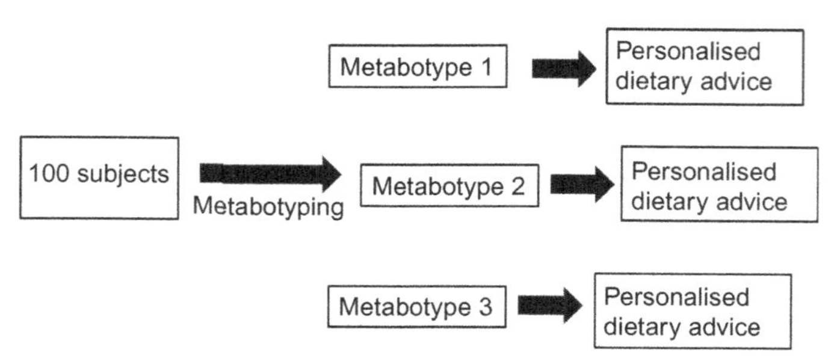

Figure 7.2 An overview of the metabotype concept. Overview of the concept of metabotyping: using the metabolic profile subjects can be classified into different metabotypes and dietary advice could then be tailored to the metabotype.

In the field of personalised medicine, the use of the baseline metabolic profiles to identify metabotypes that differentially respond to interventions has been demonstrated in a number of examples. Metabolomic analysis revealed a baseline metobotype that could predict how an individual patient with major depressive disorder would respond to treatment (Kaddurah-Daouk et al., 2011). In the future, such analysis will help define a patient's treatment strategy. Another clear example of this approach is the use of metabolomic profiles to identify metabotypes that respond to paracetamol. Clayton et al. (2006) used a combination of predose metabolic profiling and statistical analysis to predict the response of individual subjects to drug treatment. A separate study demonstrated that the metabolic profile directly after initial treatment was able to predict which subjects were susceptible to mild acetaminophen-induced liver injury (Winnike et al., 2010). These and other studies have championed the concept that metabotyping could be used to improve pharmaceutical efficacy and safety. The success of these studies in personalised medicine is encouraging for workers in the field of nutrition. Taken together with the successful metabotyping in nutrition research, an optimistic picture emerges for personalised/targeted nutrition.

7.4 Extension of metabotypes to include markers of dietary origin

Although the strict definition of metabotype is centred about the metabolic phenotype, it is possible to extend the definition to include markers of dietary origin. Focusing the metabolomic analysis on these compounds has been referred to as "nutrityping" or "phytoprofiling" (O'Sullivan et al., 2011a; Xie et al., 2013). Within this context, subjects are grouped/characterised into groups that characterise their habitual dietary intake using metabolomics-derived data. Compared to the metabotyping field, this area is in its infancy with only some proof of principles currently existing. Work in our laboratory demonstrated that using cluster analysis people could be classified into three dietary patterns based on their food intake data (O'Sullivan et al., 2011a). Examining the metabolomic profiles revealed that the dietary patterns were reflected in metabolomic urinary profiles. Resulting from this and other work, the concept of the nutritype has emerged where classification of subjects according to a dietary intake pattern is possible based on their urinary metabolomic profile. Examples from other studies also exist that support such concepts. In the KORA study, metabolomic and dietary analyses were performed on 284 subjects with significant relationships between dietary patterns and serum metabolites (Altmaier et al., 2011). Furthermore, four dietary indices were identified in the dietary data and relationships with metabolites identified. Of note was the association between the dietary fibre index and an increase in saturation of fatty acid residues of glycerophosphatidylcholines. In a recent twin study, a strong relationship between serum metabolites and nutritional patterns was also observed (Menni et al., 2013). However, other studies have reported a poor relationship between diet and serum metabolites (Floegel et al., 2013). This is in fact not surprising as the majority of metabolites measured were endogenous metabolites, which will not be hugely influenced by diet. Optimal examination of dietary intake will be obtained by measurement of metabolites originating from foods. More details on such biomarkers are given in Chapter 9. Notwithstanding this, the current evidence from published studies supports the concept of a nutritype for classification of people into groups that reflect their habitual dietary intake.

7.5 Conclusion and future trends

As clearly indicated in the above examples, metabotyping is set to play a key role in the development and delivery of personalised nutrition. In recent years, we have witnessed a shift in nutrition research away from solely treatment of diseases to prevention of disease and health promotion. Concomitant with this, there is also an expectation that nutrition advice can be delivered to individuals in a more tailored or targeted manner. The use of a metabotyping approach to identify groups of individuals that respond differentially to dietary interventions supports the concept of developing dietary advice specific to these groups. Delivery of such targeted dietary advice would be more personalised than the general dietary recommendations that are currently in place. Implementation of such a strategy would represent a significant move towards personalised dietary advice, and metabolomics is set to play a key role in defining metabotypes.

7.6 Sources of further information and advice

More information on nutrition and personalised nutrition can be obtained from the following websites:

- Personalised nutrition: www.food4me.org
- Nutrition Society: www.nutritionsociety.org
- British Nutrition Foundation: www.nutrition.org.uk
- Food Standards Agency: http://www.food.gov.uk
- European Food Safety Authority: http://www.efsa.europa.eu

Metabolomic resources are available at the following:

- www.metabolomicssociety.org
- www.nugo.org

References

Altmaier, E., Kastenmuller, G., Romisch-Margl, W., Thorand, B., Weinberger, K.M., Illig, T., Adamski, J., Doring, A., Suhre, K., 2011. Questionnaire-based self-reported nutrition habits associate with serum metabolism as revealed by quantitative targeted metabolomics. Eur. J. Epidemiol. 26, 145–156.

Claesson, M.J., Jeffery, I.B., Conde, S., Power, S.E., O'Connor, E.M., Cusack, S., Harris, H.M., Coakley, M., Lakshminarayanan, B., O'Sullivan, O., Fitzgerald, G.F., Deane, J., O'Connor, M., Harnedy, N., O'Connor, K., O'Mahony, D., van Sinderen, D., Wallace, M., Brennan, L., Stanton, C., Marchesi, J.R., Fitzgerald, A.P., Shanahan, F., Hill, C., Ross, R.P., O'Toole, P.W., 2012. Gut microbiota composition correlates with diet and health in the elderly. Nature 488, 178–184.

Clayton, T.A., Lindon, J.C., Cloarec, O., Antti, H., Charuel, C., Hanton, G., Provost, J.P., Le Net, J.L., Baker, D., Walley, R.J., Everett, J.R., Nicholson, J.K., 2006. Pharmaco-metabonomic phenotyping and personalized drug treatment. Nature 440, 1073–1077.

Clayton, T.A., Baker, D., Lindon, J.C., Everett, J.R., Nicholson, J.K., 2009. Pharmacometabonomic identification of a significant host-microbiome metabolic interaction affecting human drug metabolism. Proc. Natl. Acad. Sci. U. S. A. 106, 14728–14733.

Elnenaei, M.O., Chandra, R., Mangion, T., Moniz, C., 2011. Genomic and metabolomic patterns segregate with responses to calcium and vitamin D supplementation. Br. J. Nutr. 105, 71–79.

Floegel, A., von Ruesten, A., Drogan, D., Schulze, M.B., Prehn, C., Adamski, J., Pischon, T., Boeing, H., 2013. Variation of serum metabolites related to habitual diet: a targeted metabolomic approach in EPIC-Potsdam. Eur. J. Clin. Nutr. 67, 1100–1108.

Gibney, M.J., Walsh, M.C., 2013. The future direction of personalised nutrition: my diet, my phenotype, my genes. Proc. Nutr. Soc. 72, 219–225.

Gieger, C., Geistlinger, L., Altmaier, E., Hrabe de Angelis, M., Kronenberg, F., Meitinger, T., Mewes, H.W., Wichmann, H.E., Weinberger, K.M., Adamski, J., Illig, T., Suhre, K., 2008. Genetics meets metabolomics: a genome-wide association study of metabolite profiles in human serum. PLoS Genet. 4, e1000282.

Horigan, G., McNulty, H., Ward, M., Strain, J.J., Purvis, J., Scott, J.M., 2010. Riboflavin lowers blood pressure in cardiovascular disease patients homozygous for the 677C– >T polymorphism in MTHFR. J. Hypertens. 28, 478–486.

Illig, T., Gieger, C., Zhai, G., Romisch-Margl, W., Wang-Sattler, R., Prehn, C., Altmaier, E., Kastenmuller, G., Kato, B.S., Mewes, H.W., Meitinger, T., de Angelis, M.H., Kronenberg, F., Soranzo, N., Wichmann, H.E., Spector, T.D., Adamski, J., Suhre, K., 2010. A genome-wide perspective of genetic variation in human metabolism. Nat. Genet. 42, 137–141.

Kaddurah-Daouk, R., Boyle, S.H., Matson, W., Sharma, S., Matson, S., Zhu, H., Bogdanov, M. B., Churchill, E., Krishnan, R.R., Rush, A.J., Pickering, E., Delnomdedieu, M., 2011. Pretreatment metabotype as a predictor of response to sertraline or placebo in depressed outpatients: a proof of concept. Transl. Psychiatry 1, e26.

Li, J.V., Ashrafian, H., Bueter, M., Kinross, J., Sands, C., Le Roux, C.W., Bloom, S.R., Darzi, A., Athanasiou, T., Marchesi, J.R., Nicholson, J.K., Holmes, E., 2011. Metabolic surgery profoundly influences gut microbial-host metabolic cross-talk. Gut 60, 1214–1223.

Menni, C., Zhai, G., MacGregor, A., Prehn, C., Romisch-Margl, W., Suhre, K., Adamski, J., Cassidy, A., Illig, T., Spector, T.D., Valdes, A.M., 2013. Targeted metabolomics profiles are strongly correlated with nutritional patterns in women. Metabolomics 9, 506–514.

Nicholson, J.K., Everett, J.R., Lindon, J.C., 2012a. Longitudinal pharmacometabonomics for predicting patient responses to therapy: drug metabolism, toxicity and efficacy. Expert Opin. Drug Metab. Toxicol. 8, 135–139.

Nicholson, J.K., Holmes, E., Kinross, J., Burcelin, R., Gibson, G., Jia, W., Pettersson, S., 2012b. Host-gut microbiota metabolic interactions. Science 336, 1262–1267.

Nizel, A.E., 1972. Personalized nutrition counseling. ASDC J. Dent. Child. 39, 353–360.

Nyamundanda, G., Brennan, L., Gormley, I.C., 2010. Probabilistic principal component analysis for metabolomic data. BMC Bioinformatics 11, 571.

O'Sullivan, A., Gibney, M.J., Brennan, L., 2011a. Dietary intake patterns are reflected in metabolomic profiles: potential role in dietary assessment studies. Am. J. Clin. Nutr. 93, 314–321.

O'Sullivan, A., Gibney, M.J., Connor, A.O., Mion, B., Kaluskar, S., Cashman, K.D., Flynn, A., Shanahan, F., Brennan, L., 2011b. Biochemical and metabolomic phenotyping in the identification of a vitamin D responsive metabotype for markers of the metabolic syndrome. Mol. Nutr. Food Res. 55, 679–690.

Sha, W., da Costa, K.A., Fischer, L.M., Milburn, M.V., Lawton, K.A., Berger, A., Jia, W., Zeisel, S.H., 2010. Metabolomic profiling can predict which humans will develop liver dysfunction when deprived of dietary choline. FASEB J. 24, 2962–2975.

van Bochove, K., van Schalkwijk, D.B., Parnell, L.D., Lai, C.Q., Ordovas, J.M., de Graaf, A.A., van Ommen, B., Arnett, D.K., 2012. Clustering by plasma lipoprotein profile reveals two distinct subgroups with positive lipid response to fenofibrate therapy. PLoS One 7, e38072.

Wijeyesekera, A., Clarke, P.A., Bictash, M., Brown, I.J., Fidock, M., Ryckmans, T., Yap, I.K., Chan, Q., Stamler, J., Elliott, P., Holmes, E., Nicholson, J.K., 2012. Quantitative UPLC-MS/MS analysis of the gut microbial co-metabolites phenylacetylglutamine, 4-cresyl sulphate and hippurate in human urine: INTERMAP study. Anal. Methods 4, 65–72.

Wilson, C.P., Ward, M., McNulty, H., Strain, J.J., Trouton, T.G., Horigan, G., Purvis, J., Scott, J. M., 2012. Riboflavin offers a targeted strategy for managing hypertension in patients with the MTHFR 677TT genotype: a 4-y follow-up. Am. J. Clin. Nutr. 95, 766–772.

Winnike, J.H., Li, Z., Wright, F.A., MacDonald, J.M., O'Connell, T.M., Watkins, P.B., 2010. Use of pharmaco-metabonomics for early prediction of acetaminophen-induced hepatotoxicity in humans. Clin. Pharmacol. Ther. 88, 45–51.

Xie, G., Li, X., Li, H., Jia, W., 2013. Toward personalized nutrition: comprehensive phytoprofiling and metabotyping. J. Proteome Res. 12 (4), 1547–1559.

Using metabolomics to identify biomarkers for metabolic diseases: analytical methods and applications

8

J.-L. Sébédio[1,2], *S. Polakof*[1,2]
[1]Institut National de la Recherche Agronomique (INRA), Clermont-Ferrand, France;
[2]Clermont Université, Clermont-Ferrand, France

8.1 Introduction

Shifts in dietary pattern and food composition and processing, and a modification in physical activity collectively known as "nutritional transition", have led to an energy imbalance not only in the Western world but also in emerging countries with an increasing prevalence of overweight and obesity (Popkin, 2011) and the associated pathologies such as type 2 diabetes mellitus (T2DM). For a long time, research on the relationship between diet and health has considered the impact of isolated nutrients or food compounds and often in experimental conditions far from the complexity of the real diet. Numerous mechanistic hypotheses linking food consumption with biological effects have been generated by experiments on animal models or cells, but could not be validated in human studies.

Over the past few years, new concepts have emerged such as the "omics" technologies (transcriptomics, metabolomics, and proteomics). These have enabled an evolution from a rather reductionist approach towards a more promising integrative approach for nutrition because these technologies are capable of taking into account the multiplicity and interconnecting metabolic effects induced by diet. They have also opened a new way to analyse the effects of diets from gene to metabolites, giving unique insights into mechanisms underlying the development of chronic metabolic diseases, leading to a comprehensive phenotyping of individuals and determining biomarkers for early diagnosis of risks (screening biomarkers). Other biomarkers can also assist in the care of patients with suspected disease (diagnosis biomarkers) or with progression or remission of disease (prognostic biomarkers) (Roberts and Gerszten, 2013).

Among these new concepts, metabolomics which allows the measurement of a large fraction of the metabolites of a tissue or biofluids, is currently considered a promising approach to characterise the role of diet in the regulation of metabolic pathways underlying all biological processes. Its application to many research areas (Gika et al., 2014) has been increasing at an exponential rate since about 2005. Metabolomics has been successfully developed in pharmaceutical, medical (Armitage and Barbas, 2014;

Metabolomics as a Tool in Nutrition Research. http://dx.doi.org/10.1016/B978-1-78242-084-2.00008-3

Roux et al., 2011), and plant sciences; however, applications in nutrition are fewer. In recent years, metabolomics has been used to phenotype the nutritional status of individuals and to facilitate the discovery of new biomarkers associated with specific nutrients (food metabolome) (see Chapter 9) or metabolic dysfunctions (Herder et al., 2014).

Since 2007, several studies have shown that metabolomics analyses of biofluids could be used to distinguish individuals who are metabolically well from those who are metabolically unwell (Batch et al., 2013; Kim et al., 2010; Mihalik et al., 2012). This chapter will deal with the application of metabolomics to metabolic diseases, which are directly linked to nutritional patterns and more particularly metabolic syndrome (MetS), T2DM, and insulin resistance (IR). Both major animal and human intervention studies will be described. A section of this chapter will also deal with cohort studies, which are aiming to discover predictive biomarkers in order to identify individuals at risk for developing such pathologies.

8.2 Using metabolomics to understand the relationship between nutrition and chronic metabolic diseases

Numerous studies have been conducted in order to apply metabolomics to characterise the major metabolic-related chronic dysfunctions, including obesity, MS, IR, and T2DM. However, very few studies have applied metabolomics to elucidate the impact that nutrition may have on these diseases. Among the studies exploring the nutritionally related metabolic disorders, those using diets rich in fat (high-fat, HF) or free sugar constitute the majority, and this section will basically describe the published protocols, including a brief look at genetically modified models. Given that metabolomics can report directly the metabolic and physiological status of an organism at a given time, the number of studies employing metabolomics strategies to provide further insights into the molecular mechanisms at the basis of nutritionally related diseases has increased. Taking into account the important amount of data obtained in those studies, this section will discuss the different families of metabolites, which are currently suspected to be potential biomarker candidates of the metabolic disorders cited above.

8.2.1 *Acylcarnitines*

As stated above, metabolomics is now widely used as a tool able to put in evidence metabolic changes associated with different metabolic dysfunctions. Acylcarnitines have traditionally been used to measure inborn errors of metabolism, but in the last years, these have been shown to be markers of IR (see Table 8.1; Bain et al., 2009; Schooneman et al., 2013).

In a recent study, Barr et al. (2012) examined the plasma metabolome of individuals classified by their liver histological status (liver biopsies), including normal individuals or patients with nonalcoholic fatty liver disease (NAFLD) or with steatosis or nonalcoholic steatohepatitis (NASH). The authors found that the metabolic signature

Table 8.1 Summary of the most common metabolites discriminated in the metabolomics studies addressing differences among healthy and disturbed (metabolic perturbation) phenotypes

Molecule (biomarker)	Metabolic dysfunction	Species	Metabolic or physiological function affected	Reference
↑ Acylcarnitines	NASH (obese)	Human	Mitochondrial β-oxidation	Barr et al. (2012)
	Obesity/IR	Human/rat	BCAA metabolism	Koves et al. (2005, 2008), Newgard et al. (2009), and Sampey et al. (2012)
↑ Monoether phospholipids	NASH (obese)	Human	Peroxisome	Barr et al. (2012)
↑ Ceramides/sphingomyelin	NASH (lean)	Human	Lipotoxicity	
↓ Lysophosphocholines (16:1, 20:1, 20:1)	Obesity/IR	Mice	Insulin resistance/fat mass	Barber et al. (2012)
↓ Lysophosphocholines	T2DM	Human	Adiposity (no differences between obese and lean diabetic patients)	
↑ Valine, leucine, isoleucine	Obesity/IR	Human	Overload BCAA catabolism/ mitochondrial dysfunction	Newgard et al. (2009)
↑ Tyrosine, phenylalanine	Obesity/IR	Human		
↓ α-Ketoglutarate	Obesity/IR	Human		
↑ Valine, leucine, isoleucine	Obesity	Human	Insulin action in overweight and obese subjects	Huffman et al. (2009)
↓ Isoleucine	Overweight and obesity (weight loss protocol)	Human	Hypothetical promotion of lipolysis and suppression of lipogenesis	Perez-Cornago et al. (2014)
↑ Bile acids	NASH/steatosis	Human	Hypothetical higher bile acid pool due to a higher rate of bile acid synthesis	Kalhan et al. (2011)
↑ C3, C4, and C5 acylcarnitine	NASH/steatosis	Human	No mechanism proposed	
↓ Eicosapentaenoate, docosahexaenoate and 10-undecenoate	NASH/NAFLD	Human	No mechanism proposed	Kalhan et al. (2011) and Puri et al. (2007)

BCAA, branched chain amino acid.

was highly correlated with the body mass index (BMI) of the patients, suggesting evidence of different NAFLD as a function of the degree of obesity of the individuals. Increased levels of acylcarnitines, as biomarkers of mitochondrial β-oxidation dysfunction, were found in obese patients with NASH (Schooneman et al., 2013), but high levels of monoether phospholipids, evidencing peroxisome dysfunction, were also observed. Therefore, most of the changes evidenced in obese patients were related to the oxidation disposal of free fatty acid (FFA) routes. In a similar study, Kalham also reported that short-chain acylcarnitines were elevated in both NASH and steatotic patients when compared with the healthy control group (Kalhan et al., 2011). The profile was, however, different between both diseases, as NASH patients presented high levels of C3, C4, and C5 acylcarnitine, while in subjects suffering steatosis, only the C5 species were elevated. In the same study, some interesting changes in FFA levels were also reported, including lower levels of eicosapentaenoate (20:5*n*3), docosahexaenoate (22:6*n*3), and 10-undecenoate (11:1*n*1), in subjects with NASH, in agreement with the profile found in the hepatic tissue of NAFLD subjects (Puri et al., 2007). Unfortunately, no mechanisms explaining these changes were further studied, although the authors suggested that altered amino acid metabolism in the other peripheral tissue might contribute to the changes observed at the plasma level.

In the same line, metabolomics data from Brown et al. (2013) support this hypothesis, given that a limited capacity to oxidise fatty acid (FA) was reported when HepaRG cells develop a steatotic-like phenotype in the presence of palmitic acid. In more detail, increased levels of acetyl-CoA and reduced concentration of carnitine indicated that the mitochondrial function is impaired. Further, an altered β-oxidation capacity seems to be also reflected by the enhanced level of palmitoylcarnitine, as well as the accumulation of diacylglycerol (DAG) and monoacylglycerol (MAG), consistent with a lipotoxic phenotype and reactive oxygen species production.

Other studies also confirmed that the acylcarnitines can be potential biomarkers of the development of obesity and the associated IR. Among them, studies with obese and IR rats showed that either normal or Zucker diabetic rats when fed on an HF diet (HFD) accumulate several different species of acylcarnitines, with a possible impact on mitochondrial function, especially β-oxidation (Koves et al., 2005, 2008). This accumulation has also been observed in the muscle of HF-fed mice in parallel with a downregulation in the expression of peroxisome proliferator-activated receptor gamma coactivator 1α (PGC-1α). More interestingly, both effects were abolished by exercise (Koves et al., 2005). Together with the reduction in several TCA cycle intermediates, Muoio and Newgard suggested that the accumulation of incompletely oxidised lipid species in mitochondria (most of them being acylcarnitines) would be the result of a reduced metabolic flexibility. Further, the accumulation of incompletely oxidised substrates would cause mitochondrial stress, leading to impaired insulin action (Muoio and Newgard, 2008).

In another study, Sampey et al. (2012) revealed using a metabolomics approach that some acylcarnitines can act as biomarkers of a proinflammatory status in the context of obesity and IR. In this case, rats were fed with either a regular diet (*ad libitum*) or on a cafeteria diet (three human snack foods varied daily in addition to an *ad libitum* regular diet) for 10 weeks, and the plasma and liver metabolomes were then analysed. Rats fed with the cafeteria diet had higher levels of proinflammatory saturated fatty acids such as C12 (laurate) and C14 (myristate), as well as some acylcarnitine derivatives (lauroyl carnitine and myristoyl carnitine), compared with the control animals. Further, they demonstrated that lauroyl carnitine may act as a mediator of adipose tissue inflammation during obesity and dyslipidemic situations. Their data demonstrate that this acylcarnitine is able to inhibit the AMPK activation, a pathway known to promote an anti-inflammatory M2 macrophage phenotype (which promotes cell proliferation and tissue repair) associated with insulin sensitivity (Shah et al., 2011). Using an *in vitro* approach, they incubated bone marrow-derived macrophages in the presence of the lauroyl carnitine. The cytokine profile obtained after such exposure showed that the new phenotype corresponded to the M1 proinflammatory macrophages (which inhibits cell proliferation and causes tissue damage) and that the AMPK may be the signalling pathway responsible of such changes.

Finally, a few interventional studies in humans support the role association between the acylcarnitine metabolism and IR (Schooneman et al., 2013). In a first study on 16 obese and overweight subjects, acylcarnitine levels were followed postprandially by LC–MS/MS. The results showed that the response depended on their chain length and degree of unsaturation, with C14:0, C16:0, and C18:0 remaining unchanged, while unsaturated species (C14:1 and C14:2) falling significantly (Ramos-Roman et al., 2012). However, the magnitude of this decrease correlated with both premeal insulin-mediated glucose disposal rates and fatty acid oxidation and has been largely explained by nadir levels of C12:1, C14, and C14:1 carnitine. In another metabolomics study, 46 healthy overweight subjects were subjected to 6 months of caloric restriction (25%). The results showed that the concentrations of C2 acylcarnitine and long-chain ACs were positively associated with the amount of fat and the insulin sensitivity.

8.2.2 Branched-chain amino acids and other amino acids

Most of the data concerning the involvement of the branched-chain amino acids (BCAAs) come from the team of Christopher Newgard, who proposed in the late 2000s that these amino acids would reflect an impaired mitochondrial function, often observed during obesity and diabetes development (Table 8.1). In one of these studies, Newgard et al. (2009) reported that obese individuals, when compared with lean subjects, showed specific increases in C3 and C5 acylcarnitine levels and that this was strongly related to the metabolism of BCAAs. The authors suggested that these changes may reflect an overload of BCAA catabolism in obese subjects and explain this by changes in other metabolites, like the decreased levels of α-ketoglutarate and the increased levels of glutamate and aromatic amino acids, phenylalanine and tyrosine. In order to go further on this hypothesis, they tested if the same potential biomarkers were present in rats developing obesity and IR after feeding on an HFD supplemented with BCAAs at nutritional doses. They found that IR induced by HF/BCAA feeding was accompanied by changes in the same biomarkers, including those suggesting saturation in the capacity for mitochondrial fuel oxidation in muscle and a chronic activation of mammalian target of rapamycin and c-Jun N-terminal kinase and serine phosphorylation of IRS1 at the Ser^{307}. Among the mechanisms suggested to be responsible for such changes in plasma BCAAs, it has been proposed that the adipose tissue could play a central role, given its recently demonstrated capacity to regulate circulating BCAA levels (Herman et al., 2010; Newgard et al., 2009). BCAA levels were found to be higher in males vs. females but similar in Caucasians and African Americans (Patel et al., 2013). Furthermore, several studies have demonstrated that in obese, IR rodent models, liver and white adipose tissue branched-chain α-keto acid dehydrogenase (BCKD) abundance and/or activity is reduced when compared with lean controls (Adams, 2011). The situation in muscle is less clear, given that only small changes in some of the subunits have been reported so far. Consistent with this, using both targeted and untargeted metabolomics studies of plasma samples in humans, results seem to suggest that a reduction of BCKD activity would take place in obese, IR states. Among them, it has been demonstrated that in blood and urine of IR and T2DM subjects, the concentration of α-ketobutyrate and/or its derivate, the α-hydroxybutyrate, is enhanced (Fiehn et al., 2010; Gall et al., 2010; Salek et al., 2007). Very little is known about the changes observed at the hepatic level. Only *in vitro* data are available so far, showing that when HepaRG cells are exposed to palmitic acid for 48 h, increased accumulation of BCAA is observed, mostly in the first 24 h (Brown et al., 2013). This has been linked to the fact that the enhanced amount of BCAAs would constitute a contribution to the TCA activity that, according to this study, showed a delayed increased by the end of the incubation period (increased lactate and TCA intermediates). As a whole, this approach seems to support the idea that hepatic cells developing a steatotic phenotype would also suffer mitochondrial dysfunction.

Other trials have also confirmed that the BCAAs could act as reliable biomarkers of IR and obesity (Connell, 2013). A targeted metabolomics analysis of plasma from sedentary MetS individuals subjected to an oral glucose tolerance test revealed that 75 metabolites were associated with the disease (Huffman et al., 2009). Among them, amino acids, acylcarnitines, and FFAs revealed that large neutral amino acids, including BCAAs, were inversely associated with insulin sensitivity. Also, a recent metabolomics study in humans (UPLC/MS/MS) showed that valine, leucine, and isoleucine were elevated in the plasma of NASH in comparison with steatotic and healthy individuals (Kalhan et al., 2011), suggesting that in the first case, the hepatic damage would have already reached the mitochondria. Finally, the BCAAs have been also associated with the IR status in overweight and obese patients losing weight. Shah et al. (2012a,b) showed with a large number of participants ($n = 500$) losing about 8 kg over 6 months that the levels of BCAA and their related catabolites obtained by a targeted metabolomics approach were significantly correlated with the baseline HOMA-IR. Interestingly, this correlation was not further observed with the delta-HOMA-IR during the losing weight period. Importantly, in this trial, BCAAs and related metabolites were unique among a much larger and more diverse set of metabolites evaluated in predicting change in HOMA-IR and therefore suggest a potential mechanism for the heterogeneity in health benefits obtained from weight loss.

Other authors have also shown that other amino acids could also be considered as potential biomarkers of IR development (Table 8.1), given that their concentrations were factors that differentiate obese from lean subjects in several human studies (Fiehn et al., 2010; Newgard et al., 2009; Tai et al., 2010). In protocols developed in rodents, phenylalanine was suggested to act as biomarker of IR in obese rats, although no differences were observed between young and old animals (naturally developing IR) (Wijekoon et al., 2004). The same biomarker was found in NASH human patients (Kalhan et al., 2011), suggesting that this amino acid can be a key molecule in metabolic disorders with a common background. Similarly, other amino acids like aspartate and glutamate were also noticed as discriminant in the statistical analysis between normal and NASH individuals, which has been suggested to be related to an increased anaplerosis of amino acids into the TCA cycle, resulting in an increased cataplerosis to ensure the required removal of the resulting carbon skeletons of these amino acids from the cycle (Kalhan et al., 2011).

8.2.3 Lysophospholipids

Attention was also focused on the HF-induced metabolic disorders, like obesity, IR, and diabetes. Among the molecules frequently reported as potential biomarkers of such pathologies, lysophospholipids are the most commonly cited, especially in human studies (see Section 8.3 and Table 8.1). However, little is known about the mechanisms behind these changes. Barber et al. (2012) showed that in HF-fed mice developing obesity, higher levels of triacylglycerol (TG), DAG, and sphingolipids are observed when compared with the control group, but more interestingly, reduced levels of lysophosphatidylcholines (LysoPCs) were also reported. Strangely, no changes were observed in the most active tissues, like the liver, muscle, or adipose tissue allowing explaining those changes. However, some of the LysoPCs (16:1 and 20:1) were associated with the HOMA-IR index. The fact that after only 1 week of HFD, mice showed already reduced LysoPC levels and that those were associated with the fat mass rather than with the hyperglycaemia and hyperinsulinaemia suggest that an important nutritional component must exist. In order to complete these data, these LysoPCs were also measured in diabetic patients, and the same results were found although no differences were observed between obese and T2DM individuals. Again, the diet and adiposity seem to be at the origin of these LysoPC profiles, which were not explained in the publication.

In another intervention, Horakova et al. (2012) fed mice during 8 weeks with a HFD (35% lipids) alone or supplemented with either long-chain PUFA $n-3$, rosiglitazone, or both. Muscle homogenates were analysed by flow-injection analysis–mass spectrometry (FIA–MS), and 15 LysoPCs were quantified. Three species, LysoPC 18:0, LysoPC 18:2 and LysoPC 20:4, showed reduced levels in the group fed with the LC-PUFA-enriched diet, with the combined intervention with rosiglitazone having a stronger effect. This reduction in muscle LysoPC was suggested to be related to a reduced inflammation in the tissue, given that these molecules could be associated with obesity-induced low-grade systemic inflammation and that phospholipase A2-derived LysoPCs exert adverse effects on insulin responsiveness of myocytes (Han et al., 2011). In a very similar study, Kus et al. (2011) had already reported that the plasma levels of the same LysoPC were reduced in the obese mouse when fed with an LC-PUFA-enriched diet. The protective effect of several LysoPCs had already been suggested in humans consuming important amounts of fish. Lankinen et al. (2009) demonstrated in an interventional study that subjects consuming four portions of fish during 8 weeks had lower LysoPC plasma levels than those consuming no fish at all. They suggested that the decrease in LysoPC in the fish group may be related to anti-inflammatory effects of $n-3$ fatty acids, given that LysoPC is the major bioactive lipid component of oxidised low density lipoprotein (LDL) and may be responsible for many of the inflammatory effects of oxidised LDL (Aiyar et al., 2007). They demonstrated that EPA and DHA were related not only with the plasma long-chain TG but also with LysoPC.

8.2.4 Other metabolites

Among the other metabolites that have been reported by metabolomics as possible biomarkers of metabolic diseases (Table 8.1), we can cite taurine as one of the most popular. Also known as 2-aminoethanesulphonic acid, taurine is an organic acid participating in the conjugation of cholesterol and bile acids, and several studies have reported its possible involvement in obesity (Xie et al., 2012). Using both ^{1}H NMR and UPLC–MS approaches, metabolomics studies on urine of obese animal models showed that taurine levels were low when compared with those of normal individuals. This included Zucker rats (Waldram et al., 2009; Williams et al., 2006) and genetically modified mice. In the latter case, also, lower hepatic expression levels of the cysteine sulphinic acid dehydrogenase enzyme were reported (Schirra et al., 2008). From this study, despite the fact that other authors reported that taurine levels actually increased during obesity in the liver of rodents (Klein et al., 2011; Rubio-Aliaga et al., 2011; Schirra et al., 2008), it has been concluded that a reduction in the hepatic taurine production could be associated with obesity (Xie et al., 2012). However, the elevation of hepatic taurine and the decreased production of biosynthesised taurine in obesity induced by HFD are associated with depletion of the blood taurine concentrations. In fact, this situation was already observed in both obese rodents (Duggan et al., 2011b) and humans (Jeevanandam et al., 1991), and more interestingly, it has been shown that it could be reversed by increasing the amount of dietary taurine intake. It was proposed by Tsuboyama-Kasaoka et al. that the imbalance in taurine metabolism would modify the ability to oxidise fatty acids and then that increasing taurine intake would improve FA oxidation, counteracting the obesity-related taurine depletion (Tsuboyama-Kasaoka et al., 2006).

Kim et al. (2009) also showed that metabolomics allows discrimination between different phenotypes consuming the same deleterious diet. In this particular study, animals were classified as low- and high-weight gainers fed with either a normal diet (ND) or a HFD. Analyses were made on urine by ^{1}H NMR. The obtained data allowed discrimination between both low- and high-weight gainers, even on the ND groups fed with the same diet, suggesting that despite the same amount of food consumed, those animals were actually different metabolically. Among the metabolites allowing discrimination between these two groups, the authors cited betaine, taurine, acetone/acetoacetate, phenylacetylglycine, pyruvate, lactate, and citrate. Surprisingly, this was not the case for the low- and high-weight gainers HF-fed rats. The other two groups that were clearly discriminated by the multivariate analyses were the low-weight gainers on the ND and the high-weight gainers on the HFD, and the same metabolites were found to be responsible for the discrimination, although the relative weight was not the same.

Li et al. (2010) investigated early metabolite changes during the development of diet-induced hepatic IR using a Gpat1 −/− mouse model fed on a HFD (sunflower oil). Animals were fed during 3 weeks. Both liver and plasma samples were analysed by GC–MS and LC–MS using a nontargeted approach. In the liver, the increases in three urea cycle-related metabolites were consistent with an enhanced use of amino acids for gluconeogenesis as IR developed and were interpreted by the authors as an early symptom of hepatic IR installation. Other metabolites modified in the wild-type model were taurocholate, which reduction, in both liver and plasma, suggests a possible decrease in bile acid synthesis or an increase in bile acid secretion, yet neither of these aspects were further explored in the paper. In this sense, a recent *in vitro* study by Brown et al. (2013) confirmed that in HepaGR cells developing a steatotic phenotype, taurocholate levels were also reduced, suggesting that these cells were probably at the onset of an IR installation.

In a similar study on mice, but using ^{1}H NMR instead of LC–MS for analysing plasma metabolome, Duggan et al. (2011a) reported that metabolomics analysis of serum samples allowed differentiating the short- and long-term effects of chow and HFDs. The major finding showed that the final week's diet was the predominant contributor to the metabolic profile (stronger than obesity). In this sense, several metabolites, like valine, leucine, isoleucine, glutamine, and glutamate, responded similarly regardless of the treatment in the final week, and these were associated with obesity. Other metabolites responded differently when the final week's diet returned to a normal fat content (H–C), including glucose, creatine, ornithine, taurine, pyruvate, alanine, and lactate. The authors suggested that these changes resulted from the diet rather from obesity.

Bile acids are also a family of metabolites that has been mentioned in some studies as discriminatory molecules in several metabolic diseases, especially those when liver activity seems to be compromised. Among the data so far published, the study of Kalhan et al. (2011) showed that the concentrations of glycocholate, taurocholate, and glycochenodeoxycholate were markedly higher in subjects with NASH, while taurocholate and glycochenodeoxycholate were only significantly higher in subjects with steatosis. Although the mechanism behind these changes remains to be elucidated, mechanistic hypotheses included an increased peroxisomal and microsomal metabolism or possibly an adaptive response to the accumulation of triglycerides in the liver. In any case, it seems that a compromised hepatic function would be responsible of such altered profiles, as the healthy liver is able to efficiently capture and remove bile acids from the hepatic portal circulation. The final possibility could be the involvement of the IR condition, often reported in these patients, given that in animal models of diabetes, higher plasma bile acid levels were reported. Furthermore, this profile would be corrected by insulin therapy (Wei et al., 2009).

8.3 Cohort studies and biomarker identification

As described in Section 8.2, a large part of the data published so far on this topic was dealing with animal models using feeding studies or human-controlled interventions but often with protocols based only on the comparison between cases and control subjects. It is only recently that longitudinal observations either on small number of individuals or on large cohorts were published. When dealing with cohorts, one major problem is the sample size, which may be used especially when using UPLC–MS as a tool, and often the ongoing studies have been carried out with 400–500 individuals when using this technique (see Chapter 1 for detailed explanations). A much greater number of samples may be analysed when using NMR, and it is always difficult to find a good compromise between number of subjects, sensitivity of the technique, and chemical composition of the biological tissue. Different cohorts have been used both for determining biomarkers of metabolic dysfunctions and for providing metabolite profiles predicting the risk of developing pathologies such as T2DM.

Among these cohorts, much data have been published using the Framingham Offspring Study (http://www.framinghamheartstudy.org for more details). This cohort consisted of subjects who were 30–50 years old and free of coronary heart diseases and who were either genetic or adoptive offspring or spouses of offspring of the original Framingham Heart Study (Wilson et al., 1991). Among the normoglycaemic subjects ($n=2422$) who had a routine examination between 1991 and 1995, 201 developed diabetes during the 12-year follow-up (cases). Metabolite profiling from 189 individuals (negative for diabetes diagnosis at the time the blood was collected) (Wang et al., 2011) was performed at baseline using a targeted UPLC–MS approach. Controls (189 subjects negative for diabetes diagnosis at the time the blood was collected and who did not develop diabetes) were matched for age, BMI, and fasting glucose. The experimental protocol is described in Figure 8.1. Five branched-chain (BCAA) and aromatic amino acids, namely, isoleucine, leucine, valine, tyrosine, and phenylalanine, were found to be highly associated with the future incidence of diabetes. Further examination of the data revealed that the association of three

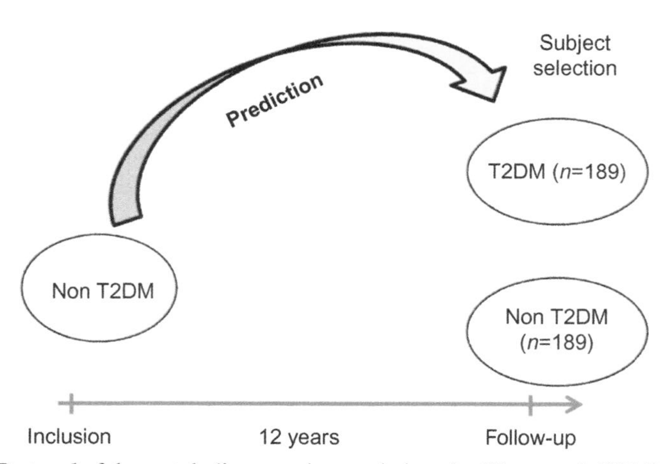

Figure 8.1 Protocol of the metabolic screening carried out by Wang et al. (2011), in the frame of the Framingham Offspring Study.

molecules (isoleucine, tyrosine, and phenylalanine) could predict that individuals in the top quartile had a five to sevenfold higher risk of developing diabetes, compared with subjects in the lowest quartile. The association of these three amino acids was also tested in another cohort, the Malmö Diet Cancer study (http://snd.gu.se/en/catalogue/study/EXT0012, for more details). Similarly, people being in the upper quartile had a fourfold higher risk compared with those in the lowest one. The strength of this study is the long period of follow-up selected (12 years using a well-known cohort), the utilisation of classical clinical biomarkers in association with a metabolomics approach, and the validation of the potential prospective biomarkers using two other cohorts. One of the weak points of using a targeted approach was the number of quantified metabolites (61). However, this targeted approach permitted a highly specific identification of metabolites, but indications of the families of molecules, which may be linked to diabetes, have already been found in case–control approaches using a limited number of subjects as described in Section 8.2. Further data using other targeted methods were recently published based on subjects from the same cohort. Using 188 case and 188 control subjects of the same cohort who did not developed diabetes, both being followed for 12 years, a UPLC targeted approach on 70 metabolites (Wang et al., 2013; Weir et al., 2013) showed that 2-aminoadipic acid, a product of lysine degradation, was increased up to 12 years before the onset of diabetes but this compound did not correlate well with the previously described amino acids suggesting an action on a distinct pathway. In the same study, this compound was also shown to modulate glucose homeostasis in mice using both a chow diet and a HFD and to enhance *in vitro* insulin secretion from a pancreatic β-cell line and in isolated islets. In this case, the replication was carried out on 162 individuals from the cohorts previously mentioned. From these data, the authors hypothesised that this amino acid product may contribute to a compensatory effect, upregulating insulin secretion to maintain glucose homeostasis.

Other studies have investigated the potential role of lipids as predictive biomarkers of developing metabolic diseases. The San Antonio Family Heart Study (http://www.txbiomed.org/departments/genetics/genetics-detail?p=24) has identified, after analyses of 300 lipid plasma species in 1000 individuals, some correlations between circulating molecular lipid species (ceramide, lysophospholipids) and common anthropometric, physiological, and lifestyle parameters such as age, sex, obesity, and smoking (Weir et al., 2013). In the population-based KORA (Cooperative Health Research in the Region of Augsburg) (http://epi.gsf.de/kora-gen/index_e.php) study, a targeted lipidomic approach (Jourdan et al., 2012) showed that a decrease in chain length or in unsaturation of the fatty acid moieties of various phosphatidylcholines (PCs) was observed with increasing the fat-free mass index. Using the same cohort and a targeted approach on 140 metabolites, a lysophospholipid-containing linoleic acid (LPL-18:2) was also found correlated with impaired glucose tolerance and T2DM (Wang-Sattler et al., 2012). In the Cancer and Nutrition (EPIC)-Potsdam study (http://www.epic-oxford.org/home/) ($n = 800$ cases with a 7-year follow-up), and using a targeted approach on 163 metabolites, with replication in the KORA cohort, Floegel et al. (2013) confirmed the role that phospholipids derivatives may play, showing that 14 metabolites were positively associated with T2DM risk. For example, diacyl-phosphatidylcholines (C32:1, C36:1, C40:5, etc.) were positive while sphingomyelin C16:1, LPC-18:2, acyl-alkyl-phosphatidylcholines and ether lipid isomers (C34:3, C40:6, etc.) were significantly inversely related to T2DM risk. Furthermore, when comparing extreme quintiles, two factors, each of them being composed of a complex set of metabolites, are positively or negatively associated with risk of T2DM. The data on amino acids also confirmed those obtained by Wang et al. (2011). Lipid profiling carried out on subjects from the Framingham Offspring Study (Rhee et al., 2011) previously described also identified a relationship between lipid acyl chain content and diabetes risk. For example, lipids with lower carbon and double-bond numbers were associated with increased risk of diabetes, and it was proposed that triacylglycerols (TAGs) profiling included in clinical models could contribute to improve diabetes prediction, and efforts will be put to further study this possibility by this research team using different cohorts. A nested case–control design (2114 participants without history of diabetes) within the Cancer and Nutrition (EPIC)-Potsdam study (27,548 subjects) has shown that fatty acid profile of erythrocyte membrane phospholipids (16:1$n-7$, 18:3$n-6$, and fatty acid ratios) and activity of desaturase enzymes (stearoyl desaturase and $\Delta 5$ and $\Delta 6$ desaturases) are also linked to the incidence of T2DM (Kröger et al., 2011). On the contrary, dietary fatty acids showed only modest to low correlation with erythrocyte fatty acids and were not associated with risk. In this study, blood was obtained at baseline between 1994 and 1998 along with a food frequency questionnaire, and follow-up questionnaires were given every 2–3 years to identify chronic diseases such as T2DM during a mean follow-up of 7 years where 673 cases of diabetes (evaluated by self-reporting under the supervision of a physician) were retained for analyses. In summary, this study suggests that low $\Delta 5$ and high $\Delta 6$ activities may predict the development of diabetes.

Metabolic profiling was also carried out using NMR on blood tests after a 12 h fasting and after a 75 g of glucose load (OGTT). This study (Würtz et al., 2012b) included a total of 1873 middle-aged participants, free of lipid-lowering medication and diabetes treatment from two Finish population-based cohorts, the Pieksamaki cohort and the Health 2000 study, and a 6.5-year follow-up (only for the Pieksamaki cohort). In both cases (with or without OGTT), 19 metabolites were associated with glycaemia. These included gluconeogenesis substrates, branched-chain and aromatic amino acids, and fatty acid species. These were associated with increased glycaemia except for glycine, ω6/total fatty acids, and double bonds/fatty acid chain. Gluconeogenesis substrates such as alanine, lactate, and pyruvate were selective predictors of 6.5-year post load of glucose indicating that these metabolites may be markers of a later deteriorating glucose tolerance. The role of BCAA was again confirmed, but none of the lipid measures predicted future glycaemia in this study.

The potential role of BCAAs as biomarkers of T2DM and impaired fasting glucose (IFG) was again confirmed in the TwinsUK (http://www.twinsuk.ac.uk) and Health Ageing Study (Menni et al., 2013; Moayyeri et al., 2013). A combination of well-established factors (such as age, BMI, and fasting glucose) with a semitargeted metabolomics approach on 447 plasma metabolites and urine samples taken at the same time as plasma was used in order to cover a broader range of metabolites than those discussed above. Female subjects ($n = 536$ with IFG and 184 control individuals) from the KORA study were used as a replication cohort. Forty-two metabolites (carbohydrates, lipids, and amino acids) (Figure 8.2) were found to be significantly correlated with T2DM, 22 of these already being reported to be associated with T2DM or IR. Fourteen metabolites were correlated with IFG and 3-methyl-2-oxovalerate, the strongest predictive biomarker for IFG after glucose (Menni et al., 2013). Furthermore, urine was also shown to be a potential biofluid to be analysed as this compound

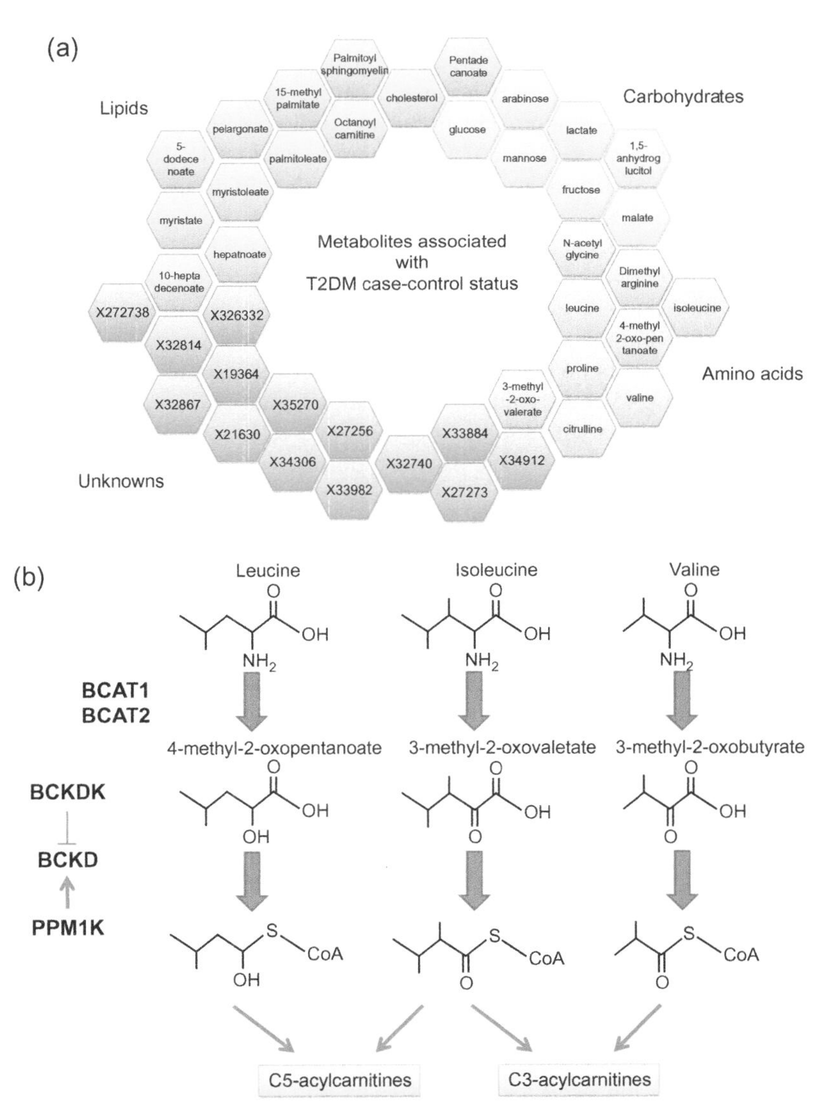

Figure 8.2 (a) Metabolites associated with the T2DM status in the TwinsUK and Health Ageing Study and (b) the BCAA catabolism with conversion to BCKAs. Adapted from Menni et al. (2013).

was significantly correlated with IFG, and this may help disease prediction and consequently early intervention. Considering that 3-methyl-2-oxovalerate is a branched-chain keto acid derivative from isoleucine (Figure 8.2), the authors consequently wondered if the products of BCAA catabolism, which primarily occurs in the mitochondria, would not be molecules that are associated with diabetes and not the elevated levels of BCAAs themselves.

High-throughput metabolite profiling on cohorts is also now being studied for evaluating the possibility of predicting more advanced cardiometabolic diseases such as atherosclerosis and coronary artery diseases (Shah et al., 2012a,b; Wurtz et al., 2012a) and also chronic kidney diseases (Rhee et al., 2013). NMR analyses of blood samples (untargeted metabolomics approach) from the Cardiovascular Risk in Young Finns Study (http://youngfinnsstudy.utu.fi, for more details) (1595 individuals aged 24–39) was combined with measurements of circulating lipids, lipoprotein subclasses, and carotid intima–media thickness (IMT), markers of subclinical atherosclerosis done at 6 years' interval. Quantification of circulating metabolites improved risk stratification of atherosclerosis in comparison with classical lipid risk factors, and systemic levels of 22:6$n-3$, glutamine, and tyrosine were identified as predictors of carotid IMT, showing the potential of this approach for strategies in the prevention of cardiovascular events (Wurtz et al., 2012a). A total of 69 metabolites (a targeted approach) including 45 acylcarnitines and 15 amino acids were quantified in plasma samples of 2023 patients with a follow-up of about 3 years undergoing cardiac catheterisation from the MURDOCK CV Study (https://www.murdock-study.com, for more details) (Shah et al., 2012a,b). The objective was to combine metabolic profiling with clinical data (LDL and HDL cholesterol, triglycerides, glucose, etc.) in order to improve risk classification. Three factors (metabolite families), fatty acids (factor 12) and short- and long-chain dicarboxylacylcarnitines (factors 2 and 3), were shown to be independently predictive of future cardiovascular events (death/myocardial infarction), and their utilisation improves risk discrimination when combined with classical clinical data. In the Malmö Diet Cancer Cardiovascular Cohort, Magnusson et al. (2013) found branched-chain and aromatic amino acids as an early link between diabetes and CVD susceptibility during 12 years of follow-up (Magnusson et al., 2013).

In order to evaluate if serum metabolomics profile alteration could be used to find early and specific markers of chronic kidney disease (CKD), which is nowadays evaluated using serum creatinine and urea, Rhee et al. (2013) followed for 8 years 1434 participants who did not have CKD at inclusion in the Framingham Heart Study. During that period, 123 individuals out of the 1434 subjects developed CKD. Metabolic profiling was achieved on plasma baseline samples and on plasma and urine samples from patients undergoing aortic and renal vein catheterisation ($n=9$). Sixteen metabolites were significantly associated with incident CKD. Among them, 13 were higher in cases compared with individuals who did not develop a CKD. These markers were tryptophan-derived metabolites, choline derivatives, citric acid cycle intermediates, purine metabolites, and two LysoPCs (18:1 and 18:2), both of them being lower in cases. Eight metabolites, namely, citrulline, choline, kynurenic acid, hydroxyindoleacetic acid, aconitate, isocitrate, xanthosine, and β-aminoisobutyric acid, were highlighted as potential candidate biomarkers of CKD risk.

The combination of clinical data obtained from cohorts follow-up with metabolomics now offers a great potential to discover novel biomarkers and to predict the evolution of health status towards chronic metabolic pathologies, and this could offer in the future the possibility of developing new nutritional strategies to delay the onset of such diseases. However, looking at studies carried out on large cohorts (Valdes et al., 2013; Yu et al., 2012), tissue metabolomics profiles are known to change with age. Consequently, the study protocol should be carefully designed in order to take into consideration the possible changes, which may occur between the baseline or intermediary measurements, and the declaration of the pathology obtained using the classical clinical biomarkers.

8.4 Isolating *in situ* biomarkers

In the last few years, the possibility to detect *in situ* a wide number of metabolites and families of compounds based on MS methods has been offered to scientists interested in obtaining the distribution of biological compounds over a tissue section with a high resolution. The two most popular approaches are matrix-assisted laser desorption/ionisation–mass spectrometry, which needs the cocrystallisation of the sample with a matrix before to be irradiated by a laser, and secondary ion mass spectrometry (SIMS), where the analyte is directly desorbed by a primary ion bombardment. As explained above, the main advantage of these techniques when compared with other chemical imaging techniques lies in the ability to acquire a large number of biological compounds in mixture with an excellent sensitivity thanks to the time-of-flight (ToF) mass analyser (Touboul et al., 2011).

Despite all the advantages offered by the metabolic imaging based on MS, only a few studies have utilised this approach in order to elaborate the metabolic *in situ* image of a tissue or organ at a given time. In this sense, most of the scientists have focused their interest on the hepatic metabolic imaging, especially related to the fatty liver. Le Naour et al. published one of the first reports based on this kind of metabolomics approach. They applied the synchrotron FTIR (Fourier transform infrared) and ToF–-SIMS microspectroscopies on hepatic biopsies from patients suffering from steatosis (Le Naour et al., 2009). Their analyses of the liver samples suggest that the lipid environment between the inside and the outside of the steatotic vesicles was actually different. The differences seemed to be based on a selective enrichment of cholesterol and DAG species carrying alkyl chains. DAG C36 were found inside the vesicles, while the DAG C30 were specifically detected outside. Much more interesting was the comparison of the same sample of the nonsteatotic part of the fatty liver with normal livers. The spectrometry data revealed that although a normal histological aspect was reported, small lipid droplets corresponding to the first steps of lipid accretion discriminate both phenotypes. Another similar study by Debois et al. in 2009 also reported important differences in the lipidomic profiles of normal and steatotic liver samples (Debois et al., 2009). The ToF–SIMS analysis showed that the normal human liver was actually zoned and that in some of these areas, very similar lipids to those detected in areas of the fatty livers were found, which was not characterised as steatotic ones by the histological control performed on serial tissue sections. Regarding the molecules characterising the metabolomics signature of the steatotic livers, the results were in accordance with those of Le Naour et al., showing the accumulation of TAG, DAG, MAG, and fatty acids, together with a dramatic depletion of vitamin E and a selective macrovacuolar localisation of cholesterol. Further, these ion species were concentrated in small vesicles of a few micrometres. A third study from a different team explored also the differential intrahepatic zonation in simple steatosis and NASH biopsies (Wattacheril et al., 2013). In this case, the authors hypothesised that specific phospholipid zonation may exist in the liver and that this specific phospholipid abundance and distribution may be associated with histological disease. Using a matrix-assisted laser desorption/ionisation–imaging mass spectrometry imaging, they found that effectively, a strong zonal distribution existed for 32, 34, and 36 carbon PCs in controls and steatotic biopsies but that this metabolic signature disappeared in NASH specimens. This was especially true for some of the lipid species such as PC 34:1 and PC 36:2. Finally, Magnusson et al. (2008) provided an example of the application of ToF–SIMS imaging on extrahepatic tissues. They used this technology to characterise the lipid distribution of the human skeletal muscle biopsies. In summary, they found that phosphocholines were located at the edge of the fibres (sarcoplasma), while DAG was reported in the intracellular areas, where low TAG and cholesterol intensities were also detected.

8.5 Conclusions and future trends

Approaches using different animal models, nutritional interventions in human, and clinical and biofluids analyses of case vs. control individuals enrolled in cohort studies have been published within the past 10 years using metabolomics and other "omics" techniques in order to find early biomarkers to identify population at risk to develop metabolic diseases. Animal studies have shown that the metabolome may change along with the development of metabolic disorders and that those changes can be reflected in specific metabolic signatures or profiles. In this sense, several families of metabolites were found to be altered at the onset of the IR and obesity of T2DM installation. Among them are several acylcarnitines and BCCA, which apparently are interconnected. Several metabolomics studies revealed that changes in those metabolites could reflect early mitochondrial dysfunction, especially at the β-oxidation capacity. Although both animal and human studies agree with the idea that these metabolites could be considered as biomarkers of some metabolic disorders, the mechanism behind these changes remains to be elucidated, although the role of BCKD enzymes at the adipose tissue levels cannot be discarded. The other big family of metabolites being strongly affected by the development of metabolic disorders and therefore susceptible to be considered as biomarkers is the LysoPCs, which seem to be rather inflammatory indicators than markers of a particular metabolic status. Despite the important volume of papers published concerning phospholipids as biomarkers, no mechanistic information is available today, and further studies would be needed in order to elucidate their role during the installation of metabolic disorders. In cohort studies, the combination of metabolomics with the classical clinical parameters permits to give a better prediction of the evolution of health status towards chronic metabolic pathologies. However, most of the studies so far published used analyses of a limited number of metabolites, which may be a limitation, compared to what may be obtained using untargeted approaches. For example, targeted studies on 257 metabolites carried out in two large cohort studies, the Nurses' Health Study and Health Professionals Follow-up Study, have shown that the majority of plasma metabolites were reproducible over a 24 h processing delay and within individual subjects over 1–2 years (Townsend et al., 2013). However, all these cohorts that have been used so far have a 7–12-year follow-up, which represents a gold asset for carrying out such studies. In general, the blood has been used as a biofluid of choice, but recent data also pointed out that urine would also give complementary information.

The recently published studies carried out using large cohorts but most of the time using targeted analyses on a small number of metabolites show strong evidence supporting the use of BCAAs as potential biomarkers of diseases such as T2DM (Batch et al., 2014). However, questions regarding the mechanisms underlying the correlation between BCAAs and diseases have to be answered before those can be used in clinical practices for disease detection.

References

Adams, S.H., 2011. Emerging perspectives on essential amino acid metabolism in obesity and the insulin-resistant state. Adv. Nutr. 2, 445–456.

Aiyar, N., Disa, J., Ao, Z., Ju, H., Nerurkar, S., Willette, R.N., MacPhee, C.H., Johns, D.G., Douglas, S.A., 2007. Lysophosphatidylcholine induces inflammatory activation of human coronary artery smooth muscle cells. Mol. Cell. Biochem. 295, 113–120.

Armitage, E.G., Barbas, C., 2014. Metabolomics in cancer biomarker discovery: current trends and future perspectives. J. Pharm. Biomed. Anal. 87, 1–11.

Bain, J.R., Stevens, R.D., Wenner, B.R., Ilkayeva, O., Muoio, D.M., Newgard, C.B., 2009. Metabolomics applied to diabetes research: moving from information to knowledge. Diabetes 58, 2429–2443.

Barber, M.N., Risis, S., Yang, C., Meikle, P.J., Staples, M., Febbraio, M.A., Bruce, C.R., 2012. Plasma lysophosphatidylcholine levels are reduced in obesity and type 2 diabetes. PLoS One 7, e41456.

Barr, J., Caballeria, J., Martinez-Arranz, I., Dominguez-Diez, A., Alonso, C., Muntane, J., Perez-Cormenzana, M., Garcia-Monzon, C., Mayo, R., Martin-Duce, A., Romero-Gomez, M., Lo Iacono, O., Tordjman, J., Andrade, R.J., Perez-Carreras, M., Le Marchand-Brustel, Y., Tran, A., Fernandez-Escalante, C., Arevalo, E., Garcia-Unzueta, M., Clement, K., Crespo, J., Gual, P., Gomez-Fleitas, M., Martinez-Chantar, M.L., Castro, A., Lu, S.C., Vazquez-Chantada, M., Mato, J.M., 2012. Obesity-dependent metabolic signatures associated with nonalcoholic fatty liver disease progression. J. Proteome Res. 11, 2521–2532.

Batch, B.C., Shah, S.H., Newgard, C.B., Turer, C.B., Haynes, C., Bain, J.R., Muehlbauer, M., Patel, M.J., Stevens, R.D., Appel, L.J., Newby, L.K., Svetkey, L.P., 2013. Branched chain amino acids are novel biomarkers for discrimination of metabolic wellness. Metabolism 62, 961–969.

Batch, B.C., Hyland, K., Svetkey, L.P., 2014. Branch chain amino acids: biomarkers of health and disease. Curr. Opin. Clin. Nutr. Metab. Care 17, 86–89. http://dx.doi.org/10.1097/MCO.0000000000000010.

Brown, M.V., Compton, S.A., Milburn, M.V., Lawton, K.A., Cheatham, B., 2013. Metabolomic signatures in lipid-loaded HepaRGs reveal pathways involved in steatotic progression. Obesity 21, E561–E570.

Connell, T., 2013. The complex role of branched chain amino acids in diabetes and cancer. Metabolites 3, 931–945.

Debois, D., Bralet, M.P., Le Naour, F., Brunelle, A., Laprevote, O., 2009. In situ lipidomic analysis of nonalcoholic fatty liver by cluster TOF-SIMS imaging. Anal. Chem. 81, 2823–2831.

Duggan, G.E., Hittel, D.S., Hughey, C.C., Weljie, A., Vogel, H.J., Shearer, J., 2011a. Differentiating short- and long-term effects of diet in the obese mouse using (1) H-nuclear magnetic resonance metabolomics. Diabetes Obes. Metab. 13, 859–862.

Duggan, G.E., Hittel, D.S., Sensen, C.W., Weljie, A.M., Vogel, H.J., Shearer, J., 2011b. Metabolomic response to exercise training in lean and diet-induced obese mice. J. Appl. Physiol. 110, 1311–1318.

Fiehn, O., Garvey, W.T., Newman, J.W., Lok, K.H., Hoppel, C.L., Adams, S.H., 2010. Plasma metabolomic profiles reflective of glucose homeostasis in non-diabetic and type 2 diabetic obese African-American women. PLoS One 5, e15234.

Floegel, A., Stefan, N., Yu, Z., Mühlenbruch, K., Drogan, D., Joost, H.-G., Fritsche, A., Häring, H.-U., De Angelis, M.H., Peters, A., 2013. Identification of serum metabolites associated with risk of type 2 diabetes using a targeted metabolomic approach. Diabetes 62, 639–648.

Gall, W.E., Beebe, K., Lawton, K.A., Adam, K.P., Mitchell, M.W., Nakhle, P.J., Ryals, J.A., Milburn, M.V., Nannipieri, M., Camastra, S., Natali, A., Ferrannini, E., Group, R.S., 2010. Alpha-hydroxybutyrate is an early biomarker of insulin resistance and glucose intolerance in a nondiabetic population. PLoS One 5, e10883.

Gika, H.G., Theodoridis, G.A., Plumb, R.S., Wilson, I.D., 2014. Current practice of liquid chromatography-mass spectrometry in metabolomics and metabonomics. J. Pharm. Biomed. Anal. 87, 12–25.

Han, M.S., Lim, Y.M., Quan, W., Kim, J.R., Chung, K.W., Kang, M., Kim, S., Park, S.Y., Han, J.S., Park, S.Y., Cheon, H.G., Dal Rhee, S., Park, T.S., Lee, M.S., 2011. Lysophosphatidylcholine as an effector of fatty acid-induced insulin resistance. J. Lipid Res. 52, 1234–1246.

Herder, C., Kowall, B., Tabak, A.G., Rathmann, W., 2014. The potential of novel biomarkers to improve risk prediction of type 2 diabetes. Diabetologia 57, 16–29.

Herman, M.A., She, P., Peroni, O.D., Lynch, C.J., Kahn, B.B., 2010. Adipose tissue branched chain amino acid (BCAA) metabolism modulates circulating BCAA levels. J. Biol. Chem. 285, 11348–11356.

Horakova, O., Medrikova, D., VAN Schothorst, E.M., Bunschoten, A., Flachs, P., Kus, V., Kuda, O., Bardova, K., Janovska, P., Hensler, M., Rossmeisl, M., Wang-Sattler, R., Prehn, C., Adamski, J., Illig, T., Keijer, J., Kopecky, J., 2012. Preservation of metabolic flexibility in skeletal muscle by a combined use of n-3 PUFA and rosiglitazone in dietary obese mice. PLoS One 7, e43764.

Huffman, K.M., Shah, S.H., Stevens, R.D., Bain, J.R., Muehlbauer, M., Slentz, C.A., Tanner, C. J., Kuchibhatla, M., Houmard, J.A., Newgard, C.B., Kraus, W.E., 2009. Relationships between circulating metabolic intermediates and insulin action in overweight to obese, inactive men and women. Diabetes Care 32, 1678–1683.

Jeevanandam, M., Ramias, L., Schiller, W.R., 1991. Altered plasma free amino acid levels in obese traumatized man. Metabolism 40, 385–390.

Jourdan, C., Petersen, A.-K., Gieger, C., Döring, A., Illig, T., Wang-Sattler, R., Meisinger, C., Peters, A., Adamski, J., Prehn, C., 2012. Body fat free mass is associated with the serum metabolite profile in a population-based study. PLoS One 7, e40009.

Kalhan, S.C., Guo, L., Edmison, J., Dasarathy, S., McCullough, A.J., Hanson, R.W., Milburn, M., 2011. Plasma metabolomic profile in nonalcoholic fatty liver disease. Metabolism 60, 404–413.

Kim, S.H., Yang, S.O., Kim, H.S., Kim, Y., Park, T., Choi, H.K., 2009. 1H-nuclear magnetic resonance spectroscopy-based metabolic assessment in a rat model of obesity induced by a high-fat diet. Anal. Bioanal. Chem. 395, 1117–1124.

Kim, J.Y., Park, J.Y., Kim, O.Y., Ham, B.M., Kim, H.J., Kwon, D.Y., Jang, Y., Lee, J.H., 2010. Metabolic profiling of plasma in overweight/obese and lean men using ultra performance liquid chromatography and Q-TOF mass spectrometry (UPLC-Q-TOF MS). J. Proteome Res. 9, 4368–4375.

Klein, M., Dorn, C., Saugspier, M., Hellerbrand, C., Oefner, P., Gronwald, W., 2011. Discrimination of steatosis and NASH in mice using nuclear magnetic resonance spectroscopy. Metabolomics 7, 237–246.

Koves, T.R., Li, P., An, J., Akimoto, T., Slentz, D., Ilkayeva, O., Dohm, G.L., Yan, Z., Newgard, C.B., Muoio, D.M., 2005. Peroxisome proliferator-activated receptor-gamma co-activator 1alpha-mediated metabolic remodeling of skeletal myocytes mimics exercise training and reverses lipid-induced mitochondrial inefficiency. J. Biol. Chem. 280, 33588–33598.

Koves, T.R., Ussher, J.R., Noland, R.C., Slentz, D., Mosedale, M., Ilkayeva, O., Bain, J., Stevens, R., Dyck, J.R., Newgard, C.B., Lopaschuk, G.D., Muoio, D.M., 2008. Mitochondrial overload and incomplete fatty acid oxidation contribute to skeletal muscle insulin resistance. Cell Metab. 7, 45–56.

Kröger, J., Zietemann, V., Enzenbach, C., Weikert, C., Jansen, E.H., Döring, F., Joost, H.-G., Boeing, H., Schulze, M.B., 2011. Erythrocyte membrane phospholipid fatty acids, desaturase activity, and dietary fatty acids in relation to risk of type 2 diabetes in the European Prospective Investigation into Cancer and Nutrition (EPIC)-Potsdam study. Am. J. Clin. Nutr. 93, 127–142.

Kus, V., Flachs, P., Kuda, O., Bardova, K., Janovska, P., Svobodova, M., Jilkova, Z.M., Rossmeisl, M., Wang-Sattler, R., Yu, Z., Illig, T., Kopecky, J., 2011. Unmasking differential effects of rosiglitazone and pioglitazone in the combination treatment with $n-3$ fatty acids in mice fed a high-fat diet. PLoS One 6, e27126.

Lankinen, M., Schwab, U., Erkkila, A., Seppanen-Laakso, T., Hannila, M.L., Mussalo, H., Lehto, S., Uusitupa, M., Gylling, H., Oresic, M., 2009. Fatty fish intake decreases lipids related to inflammation and insulin signaling – a lipidomics approach. PLoS One 4, e5258.

Le Naour, F., Bralet, M.-P., Debois, D., Sandt, C., Guettier, C., Dumas, P., Brunelle, A., Laprévote, O., 2009. Chemical imaging on liver steatosis using synchrotron infrared and TOF-SIMS microspectroscopies. PLoS One 4, e7408.

Li, L.O., Hu, Y.F., Wang, L., Mitchell, M., Berger, A., Coleman, R.A., 2010. Early hepatic insulin resistance in mice: a metabolomics analysis. Mol. Endocrinol. 24, 657–666.

Magnusson, Y., Friberg, P., Sjövall, P., Dangardt, F., Malmberg, P., Chen, Y., 2008. Lipid imaging of human skeletal muscle using TOF-SIMS with bismuth cluster ion as a primary ion source. Clin. Physiol. Funct. Imaging 28, 202–209.

Magnusson, M., Lewis, G.D., Ericson, U., Orho-Melander, M., Hedblad, B., Engström, G., Östling, G., Clish, C., Wang, T.J., Gerszten, R.E., 2013. A diabetes-predictive amino acid score and future cardiovascular disease. Eur. Heart J. 34, 1982–1989.

Menni, C., Fauman, E., Erte, I., Perry, J.R., Kastenmüller, G., Shin, S.-Y., Petersen, A.-K., Hyde, C., Psatha, M., Ward, K.J., 2013. Biomarkers for type 2 diabetes and impaired fasting glucose using a nontargeted metabolomics approach. Diabetes 62, 4270–4276.

Mihalik, S.J., Michaliszyn, S.F., de las Heras, J., Bacha, F., Lee, S., Chace, D.H., DeJesus, V.R., Vockley, J., Arslanian, S.A., 2012. Metabolomic profiling of fatty acid and amino acid metabolism in youth with obesity and type 2 diabetes: evidence for enhanced mitochondrial oxidation. Diabetes Care 35, 605–611.

Moayyeri, A., Hammond, C.J., Valdes, A.M., Spector, T.D., 2013. Cohort profile: TwinsUK and healthy ageing twin study. Int. J. Epidemiol. 42, 76–85.

Muoio, D.M., Newgard, C.B., 2008. Fatty acid oxidation and insulin action: when less is more. Diabetes 57, 1455–1456.

Newgard, C.B., An, J., Bain, J.R., Muehlbauer, M.J., Stevens, R.D., Lien, L.F., Haqq, A.M., Shah, S.H., Arlotto, M., Slentz, C.A., Rochon, J., Gallup, D., Ilkayeva, O., Wenner, B. R., Yancy JR., W.S., Eisenson, H., Musante, G., Surwit, R.S., Millington, D.S., Butler, M.D., Svetkey, L.P., 2009. A branched-chain amino acid-related metabolic signature that differentiates obese and lean humans and contributes to insulin resistance. Cell Metab. 9, 311–326.

Patel, M.J., Batch, B.C., Svetkey, L.P., Bain, J.R., Turer, C.B., Haynes, C., Muelhbauer, M.J., Steven, R.D., Newgard, C.B., Shah, S.H., 2013. Race and sex differences in small-molecules metabolites and metabolic hormones in overweight and obese adults. OMICS 17, 627–635.

Perez-Cornago, A., Brennan, L., Ibero-Baraibar, I., Hermsdorff, H.H., O'Gorman, A., Zulet, M. A., Martinez, J.A., 2014. Metabolomics identifies changes in fatty acid and amino acid profiles in serum of overweight older adults following a weight loss intervention. J. Physiol. Biochem. 70 (2), 593–602.

Popkin, B.M., 2011. Is the obesity epidemic a national security issue around the globe? Curr. Opin. Endocrinol. Diabetes Obes. 18, 328–331.

Puri, P., Baillie, R.A., Wiest, M.M., Mirshahi, F., Choudhury, J., Cheung, O., Sargeant, C., Contos, M.J., Sanyal, A.J., 2007. A lipidomic analysis of nonalcoholic fatty liver disease. Hepatology 46, 1081–1090.

Ramos-Roman, M.A., Sweetman, L., Valdez, M.J., Parks, E.J., 2012. Postprandial changes in plasma acylcarnitine concentrations as markers of fatty acid flux in overweight and obesity. Metabolism 61, 202–212.

Rhee, E.P., Cheng, S., Larson, M.G., Walford, G.A., Lewis, G.D., McCabe, E., Yang, E., Farrell, L., Fox, C.S., O'Donnell, C.J., 2011. Lipid profiling identifies a triacylglycerol signature of insulin resistance and improves diabetes prediction in humans. J. Clin. Invest. 121, 1402.

Rhee, E.P., Clish, C.B., Ghorbani, A., Larson, M.G., Elmariah, S., McCabe, E., Yang, Q., Cheng, S., Pierce, K., Deik, A., 2013. A combined epidemiologic and metabolomic approach improves CKD prediction. J. Am. Soc. Nephrol. 24, 1330–1338.

Roberts, L.D., Gerszten, R.E., 2013. Toward new biomarkers of cardiometabolic diseases. Cell Metab. 18, 43–50.

Roux, A., Lison, D., Junot, C., Heilier, J.F., 2011. Applications of liquid chromatography coupled to mass spectrometry-based metabolomics in clinical chemistry and toxicology: a review. Clin. Biochem. 44, 119–135.

Rubio-Aliaga, I., Roos, B.D., Sailer, M., McLoughlin, G.A., Boekschoten, M.V., van Erk, M., Bachmair, E.-M., van Schothorst, E.M., Keijer, J., Coort, S.L., Evelo, C., Gibney, M.J., Daniel, H., Muller, M., Kleemann, R., Brennan, L., 2011. Alterations in hepatic one-carbon metabolism and related pathways following a high-fat dietary intervention. Physiol. Genomics 43, 408–416.

Salek, R.M., Maguire, M.L., Bentley, E., Rubtsov, D.V., Hough, T., Cheeseman, M., Nunez, D., Sweatman, B.C., Haselden, J.N., Cox, R.D., Connor, S.C., Griffin, J.L., 2007. A metabolomic comparison of urinary changes in type 2 diabetes in mouse, rat, and human. Physiol. Genomics 29, 99–108.

Sampey, B.P., Freemerman, A.J., Zhang, J., Kuan, P.F., Galanko, J.A., O'Connell, T.M., Ilkayeva, O.R., Muehlbauer, M.J., Stevens, R.D., Newgard, C.B., Brauer, H.A., Troester, M.A., Makowski, L., 2012. Metabolomic profiling reveals mitochondrial-derived lipid biomarkers that drive obesity-associated inflammation. PLoS One 7, e38812.

Schirra, H.J., Anderson, C.G., Wilson, W.J., Kerr, L., Craik, D.J., Waters, M.J., Lichanska, A. M., 2008. Altered metabolism of growth hormone receptor mutant mice: a combined NMR metabonomics and microarray study. PLoS One 3, e2764.

Schooneman, M.G., Vaz, F.M., Houten, S.M., Soeters, M.R., 2013. Acylcarnitines: reflecting or inflicting insulin resistance? Diabetes 62, 1–8.

Shah, S.H., Svetkey, L.P., Newgard, C.B., 2011. Branching out for detection of type 2 diabetes. Cell Metab. 13, 491–492.

Shah, S.H., Sun, J.L., Stevens, R.D., Bain, J.R., Muehlbauer, M.J., Pieper, K.S., Haynes, C., Hauser, E.R., Kraus, W.E., Granger, C.B., Newgard, C.B., Califf, R.M., Newby, L.K., 2012a. Baseline metabolomic profiles predict cardiovascular events in patients at risk for coronary artery disease. Am. Heart J. 163, 844–850e1.

Shah, S.H., Crosslin, D.R., Haynes, C.S., Nelson, S., Turer, C.B., Stevens, R.D., Muehlbauer, M.J., Wenner, B.R., Bain, J.R., Laferrere, B., Gorroochurn, P., Teixeira, J., Brantley, P.J., Stevens, V.J., Hollis, J.F., Appel, L.J., Lien, L.F., Batch, B., Newgard, C.B., Svetkey, L.P., 2012b. Branched-chain amino acid levels are associated with improvement in insulin resistance with weight loss. Diabetologia 55, 321–330.

Tai, E.S., Tan, M.L., Stevens, R.D., Low, Y.L., Muehlbauer, M.J., Goh, D.L., Ilkayeva, O.R., Wenner, B.R., Bain, J.R., Lee, J.J., Lim, S.C., Khoo, C.M., Shah, S.H., Newgard, C.B., 2010. Insulin resistance is associated with a metabolic profile of altered protein metabolism in Chinese and Asian-Indian men. Diabetologia 53, 757–767.

Touboul, D., Brunelle, A., Laprevote, O., 2011. Mass spectrometry imaging: towards a lipid microscope? Biochimie 93, 113–119.

Townsend, M.K., Clish, C.B., Kraft, P., Wu, C., Souza, A.L., Deik, A.A., Tworoger, S.S., Wolpin, B.M., 2013. Reproducibility of metabolomic profiles among men and women in 2 large cohort studies. Clin. Chem. 59, 1657–1667.

Tsuboyama-Kasaoka, N., Shozawa, C., Sano, K., Kamei, Y., Kasaoka, S., Hosokawa, Y., Ezaki, O., 2006. Taurine (2-aminoethanesulfonic acid) deficiency creates a vicious circle promoting obesity. Endocrinology 147, 3276–3284.

Valdes, A.M., Glass, D., Spector, T.D., 2013. Omics technologies and the study of human ageing. Nat. Rev. Genet. 14, 601–607.

Waldram, A., Holmes, E., Wang, Y., Rantalainen, M., Wilson, I.D., Tuohy, K.M., McCartney, A.L., Gibson, G.R., Nicholson, J.K., 2009. Top-down systems biology modeling of host metabotype – microbiome associations in obese rodents. J. Proteome Res. 8, 2361–2375.

Wang, T.J., Larson, M.G., Vasan, R.S., Cheng, S., Rhee, E.P., McCabe, E., Lewis, G.D., Fox, C. S., Jacques, P.F., Fernandez, C., 2011. Metabolite profiles and the risk of developing diabetes. Nat. Med. 17, 448–453.

Wang, T.J., Ngo, D., Psychogios, N., Dejam, A., Larson, M.G., Vasan, R.S., Ghorbani, A., O'Sullivan, J., Cheng, S., Rhee, E.P., 2013. 2-Aminoadipic acid is a biomarker for diabetes risk. J. Clin. Invest. 123, 4309.

Wang-Sattler, R., Yu, Z., Herder, C., Messias, A.C., Floegel, A., He, Y., Heim, K., Campillos, M., Holzapfel, C., Thorand, B., 2012. Novel biomarkers for pre-diabetes identified by metabolomics. Mol. Syst. Biol. 8, 615.

Wattacheril, J., Seeley, E.H., Angel, P., Chen, H., Bowen, B.P., Lanciault, C., Caprioli, R.M., Abumrad, N., Flynn, C.R., 2013. Differential intrahepatic phospholipid zonation in simple steatosis and nonalcoholic steatohepatitis. PLoS One 8, e57165.

Wei, J., Qiu, D.K., Ma, X., 2009. Bile acids and insulin resistance: implications for treating nonalcoholic fatty liver disease. J. Dig. Dis. 10, 85–90.

Weir, J.M., Wong, G., Barlow, C.K., Greeve, M.A., Kowalczyk, A., Almasy, L., Comuzzie, A. G., Mahaney, M.C., Jowett, J.B., Shaw, J., 2013. Plasma lipid profiling in a large population-based cohort. J. Lipid Res. 54, 2898–2908.

Wijekoon, E.P., Skinner, C., Brosnan, M.E., Brosnan, J.T., 2004. Amino acid metabolism in the Zucker diabetic fatty rat: effects of insulin resistance and of type 2 diabetes. Can. J. Physiol. Pharmacol. 82, 506–514.

Williams, R., Lenz, E.M., Wilson, A.J., Granger, J., Wilson, I.D., Major, H., Stumpf, C., Plumb, R., 2006. A multi-analytical platform approach to the metabonomic analysis of plasma from normal and zucker (fa/fa) obese rats. Mol. Biosyst. 2, 174–183.

Wilson, P.W., Anderson, K.M., Castelli, W.P., 1991. Twelve-year incidence of coronary heart disease in middle-aged adults during the era of hypertensive therapy: the Framingham offspring study. Am. J. Med. 90, 11–16.

Wurtz, P., Raiko, J.R., Magnussen, C.G., Soininen, P., Kangas, A.J., Tynkkynen, T., Thomson, R., Laatikainen, R., Savolainen, M.J., Laurikka, J., Kuukasjarvi, P., Tarkka, M., Karhunen, P.J., Jula, A., Viikari, J.S., Kahonen, M., Lehtimaki, T., Juonala, M., Ala-Korpela, M., Raitakari, O.T., 2012a. High-throughput quantification of circulating metabolites improves prediction of subclinical atherosclerosis. Eur. Heart J. 33, 2307–2316.

Würtz, P., Tiainen, M., Mäkinen, V.-P., Kangas, A.J., Soininen, P., Saltevo, J., Keinänen-Kiukaanniemi, S., Mäntyselkä, P., Lehtimäki, T., Laakso, M., 2012b. Circulating metabolite predictors of glycemia in middle-aged men and women. Diabetes Care 35, 1749–1756.

Xie, B., Waters, M.J., Schirra, H.J., 2012. Investigating potential mechanisms of obesity by metabolomics. J. Biomed. Biotechnol.. 2012, 805683.

Yu, Z., Zhai, G., Singmann, P., He, Y., Xu, T., Prehn, C., Römisch-Margl, W., Lattka, E., Gieger, C., Soranzo, N., 2012. Human serum metabolic profiles are age dependent. Aging Cell 11, 960–967.

Using metabolomics to evaluate food intake: applications in nutritional epidemiology

C. Manach[1], *L. Brennan*[2], *L.O. Dragsted*[3]
[1]Institut National de la Recherche Agronomique (INRA), Clermont-Ferrand, France; [2]University College Dublin, Dublin, Ireland; [3]University of Copenhagen, Copenhagen, Denmark

9.1 Introduction

Nutritional epidemiology is a central discipline in the development of public health policies aiming at promoting and maintaining healthful dietary patterns in general or for specific populations. The main purposes of nutritional epidemiology are (i) to explore diet–health relationships and determine the dietary factors involved and (ii) to monitor the nutritional status of populations and identify their major determinants for the development and evaluation of public health interventions. Numerous studies from basic, clinical, and epidemiological research sought to identify and clarify the role of dietary factors in affecting well-being and increasing or decreasing the risk of chronic diseases. This research has highlighted, with varying degrees of certainty, the role of some dietary factors in the incidence of chronic diseases such as cancer, cardiovascular disease, obesity, diabetes, and osteoporosis. However, there are still many unresolved questions in nutrition, and literature is still full of inconsistencies. A number of reasons contribute to this including the following two. First, the number of dietary factors considered so far is very restricted compared to the wide range of chemical constituents, additives, and contaminants supplied by food. Second, important disparities exist in individual phenotypes, thus in individual nutritional requirements for optimal health, which has substantiated the concept of personalised nutrition (Gibney and Walsh, 2013; Kaput, 2008). Nutrition research has recently entered a new era, where the complexity of the diet and of its relationships with genotype, lifestyle, and diseases is appraised with new methodological approaches, including "omics" technologies, to resolve questions that were not answered with classical approaches (Afman and Muller, 2006; Trujillo et al., 2006). Genome-wide association studies (GWAS) have shown that genetic polymorphisms are poor predictors of disease risks, and this has reinforced the need to understand the gene–environment (including diet)–health relationships (Corella et al., 2009; Minihane, 2013). On the other hand, large interindividual variations are observed in response to nutritional challenges, due to differences in gene polymorphisms, epigenetic patterns, or gut microbiota composition (Lampe et al., 2013; Zeisel, 2007; Zivkovic et al., 2009). These findings raised the need for large-scale prospective studies on multiethnic cohorts with genotyping and extensive phenotyping of individuals based on biochemical, functional, imaging, and

Metabolomics as a Tool in Nutrition Research. http://dx.doi.org/10.1016/B978-1-78242-084-2.00009-5

omic measurements. But in contrast with the huge investment in cutting-edge technologies to analyse genotype and health phenotype, the methods and tools available to characterise and quantify dietary intakes of individuals are far from offering the accuracy and level of detail required for modern nutritional epidemiology.

The purpose of dietary assessment is to estimate intakes of foods, nutrients, and bioactive compounds and to assess individuals' nutritional exposures for the exploration of associations with health outcomes and the monitoring of population nutritional status. These data are still extremely difficult to obtain, especially at the individual level, due to the wide range of foods consumed and the high heterogeneity and variability of human dietary choices. Methods currently used to assess food intake are based on self-reporting instruments such as dietary records, 24 h recalls, or food frequency questionnaires (FFQs). The advantages and limitations of these methods have been recently described in detail (Tucker et al., 2013). With all self-reporting instruments, individuals may misreport dietary intakes because of memory or literacy problems and because of a desire to be perceived as compliant to a socially desirable behaviour or to reduce the inconvenience of burdensome reporting (Macdiarmid and Blundell, 1998). Diet records showed acceptable accuracy in small- or medium-sized studies with motivated volunteers, although some subjects still tend to modify their food intake, eating less and avoiding complex dishes on recording days. However, dietary records are considered too costly and burdensome for application in large cohorts. The method of 24 h recalls is appropriate for dietary assessment at the population level. But due to the wide day-to-day variability in food choices, there is a high risk that individuals can be misclassified in quintiles of intakes where only one 24 h recall is considered. Multiple 24 h recalls are thus necessary to correctly reflect habitual intakes of foods or nutrients for individuals, which increases the cost and burden of assessment. A Finnish study estimated that between 7 and 14 24 h recalls would be required to accurately assess most common nutrients and up to 21 repetitions would be necessary for more variable nutrients such as vitamin A (Hartman et al., 1990). Although statistical algorithms have been developed to estimate usual intake of episodically consumed foods with a reduced number of 24 h recalls (Kipnis et al., 2009), obviously multiple 24 h recalls cannot provide precise data for all foods. FFQs, which retrospectively record dietary habits over periods as long as 1 year, are still the most cost-effective tools in cohort studies. However, their reliability has been challenged in the past decade in publications reporting much stronger associations between health outcomes and food intakes when multiple dietary records or biomarkers were used rather than FFQs (Bingham et al., 2003, 2008; Freedman et al., 2006; Kristal et al., 2005). Limitations of FFQs have long been recognised: recall errors and misreporting inherent to self-reporting, failure to capture a large spectrum of dietary diversity due to food grouping, and imprecision due to difficulty to assess portion sizes. Measurement errors are a real concern in nutritional epidemiology since even modest errors in classification of volunteers into quintiles of intake may greatly attenuate the observed relative risks. Marshall and Chen (1999) estimated that with a 30% misclassification for intake, which is common in observational studies, a true relative risk of 5 would be observed as equivalent to 1.8. Evidence is mounting that misclassification of volunteers with FFQ data led to the attenuation of associations between diet and diseases, especially for diet–cancer associations, in large cohort studies conducted so far (Schatzkin and Kipnis, 2004).

Beyond imprecision attached to food intake data obtained with questionnaires, concern also exists for the conversion into nutrient/micronutrient intake using tables of food composition. Food databases usually compile food contents for 20–60 nutrients and micronutrients in hundreds of foods and dishes (Champagne and Wroten, 2012). Many nonnutrients are not covered yet, and although the situation will certainly improve within 5–10 years, comprehensive coverage of all nonnutrients for the hundreds of thousands of existing foods is unrealistic. For nutrients present in food databases, a source of imprecision is the high content variability that may exist within foods depending, for example, on the mode of production, processing, and preservation or on varieties/cultivars for plant foods. This variability is not reflected in the mean values provided by databases; therefore, calculations of nutrient/nonnutrient intakes can lack precision and accuracy in some cases. Since the mean values can differ between databases depending on the raw data aggregated, the calculated nutrient/nonnutrient intake can also differ according to the database used.

To overcome some of the problems (imprecision, cost, and burden) associated with dietary assessment using questionnaires, new tools have been developed, thanks to information and communication technology advances. Internet-based 24 h recalls are now applied in large cohort studies, which reduces the logistic burden compared to classical methods based on dieticians' interviews (Hercberg, 2012; Subar et al., 2012). With user-friendly interfaces, warning and help messages, and flexibility in time for questionnaire filling, the self-administered online questionnaires reduce the completion time and allow a greater level of details. Mobile phone applications are under development for self-monitoring of dietary intake (Six et al., 2010). The use of integrated digital camera with image processing software allows identification of foods and estimation of portion size (Stumbo, 2013). These tools are particularly promising to assist dietary information collection in some specific populations such as adolescents. However, even with these technological innovations and wise combination of instruments, self-reporting methods still hold inherent limitations. They are unlikely to meet alone the challenges of dietary assessment for modern nutritional epidemiology, among which are as follows:

- High-throughput assessment of individual dietary intakes for very large-scale population studies, including GWAS.
- Applicability to all types of populations including infants, older people, obese adolescents, men, and women for various geographic origins, immigrants, and low-income populations.
- Comparability across populations and across studies to allow meta-analyses.
- High-level accuracy for a wide range of dietary factors: consumption of food groups such as plant foods, cereals, meat, and dairy products or specific foods including some infrequently consumed and intake not only of energy, proteins, fats, sugars, minerals, and vitamins but also of food bioactives, additives, and contaminants.
- Ability to characterise dietary behaviours beyond food intakes: dietary patterns, level of adherence to dietary recommendations, food purchase habits, and culinary habits.
- Assessment of physiological exposures of individuals to a large panel of food nonnutrients likely to exert beneficial or detrimental effects on human health, including some still unknown compounds.

9.2 Biomarkers as a complementary approach to questionnaires

The complementary approach to questionnaires is the use of biochemical indicators, the so-called biomarkers. Biomarkers may reveal physiological exposure to nutrients and nonnutrients and can also indirectly reflect food intake. Biomarkers represent objective phenotypic assessments, typically based on a blood or urine sample, but they may also use other samples or whole-body measurements. Errors associated with biomarker measurements are strictly independent from measurement errors associated with questionnaires. Biomarkers are useful at different levels in nutritional epidemiology. Intake (and exposure) biomarkers can be used to validate FFQs though comparison of intake data obtained by both methods for representative foods. They provide independent data to complement questionnaires for the stratification of subjects into quintiles of consumers. Biomarkers are expected to assess individuals' dietary intake and nutritional exposures with a high precision allowing comparison of subjects on a continuous scale of values instead of using stratification into quintiles. Beyond observational studies, biomarkers are often used to monitor subject compliance in nutritional intervention studies. A key attribute of biomarkers is that they measure the physiological exposure of individuals to nutrient and nonnutrient metabolites, reflecting not only the food intakes but also the bioavailability of the food components.

There are several different kinds of biomarkers and their use has a range of strengths and limitations (Jenab et al., 2009). Nutritional or dietary biomarkers are used for assessing nutrient status or food intake. This may be the more recent or the longer-term food intake, or both, and each biomarker is typically related to a specific food item, food component, or nutrient. Recovery biomarkers represent the balance between total intake and excretion/degradation over a defined time period, whereas prediction biomarkers measure a fraction of the analyte proportional to the total intake. To be classified in these categories, the correlation with the true intake should be >0.8 (Jenab et al., 2009). The short-term nutritional biomarkers typically represent food-derived compounds with short half-lives, and these compounds are measures of recent food intake. Examples include blood plasma caffeine as a measure of caffeine intake (Kamimori et al., 2002), breath ethanol for recent alcohol intake (Friel et al., 1995), and total urine proline betaine as a marker of orange juice intake (Heinzmann et al., 2010). These compounds are intake biomarkers in the sense that they come directly from the food and therefore represent directly the consumption and may turn out to be replacement biomarkers, always representing a small but fixed fraction of the intake, upon thorough validation. However, host factors play a role at least for the first two of these compounds since they are metabolised and the derived metabolites may represent to some extent the same intakes, e.g., paraxanthine (Klebanoff et al., 1998) and ethyl glucuronide (Hoiseth et al., 2010). The latter is used in forensics as a prediction biomarker because it lingers in plasma and urine for some additional hours when ethanol itself cannot be measured anymore. For some groups of compounds, methodologies exist to cover all in a single biomarker, for example, isothiocyanate mercapturic acids as measures of total crucifer intakes (Vermeulen et al., 2003). However, more detail may be gained by measuring specific mercapturic acids (Andersen et al., 2013). All of these markers may be seen as concentration biomarkers that are useful to assess the actual recent dietary intakes and to predict measurement errors by the 24 h assessment methods. The metabolically derived markers may also be seen as markers of the efficiency of host metabolism, and ratios between metabolites may reflect individual capacity or susceptibility. For example, the ratio between certain caffeine metabolites has been used as a phenotypic measure of hepatic CYP1A2 metabolism (Kall and Clausen, 1995). Most currently known short-term biomarkers of food intake have this inherent duality, which adds to the biological variability between individuals eating the same food items. Many nutritional biomarkers with short half-lives are continuously present in body fluids because they are also formed endogenously. For instance, plasma trimethylamine oxide as a marker of recent fish intake (Andersen et al., 2014b; Wang et al., 2014) or urinary methylhistidines as markers of animal protein intakes (Dragsted, 2010) are marker compounds that are also formed endogenously from cholines by our gut microbiota and from restructuring of our muscle proteins, respectively. A background level must therefore be known or estimated and subtracted for their application in food intake assessment. There are therefore few perfect biomarkers of recent intake; however, a large number of compounds are now known to reflect recent food intakes (Scalbert et al., 2014), and they may therefore be used in combination to roughly assess the compliance in intervention studies and/or the validity of dietary recall information. They may also be used in observational studies for foods that are consumed on a daily basis, but because of their reflection of short-term intakes, they are not accurate markers at the individual level of less commonly ingested foods. However, they may still be used to assess differences in intakes at the group level, e.g., between quintiles of subjects with different waist circumferences or between genders.

Several foods contain characteristic substances that have longer half-lives and therefore accumulate as a function of average intake over a more extended period of time. These compounds are often more lipophilic, or they are degraded or excreted more slowly due to specific affinities or transporters. Markers of food intakes in this category include long-chain omega-3 fatty acids in blood as a measure of seafood intakes, alkylresorcinols as markers of specific whole grain intakes, and total plasma carotenoids as measures of average fruit and vegetable intakes (Baldrick et al., 2011; Marklund et al., 2013; Silva et al., 2014). These markers may in general represent the balance between average intake and excretion over several days or even weeks and may therefore be seen as recovery dietary biomarkers; however, they all have flaws related to special groups such as vegans, subjects eating whole-grain oat or maize, and supplement users (Garcia et al., 2010; Johansson-Persson et al., 2013; Silva et al., 2014). Nutritional biomarkers representing a longer-term balance may also be measures of nutrients actively retained by our organism, for example, many micronutrients such as potassium and vitamin C as well as endogenous compounds such as steroids. Such compounds may be good markers for longer-term intake, representing days, weeks, or even months provided they have not reached a level where active transport out of the body is triggered. For instance, vitamin C is lost slowly when body stores are low, whereas almost 100% of a dose may be quickly eliminated in case of sufficient stores (Levine et al., 1996). In some cases, these markers may be used as nutritional status biomarkers (typically concentration biomarkers) to assess the actual status for a nutrient in order to evaluate whether it is adequate or points to a deficiency. Only targeted methods of analysis may cover some of the established biomarkers in this category, but many new biomarkers representing longer-term exposures are likely to surface from the explorative (untargeted metabolomics) applications in the near future.

9.3 Definition of the food metabolome

The "food metabolome" has been defined as the sum of metabolites directly derived from the digestion of foods, their absorption in the gut, and biotransformation by the host tissues and the microbiota (Manach et al., 2009; Scalbert et al., 2014). In nutritional studies, the food metabolome is the sum of metabolites that reflect the intake of any specific food. The emphasis is often put on those compounds that are specific to the food, because they are common to either the food class, a specific food, or a component present in that food. For instance, metabolites of flavonoids in general reflect plant-derived foods and beverages; but some flavonoid classes mainly reflect a single group of plant foods, for example, isoflavonoids mainly reflect soy food intakes and anthocyanins the berry-derived foods and drinks with few exceptions. Metabolites from a specific anthocyanin, for example, pelargonidin, may mainly derive from strawberry and therefore be a part of the strawberry food metabolome together with qualifier compounds such as strawberry aroma furaneols (Andersen et al., 2014a). The food metabolome is still only partially known for any food, and for the majority of food items, there is still very limited data originating from single-compound biomarker studies of the past. Large groups of important foods are still not well covered and probably will need to await more sensitive instrumentation to map the more unique characteristics of their food metabolomes. This is, for instance, the case for most kinds of meats, oils, and spices and for refined foods based on potato, corn, and wheat starches. So it may be estimated that it will take at least another 5–10 years before we have a first reasonable coverage of the food metabolome.

9.4 Metabolomics as a tool for dietary biomarker discovery

The realisation that the metabolomic profile was strongly influenced by recent dietary intake sparked an interest in the use of this approach for the identification of novel dietary biomarkers of intake. Nontargeted metabolomics is a data-driven approach; thus, prior knowledge of food components and their metabolic fate is not required. Candidate biomarkers are discovered on the basis of their appearance or increased concentration in biofluids after consumption of the food. Applications of metabolomics in this field in general fall into three different study design approaches:

(i) Specific interventions to identify food markers in biofluids following consumption of the foods of interest.
(ii) Use of cohort studies to search for biomarkers of specific foods by comparing consumers and nonconsumers.
(iii) Analysis of dietary patterns in conjunction with metabolomic profiles to identify nutritypes and biomarkers.

In recent years, the application of metabolomics has identified a number of putative biomarkers of intake of certain foods including salmon, whole-grain wheat cereal, berries, cruciferous vegetables, citrus fruits, nuts, coffee, cocoa, and red meat (Table 9.1). One of the earliest biomarkers of dietary intake to be identified using a metabolomics-based approach was trimethylamine *N*-oxide (TMAO): many metabolomic studies have reported high levels in urine samples following fish consumption (Lee et al., 2006; Lenz et al., 2004; Lloyd et al., 2011b). However, it should be noted that TMAO can be produced endogenously and has also been reported as a marker of meat intake in a number of studies (Dragsted, 2010; Stella et al., 2006). As a result, further work is needed to assess its specificity, and it may be possible that TMAO may be more useful as a dietary biomarker of protein as opposed to a specific food, i.e., meat/fish. Moreover, a recent study assessing the effect of high- or low-protein diets found that urinary TMAO was highly correlated to daily urinary nitrogen excretion ($r = 0.89$) and thereby consumed protein (Rasmussen et al., 2012). Finally, a number of metabolomics-based studies have confirmed the use of 1-methylhistidine as a biomarker of meat consumption (Cross et al., 2011; Dragsted, 2010; Stella et al., 2006). The robust data consistently presented for 1-methylhistidine as a marker of red meat support its further development for use in nutrition.

With respect to citrus fruits, a number of controlled interventions and cross-sectional studies have independently identified proline betaine as a marker of citrus fruit intake (Andersen et al., 2014a; Heinzmann et al., 2010; Lloyd et al., 2011a; May et al., 2013; Pujos-Guillot et al., 2013). Heinzmann and co-workers performed an acute intervention approach where eight volunteers consumed a standardised breakfast, lunch, and dinner from day 0 until lunch on day 3. In the evening of day 2, a supplementary mixed-fruit meal (apple, orange, grapefruit, and grapes) was introduced. Urine was collected four times a day from the morning of day 1 until the evening of day 3. Metabolomic analysis of the urine revealed urinary excretion of proline betaine as a biomarker of citrus fruit intake. Using participants of the INTERMAP UK cohort, this biomarker was confirmed as a marker of citrus fruit: a receiver operating characteristic curve resulted in an AUC of 92.3% with a sensitivity and a specificity of 90.6% and 86.3%, respectively. In the study performed by Lloyd and colleagues, an acute breakfast challenge approach was used. Acute exposure of volunteers to orange juice resulted in the appearance of proline betaine and a number of biotransformed products in postprandial urine samples (Lloyd et al., 2011a). More recently, another study confirmed proline betaine as a marker of citrus intake by using a number of different study approaches including an acute intervention and examination of low and high consumers in a cohort study (Pujos-Guillot et al., 2013).

Table 9.1 List of candidate biomarkers of intake identified using a metabolomic approach

Dietary factor	Study design	Number of subjects	Sample type	Analytical method	Discriminating metabolites/ candidate biomarkers	References
Fruits						
Mixed fruit meal (apple, orange, grapes, and grapefruit)	Acute study	8	Urine (4.5 h postprandial)	NMR	Proline betaine	Heinzmann et al. (2010)
Citrus fruits	Cross-sectional	499	Urine (24 h)			
Citrus fruits	Acute study	12	Urine (fasting)	FIE-FTICR-MS	Proline betaine, hydroxyproline betaine*	Lloyd et al. (2011a)
Citrus fruits	Cross-sectional	80	Urine (morning spot)	LC–ESI–QTof; LTQ-Orbitrap	Proline betaine; hydroxyproline betaine, limonene 8,9-diol glucuronide*, nootkatone 13,14-diol glucuronide*, *N*-methyltyramine sulphate*, naringenin 7-*O*-glucuronide, hesperetin 3′-*O*-glucuronide	Pujos-Guillot et al. (2013)
Orange juice	Acute study	4	Urine (kinetics)			
Orange juice	Cross-over intervention	12	Urine (24 h)			
Apple	Cross-over intervention	24	Plasma (fasting)	LC–ESI–Qtof	3-Hydroxyisobutyric acid, proline betaine, *p*-cresol sulphate, bile acids, lyso-PCs, acyl-carnitines	Rago et al. (2013)
Orange/citrus	Intervention	107	Urine (24 h)	LC–ESI–QTof; LTQ-Orbitrap	Proline betaine, hesperetin glucuronide	Andersen et al. (2014a)
Aronia-citrus juice	Intervention	51	Urine (morning spot)	LC–ESI–QTof	Proline betaine*, ferulic acid*	Llorach et al. (2014)

Strawberry	Intervention	107	Urine (24 h)	LC–ESI–QTof; LTQ-Orbitrap	2.5-Dimethyl-4-methoxy-3(2H)-furanone sulphate*	Andersen et al. (2014a)
Raspberries	Acute study	24	Urine (kinetics)	FIE-FTICR-MS; GC–Tof-MS	Caffeic acid sulphate; methyl-epicatechin sulphate; 3-hydroxyhippuric acid	Lloyd et al. (2011b)
Lingonberries	Acute study	14	Urine (3 h postprandial)	NMR	Hippuric acid, 4-hydroxyhippuric acid	Lehtonen et al. (2013)
Cruciferous vegetables, citrus and soya	2 week-cross-over intervention	10	Urine (fasting)	LTQ-FT LC–MS/MS	Proline betaine*, sulforaphane*, hippuric acid*, genistein*, daidzein*, equol*, glycitein*, *O*-desmethylangolensin*, trigonelline*, (iso)valerylglycine*, hydroxyphenylacetyl-glycine*, nicotinuric acid*	May et al. (2013)
Cruciferous vegetables, citrus, and soya	Cross-sectional	93	Urine (fasting)	LTQ-FT LC–MS/MS	Proline betaine	
Vegetables						
Broccoli	Acute study	24	Urine (kinetics)	FIE-FTICR-MS	Tetronic acid*, L-xylonate/L-lyxonate*, erythritol*	Lloyd et al. (2011b)
Cruciferous vegetables	Intervention	20	Urine (kinetics)	NMR	*S*-Methyl-L-cysteine sulphoxide	Edmands et al. (2011)
Cruciferous vegetables	Acute study	17	Urine (kinetics)	LC–ESI–QTof	Sulforaphane *N*-acetyl-cysteine, Iberin *N*-acetyl-cysteine*, *N*-acetyl-(*N*′-benzylthiocarbamoyl)-cysteine, sulforaphane *N*-cysteine*, *N*-acetyl-*S*-(*N*-3-methylthiopropyl)cysteine*,	Andersen et al. (2013)

Continued

Table 9.1 Continued

Dietary factor	Study design	Number of subjects	Sample type	Analytical method	Discriminating metabolites/ candidate biomarkers	References
					N-acetyl-*S*-(*N*-allylthiocarbamoyl) cysteine (AITN-NAC)*, 4-iminopentylisothiocyanate*, erucin *N*-acetyl-cysteine*	
Beetroot	Intervention	107	Urine (24 h)	LC–ESI–QTof; LTQ-Orbitrap	4-Ethyl-5-amino-pyrocatechol sulphate*, 4-ethyl-5-methylamino-pyrocatechol sulphate*, 4-methylpyridine-2-carboxylic acid glycine conjugate*	Andersen et al. (2014a)
Cruciferous vegetables	Intervention	107	Urine (24 h)	LC–ESI–QTof; LTQ-Orbitrap	Sulforaphane *N*-acetyl-cysteine, Iberin *N*-acetyl-cysteine*, *N*-acetyl-*S*-(*N*-3-methylthiopropyl)cysteine*, *N*-acetyl-*S*-(*N*-allylthiocarbamoyl)cysteine (AITN-NAC)*	
Red cabbage	Intervention	107	Urine (24 h)	LC–ESI–QTof; LTQ-Orbitrap	3-Hydroxy-3-(methyl-sulphinyl) propanoic acid*, 3-hydroxy-hippuric acid sulphate*, 3-hydroxy-hippuric acid*	
Cereals						
Whole rye grain	Cross-over intervention	20	Urine (24 h)	LC–ESI–QTof	3,5-Dihydroxycinnamic acid sulphate*, 2-aminophenol sulphate*, azelaic acid*, 3-(3,5-dihydroxyphenyl)-1-propanoic acid sulphate* and glucuronide*, enterolactone glucuronide*, indolylacryloylglycine*, ferulic acid-4-*O*-sulphate*, 2-4-dihydroxy-1,4-benzoxazin-3-one sulphate*, 3,5-dihydroxyphenylethanol sulphate*	Bondia-Pons et al. (2013)

Whole-grain sourdough rye bread	Intervention	28	Urine (24 h)	FIE-FTICR-MS	2-Hydroxy-*N*-(2-hydroxyphenyl) acetamide (HHPAA) glucuronide*, *N*-(2-hydroxyphenyl)acetamide (HPAA) sulphate*, 2-hydroxy-1,4-benzoxazin-3-one (HBOA) glucuronide*, *N*-feroylglycine sulphate*, 2-hydroxy-*N*-(2-hydroxyphenyl)acetamide (HHPAA) sulphate*	Beckmann et al. (2013)
Beverages						
Coffee		18	Urine (fasting)	HILIC–UPLC–ESI–QTof	*N*-Methylpyridinium, trigonelline	Lang et al. (2011)
Coffee		9	Urine (kinetics)			
Coffee		68	Urine (morning spot, 24 h, fasting)	FIE-FTICR-MS	Dihydrocaffeic acid	Lloyd et al. (2013)
Coffee	Cross-sectional	39	Urine (morning spot)	LC–ESI–QTof; LTQ-Orbitrap	Atractyligenin glucuronide*, cyclo (isoleucyl-prolyl)*, 1-methylxanthine, 1,7-dimethyluric acid, kahweol oxide glucuronide*, 1-methyluric acid, trigonelline, dimethylxanthine glucuronide*, 5-acetylamino-6-formylamino-3-methyluracil (AFMU), hippuric acid, trimethyluric acid*, paraxanthine, 3-hydroxyhippuric acid, 1,3 or 3,7-dimethyluric acid*, caffeine	Rothwell et al. (2014)
Black tea	Acute study	3	Urine (24 h)	NMR	Hippuric acid*, gallic acid, 1,3-dihydroxyphenyl-2-*O*-sulphate*	Daykin et al. (2005)
Black tea	Acute study	20	Urine (kinetics)	NMR	Hippuric acid*, 4-hydroxyhippuric acid*, 1,3-dihydrophenyl-2-*O*-sulphate*	van Velzen et al. (2009)

Continued

Table 9.1 Continued

Dietary factor	Study design	Number of subjects	Sample type	Analytical method	Discriminating metabolites/ candidate biomarkers	References
Tea (green and black)	Cross-over intervention	17	Urine (24 h)	NMR	Hippuric acid*, 1,3-dihydrophenyl-2-*O*-sulphate*	van Dorsten et al. (2006)
Chamomile tea	Intervention	14	Urine (morning spot)	NMR	Hippuric acid*	Wang et al. (2005)
Wine	Intervention	61	Urine (24 h)	NMR	Tartrate*, 4-hydroxyphenylacetate*, mannitol*, ethanol*	Vazquez-Fresno et al. (2012)
Mixed red wine and grape juice extracts	Intervention	58	Urine (24 h)	NMR, GC–Tof–MS	Syringic acid, 3-hydroxyhippuric acid, 4-hydroxyhippuric acid, 3-hydroxyphenylacetic acid*, 4-hydroxymandelic acid, vanilmandelic acid, hippuric acid, 3-hydroxyphenylpropionic acid, 1,2,3-trihydroxybenzene, 4-hydroxybenzoic acid, homovanillic acid, dihydroferulic acid, phenylacetylglutamine	van Dorsten et al. (2010)
Mixed red wine and grape juice extracts	Intervention	35	Urine (24 h)	GC–MS, LC–MS	3-Hydroxyhippuric acid*, syringic acid*, pyrogallol*, 3-hydroxyphenylacetic acid*, 3-hydroxyphenylpropionic acid*, 3,4-dihydroxyphenylpropionic acid*, indole-3-lactic acid*, hippuric acid*, catechol*, 4-hydroxyhippuric acid*, 3,4-dihydroxyphenylacetic acid*, vanillic acid*	Jacobs et al. (2012)

Animal products						
Salmon	Acute study	24	Urine (kinetics)	FIE-FTICR-MS	Anserine, methylhistidine, trimethylamine-*N*-oxide	Lloyd et al. (2011b)
Mixed fish	Meal study	17	Urine (kinetics)	UPLC–ESI–QTof	Trimethylamine-*N*-oxide	Andersen et al. (2014b)
Oily fish		67	Urine (morning spot, 24 h, fasting)	FIE-FTICR-MS	Methylhistidine	Lloyd et al. (2013)
Cod	Meal study	10	Urine (kinetics)	UPLC–ESI–QTof	Trimethylamine-*N*-oxide, arsenobetaine, methylhistidines, 1,2,3,4-tetrahydro-β-carboline-3-carboxylic acid, N^6,N^6,N^6-trimethyl-lysine	Stanstrup et al. (2014)
Cod	Meal study	11	Plasma (kinetics)	UPLC–ESI–QTof	Trimethylamine-*N*-oxide, arsenobetaine, creatine, methylhistidines, 1,2,3,4-Tetrahydro-β-carboline-3-carboxylic acid, docosahexaenoic acid, taurine, proline, phenylalanine	Stanstrup et al. (2014)
Dairy products						
Whey protein	Meal study	12	Plasma (kinetics)	UPLC–ESI–QTof	Branched-chain amino acids, phenylalanine threonine, methionine, kynurenine, gamma-glutamyl-leucine, gamma-glutamyl-methionine	Stanstrup et al. (2014)
Whey protein	Meal study	11	Plasma (kinetics)	UPLC–ESI–QTof	Branched-chain amino acids, phenylalanine, threonine, methionine,	Stanstrup et al. (2014)

Continued

Table 9.1 **Continued**

Dietary factor	Study design	Number of subjects	Sample type	Analytical method	Discriminating metabolites/ candidate biomarkers	References
					glutamic acid, kynurenine, citrulline, α-keto-3-methylvaleric acid, 3-hydroxy-2-methylbutyric acid, hydroxybutyric acids, α-hydroxydecanoic acid, lauric acid, myristic acid, propionyl carnitine	
Casein	Meal study	11	Plasma (kinetics)	UPLC–ESI–QTof	*N*-phenylacetyl-methionine, methionine sulphoxide	Stanstrup et al. (2014)
Casein	Meal study	11	Urine (kinetics)	UPLC–ESI–QTof	*N*-phenylacetyl-methionine, beta-Asp-Leu	Stanstrup et al. (2014)
Cheese	Cross-over intervention		Urine (kinetics)	UPLC–ESI–QTof	Tyramine sulphate, isobutyryl glycine (and other acyl glycines), xanthurenic acid, 4-hydroxyphenylacetic acid	Hjerpsted et al. (2014)
Other foods						
Cocoa powder	Acute study	10	Urine (kinetics)	LC–ESI–QTof	Vanilloylglycine*, 6-amino-5-[*N*-methylformylamino]-1-methyluracil*, 3-methyluric acid*, 7-methyluric acid*, 3-methylxanthine*, 7-methylxanthine*, 3,7-dimethyluric acid*, theobromine, caffeine, trigonelline*, hydroxynicotinic acid*, tyrosine, 3,5-diethyl-2-methylpyrazine*, hydroxyacetophenone*, cyclo(Ser-Tyr)*, cyclo (Pro-Pro)*, epicatechin-*O*-Sulf*, *O*-methylepicatechin*, vanillic acid, 4-hydroxy-5-(3,4-dihydroxyphenyl)-valeric acid*, 5-(3′,4′-dihydroxyphenyl)-	Llorach et al. (2009)

					valerolactone glucuronide* and sulphate*, 3′-methoxy-4′-hydroxyphenylvalerolactone* and glucuronide*	
Cocoa powder	Acute study	10	Urine (24 h)	LC–ESI–QTof	Hydroxynicotinic acid*, 6-amino-5-[*N*-methylformylamino]-1-methyluracil*, 7- and 3-methyluric acid*, 7- and 3-methylxanthine*, 3,7-dimethylruric acid*, cyclo(propylalanyl)*, 3,5-diethyl-2-methylpyrazine*, theobromine*, vanillic acid-Gluc* and -Sulf-Gluc*, vanilloylglycine*, 4-hydroxy-5-(dihydroxyphenyl)-valeric acid-Glucs* and -Sulf*, 3′-methoxy-4′-hydroxyphenylvalerolactone*, 4′-hydroxy-5-(hydroxymethoxyphenyl) valeric acid-Gluc*, 5-(3′,4′-dihydroxyphenyl)-γ-valerolactone-Gluc* and -Sulf* and -SulfGluc*, (epi) catechin-Gluc* and -SulfGluc*, methyl-(epi)catechin-Sulf*, *N*-[4′-hydroxy-3′-methoxy-E-cinnamoyl]-laspartic acid*, *N*-[4′-hydroxycinnamoyl]-L-aspartic acid*, methoxyhydroxyphenylvalerolactone-Glucs*, hydroxyphenylvalerolactone-Gluc* and -Sulf*, 5-(hydroxymethoxyphenyl)valeric acid-Sulf*, 4-hydroxy-5-(phenyl)valeric acid-Sulf*	Llorach et al. (2013)
Chocolate	Intervention	107	Urine (24 h)	LC–ESI–QTof; LTQ-Orbitrap	6-Amino-5-[*N*-methylformylamino]-1-methyluracil (6-AMMU)*, theobromine, 7-methyluric acid	Andersen et al. (2014a)

Continued

Table 9.1 **Continued**

Dietary factor	Study design	Number of subjects	Sample type	Analytical method	Discriminating metabolites/ candidate biomarkers	References
Almond skin extract	Acute study	24	Urine (kinetics)	LC–ESI–QTof	(Epi)catechin-Sulf*, *O*-methyl-(epi) catechin-Sulf*, naringenin-*O*-Gluc*, 5-(hydroxyphenyl)-γ-valerolactone-Gluc* and -Sulf*, 5-(dihydroxyphenyl)-γ-valerolactone-Gluc*, -SulfGluc* and -Sulf*, 5-(trihydroxyphenyl)-γ-valerolactone-Gluc*, 5-(hydroxymethoxyphenyl)-γ-valerolactone-Gluc* and Sulf*, 4-hydroxy-5-(dihydroxyphenyl)-valeric acid-Gluc* and Sulf*, 4-hydroxy-5-(hydroxymethoxyphenyl)valeric acid-Gluc*, 4-hydroxy-5-(methoxyphenyl) valeric acid-Gluc*, 4-hydroxy-5-(hydroxyphenyl)valeric acid-Gluc and -Sulf*, 4-hydroxy-5-(phenyl)valeric acid-Sulf*, 2-(dihydroxyphenyl)acetic acid-Gluc*, -SulfGluc* and -Sulf*, 2-(hydroxymethoxyphenyl)acetic acid-Gluc*, 2-(hydroxyphenyl)acetic acid-Sulf*, 3-(hydroxyphenyl)propionic acid-Gluc*, 3-(dihydroxyphenyl) propionic acid-Sulf*, vanillic acid-Gluc*, hydroxyhippuric acid*, ferulic acid-Gluc*	Llorach et al. (2010)

Nuts	Intervention	42	Urine (24 h)	LC–ESI–QTof; LTQ-Orbitrap	10-Hydroxydecene-4,6-diynoic acid-Sulf*, tridecadienoic/tridecynoic acid-Gluc*, dodecanedioic acid*, 1,3-dihydroxyphenyl-2-*O*-Sulf*, *p*-coumaroyl alcohol-Gluc* and -Sulf*, *N*-acetylserotonine-Sulf*, 5-hydroxyindoleacetic acid*, urolitin A-Gluc, Sulf*and SulfGluc*	Tulipani et al. (2011)
Spray-dried proteins (whey, casein, gluten)	Meal studies	23	Plasma (kinetics)	UPLC–ESI–QTof	Cyclic gamma-glutamyl amino acids; cyclic dipeptides (3,6-dialkyl-2,5-diketopiperazines)	Stanstrup et al. (2014)
Walnut	Intervention	107	Urine (24 h)	LC–ESI–QTof; LTQ-Orbitrap	5-Hydroxyindole-3-acetic acid	Andersen et al. (2014a)
Dietary fibres (oat bran, rye bran, sugar beet fibres)	Cross-over intervention	25	Plasma (fasting)	LC–ESI–QTof	2-Aminophenol sulphate, 2,6-dihydroxybenzoic acid, hydroxylated and glucuronidated nuatigenin*	Johansson-Persson et al. (2013)

Asterisk means tentative identification, not confirmed by analysis of authentic standard.
NMR, nuclear magnetic resonance; FIE-FTICR-MS, flow infusion electrospray-Fourier transform ion cyclotron resonance-mass spectrometry; LC–ESI-QTof, liquid chromatography–electrospray ionisation-quadrupole time-of-flight mass spectrometer; LTQ–Orbitrap, linear ion trap–orbitrap mass spectrometer; GC–Tof-MS, gas chromatography–time-of-flight-mass spectrometry; LTQ–FT, linear ion trap–Fourier transform mass spectrometer; LC–MS/MS, liquid chromatography–tandem mass spectrometry; HILIC–UPLC–ESI–QTof, hydrophilic interaction liquid chromatography–ultra performance liquid chromatography–electrospray ionization–quadrupole time-of-flight mass spectrometer.

Table 9.1 shows that many metabolites of phytochemicals, including polyphenols, terpenes, glucosinolates, and alkaloids, have been suggested as biomarkers of various plant foods intake. Some are present exclusively in the target foods, for example, flavanones in citrus fruits or glucosinolates in cruciferous vegetables. However, others of the discriminant metabolites associated with the consumption of a particular food in a controlled study design are actually not specific enough for this food and may not be confirmed as biomarkers of intake usable in populations in a free-living situation. For example, hippuric acid was found discriminant for the consumption of coffee, black tea, chamomile tea, lingonberries, mixed red wine and grape juice extract, and mixed supplementation with cruciferous vegetables, citrus, and soya in independent studies (Table 9.1). This metabolite is a final product of gut microbiota degradation of quinic acid; of many polyphenols, such as catechin and chlorogenic acid; and of the aromatic amino acids phenylalanine, tyrosine, and tryptophan (Spencer et al., 2008). It was also described as a potential biomarker of toluene exposure and is used as a measure of renal clearance (Lees et al., 2013). Therefore, hippuric acid should not be considered as a reliable biomarker of intake of any food, although it might be used as a complementary indicator, whose concentration changes must be coherent with dietary intakes.

Foods are composed of a range of chemical compounds, many of which vary due to factors such as variety and seasonality of food processing. Therefore, we need to exert a certain amount of caution when proposing single biomarkers of certain foods. If we are to move to the situation where biomarkers are to be used as an objective measure of dietary intake, then a combination of markers may be more useful. Metabolomics is particularly appropriate for providing combination of markers. While conceptually this makes sense, it should be noted that there are currently, to the best of our knowledge, no clear examples that demonstrate that combinations of biomarkers improve sensitivity and specificity with respect to dietary intake. However, in the biomedical field, it is becoming increasingly evident that combinations or panels of biomarkers are more effective as disease diagnosis and have improved sensitivity and specificity (Fan et al., 2011).

9.5 Dietary patterns and metabolomic profiles: potential use of nutritypes

In nutrition epidemiology, there is a growing interest in assessing dietary patterns and linking these to health outcomes. Stemming from this work, a number of studies have emerged demonstrating the link between dietary patterns and metabolomic profiles. In a recent study, the application of dietary pattern analysis to 125 subjects revealed three cluster groups that were associated with unique food intakes and differed significantly in the nutrient intake profiles (O'Sullivan et al., 2011). Assessment of the metabolomic profiles revealed that the cluster groups were reflected in the urinary metabolomic profiles. The novelty of this work lies in the fact that the identification of nutritypes (i.e. metabolic profiles that reflect dietary intake) has the potential to aid dietary assessment by unobjectively classifying people into certain dietary patterns.

Peré-Trepat and colleagues also developed a strategy for assessing links between dietary data (FFQ) and metabolomic profiles (Pere-Trepat et al., 2010). In this work, dietary patterns were defined by principal component analysis and then regressed against NMR metabolic profiles to identify metabolites associated with dietary patterns. This study adds further support to the concept of nutritypes.

Using the KORA (Cooperative Health Research in the Region of Augsburg) study population, seven dietary patterns were observed (Altmaier et al., 2011). Statistical analysis revealed that certain dietary patterns were highly associated with serum metabolite concentrations. Focusing on lipids, O'Gorman et al. recently demonstrated that certain dietary patterns are highly associated with the lipidome profile (O'Gorman et al., 2014).

Overall, these studies provide good evidence for the potential use of metabolomics in the characterisation of subjects according to their habitual dietary pattern.

9.6 Validation of putative biomarkers

Untargeted metabolomics has led to the discovery of a wealth of putative new biomarkers of specific food intake. Most of them are short-term markers observed in meal studies or controlled interventions, and their validation for use in observational studies will be a high priority in the coming years. In a cross-sectional analysis of a dietary intervention study, it was found that only around 20% of the markers found in meal studies could be confirmed in a more complex setting where subjects were choosing their own food items (Andersen et al., 2014a). Part of this failure was due to lack of sensitivity, and more targeted analysis may show that additional biomarkers could actually be useful. However, part of the failures was due to other foods containing metabolites that interfere or add to the marker measurement. For instance, several citrus terpenoids, including limonene, are found in a wealth of citrus-flavoured foods such as sweets, soft drinks, and bakery products (Andersen et al., 2014b). This underlines the need for validation of the novel putative markers from metabolomics under several study design conditions, including observational settings. The new multitargeted analytic methods open also for the use of combination markers so that certain markers act as qualifiers. For instance, if proline betaine is observed together with limonene metabolites, that would confirm citrus exposure; the lack of concomitant proline betaine may indicate intake of citrus-flavoured foods or soft drinks.

Clearly, the quality of a biomarker is a central issue. Biomarkers must be specific, accurate, and sensitive enough to detect small changes. The choice of biomarker is highly dependent on the study design and sampling strategy because different qualities may be more useful for the research questions posed. But first and foremost, there is a requirement for the validation of all putative biomarkers before they can be applied in a targeted fashion. No consensus criteria exist yet for the validation of nutritional biomarkers. Validation should include analytic assessment of precision and accuracy. Preferably, the marker should be validated against other markers for the same food intake, if such markers exist. Efforts should also include biological validation to assure dynamic dose–response and time–response in relation to intakes of the targeted food component; finally, it should be assessed that the marker is not influenced by unrelated compounds. Analytic validation is well described and is similar for biomarkers and for clinical chemistry (Rozet et al., 2011). Dose–response and time–response are important for interpretation and must be validated in study designs that resemble those that the marker is intended for, i.e., reflecting shorter- or longer-term food intakes. Biomarkers are dependent on how representative the sample is, for example, a blood draw may only represent a limited time span for a marker of food intake having a short half-life. However, a 24-h urine sample may be useful to monitor if a specific food was ingested at any time during that period. The question of whether a biomarker is valid would therefore depend very much on the purpose of the study. If the purpose is to determine the relationship of individual intakes of a specific food with disease risk, then it would be necessary to have a marker and a sampling scheme that represents longer-term average intakes or balances. This could be a validated recovery, prediction, or perhaps even concentration/replacement dietary biomarkers. If the purpose is to validate an FFQ in a controlled setting, it may be acceptable to use a validated shorter-term biomarker in order to check that reported and observed frequencies correlate.

The limitation of many emerging biomarkers from metabolomics is that we have little indication of their variability, e.g., their applicability to different populations, questions of interindividual variation in absorption and metabolism, and gene–diet interactions, just to mention a few host factors. Additional factors relate to food cultures, effects of cooking practices, variable bioaccessibility in different foods, etc. The best emerging biomarkers will have to be robust to these factors and have high correlations with true exposures, whereas others will have limitations that make them useful only under specific conditions.

9.7 The future of metabolomics in dietary assessment

9.7.1 Overcoming methodological bottlenecks in marker identification

Table 9.1 shows that metabolomics studies based on high-resolution mass spectrometry provided more candidate biomarkers than NMR. This is due to the higher sensitivity of mass spectrometry compared to NMR, which ensures the detection of nonnutrient metabolites present in biofluids in nano- or micromolar concentrations. However, mass spectrometry does not allow routine identification of the discriminant metabolites, and one of the major challenges is the identification of features emerging from the studies as putative biomarkers. Only 10–15% of the ions observed by high-resolution MS can generally be identified by screening exact masses in metabolite databases (Wishart, 2008). The situation is even worse for food metabolome studies since many food component metabolites are not described in chemical databases and not commercially available as standards. The multistep workflow for the

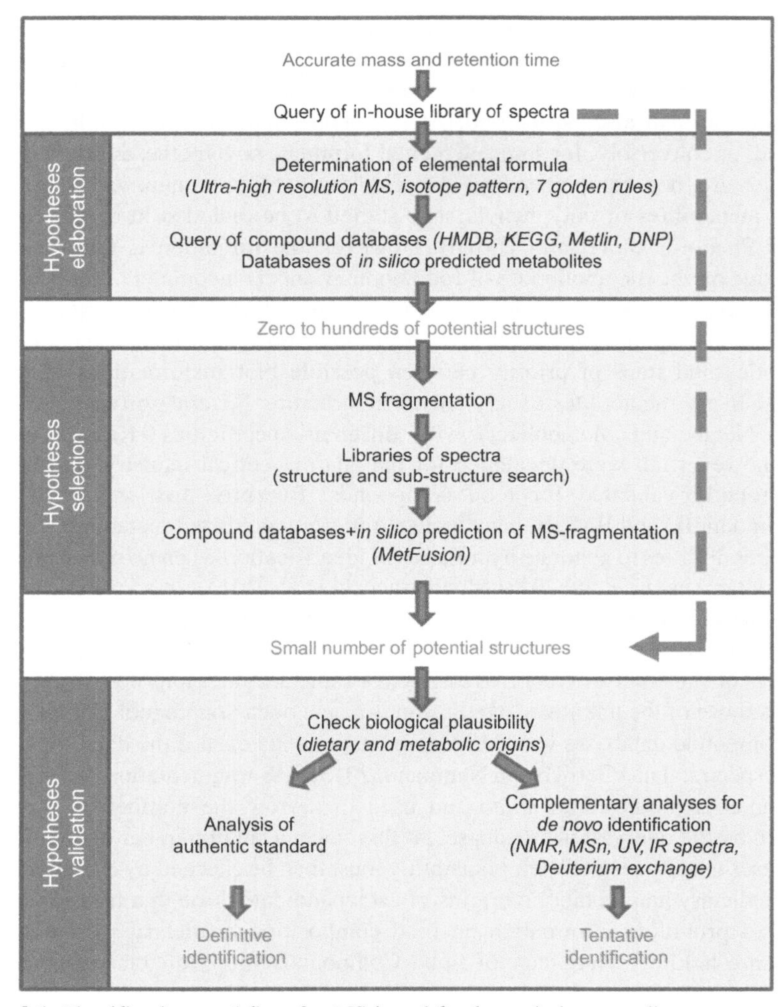

Figure 9.1 Identification workflow for MS-based food metabolome studies.

identification of discriminating ions in food metabolome studies is summarised in Figure 9.1. Identification of an unknown discriminant ion starts with the comparison of acquired analytic data (accurate mass and retention time) and with those of standards available in the in-house library of spectra. When no match is found, the elemental formula is determined using ultrahigh-resolution MS (Orbitrap and FTICR instruments) and isotope patterns, taking into account the seven golden rules (Kind and Fiehn, 2007; Stanstrup et al., 2013). When organic compounds are suspected, the number of possible elemental formulas can be restricted to those existing in natural products, through online query of the Dictionary of Natural Products with the accurate mass of the unknown (http://dnp.chemnetbase.com). The elemental formula, or the accurate mass, is then used to query several other compound databases to find hypotheses of identification. The main databases used in metabolomics are HMDB, METLIN, and LIPID MAPS, but more generalist databases such as ChEBI, KEGG, and PubChem can also be queried. At this stage, hundreds of hypotheses can be retrieved, or conversely, for some elemental formulas, no hypotheses are found since databases are not comprehensive, especially regarding nonnutrient metabolites. Known metabolites of polyphenols have started to be included in online databases such as Phenol-Explorer and HMDB. However, the limitation is that our current knowledge on the metabolic fate of food nonnutrients is incomplete. Initiatives have emerged to use *in silico* prediction of metabolism in in-house databases (Pujos-Guillot et al., 2013). Expert systems integrating current knowledge on the metabolism of xenobiotics and rules of priority between possible biotransformations can predict the most likely metabolites of any chemical structure. Several softwares exist (e.g. Meteor Nexus and Metabolizer) with different specificities (Kirchmair et al., 2012); however, all were developed for the pharmaceutical industry, and none has been properly validated for food compounds. Recently, two online databases, MyCompoundID and IIMDB, have included *in silico* predicted metabolites and offer further possibilities to generate hypotheses of identification when no match is found in classic databases (Li et al., 2013; Menikarachchi et al., 2013). In addition to database queries, MS fragmentation is very often carried out in the process of marker identification. Libraries of spectra such as MassBank and METLIN can be queried to find structures or substructures reported to give the same daughter ions upon MS fragmentation as those of the unknown. MetFusion is a new open-source tool that allows querying compound databases with MS fragmentation data even if the database does not contain spectral data (Gerlich and Neumann, 2013). MS fragmentation of the database compounds is predicted *in silico* and used to narrow the number of hypotheses retrieved by the query of the database. At this stage, a small number of identification hypotheses usually result. Their plausibility must then be checked by documenting the possible dietary and metabolic origins of each candidate through a literature survey. Databases providing information on food composition or dietary sources of compounds are helpful: Dictionary of Food Compounds (http://dfc.chemnetbase.com), Phenol-Explorer (www.phenol-explorer.eu), Dr. Duke's Phytochemical and Ethnobotanical Databases (www.ars-grin.gov/duke), and KNApSAcK (http://kanaya.naist.jp/knapsack_jsp/top.html). Two new databases FooDB (www.foodb.ca) and PhytoHub (www.phytohub.eu) are being developed with contents and functionalities specifically designed for metabolomics studies, as they will integrate for each compound spectral data, information on dietary origins, and known and predicted metabolic fate. PhytoHub will be focused on dietary phytochemicals, whereas FooDB will have a very wide coverage of all food constituents. When plausible hypotheses are obtained, they must be validated by the analysis of authentic standards. However, for nonnutrient metabolites, the standards are often not commercially available. Some metabolites can be synthesised by *in vitro* enzymatic synthesis or extracted by preparative chromatography from biological samples; however, identifications often remain tentative when the authentic standard is lacking. The complementary analyses necessary for *de novo* elucidation of the chemical structure (NMR, UV, IR spectra, deuterium exchanges, etc.)

can be very burdensome, and identification of one compound can sometimes take several weeks or more.

The difficulties encountered in marker identification should be reduced in the near future, thanks to technological advances. Mass spectrometry instruments are continuously evolving in terms of sensitivity and mass accuracy, and in parallel, there is a very active development of new bioinformatics tools to improve and automatise the process of marker identification (Scalbert et al., 2014; Xia et al., 2012). This should markedly accelerate the discovery of dietary biomarkers with nontargeted metabolomics.

9.7.2 Sharing of resources (databases, standard original procedures (SOPs), chemical standards, and raw data)

Large databases of compounds such as the Human Metabolome Database (www.hmdb.ca), METLIN (http://metlin.scripps.edu/index.php), LIPID MAPS (http://www.lipidmaps.org/), and several others are helping the community for the identification of markers; however, there are still a majority of unknown features in many food metabolomics studies. This is because the food metabolomes contain hitherto unknown metabolites of food components that may themselves not even be structurally elucidated. In that sense, the development of *in silico* tools for prediction of food component metabolism, also integrating gut microbiota metabolism, would greatly help to complement compound databases. Even for well-known candidate compounds, there is often no published spectral data, and a very large number of food metabolites are not commercially available, so that standards are not available for validation of feature assignments. This calls for additional sharing of compound features such as spectral data into public data repositories in formats where spectral details may be queried online by automated annotation programmes. Even so, the spectral data for some platforms such as LC–MS may be context specific so that they vary with solvent, instrumental setup, etc. Access to authentic standards is therefore a prerequisite for the best possible level of identification. A repository of human metabolites or a site offering increased exchange of custom synthesised metabolites between laboratories would therefore be additional tools to further food metabolomics.

The metabolomes recorded are highly dependent on the procedures used. No technique is able to cover the full human metabolome, so changes in pH, solvents, instrumental settings, and any other characteristic of the profiling procedure may cause major changes in metabolite coverage. This is also true for the software tools currently available for data preprocessing; and the statistical strategy to find markers is still another factor that may influence the metabolite set eventually recorded as the most important for food intake. The procedures used must therefore be carefully described for any metabolomics study, and standard operational procedures (SOPs) for good profiling, preprocessing, and data analysis should be shared more actively by the actors in the field. Some detailed procedures have been posted on Internet sites such as the NuGO (http://www.nugo.org) project homepage and by some of the research laboratories; however, there is no consensus set of "good practice SOPs" on the Internet.

9.7.3 Databasing of biomarkers: development of tools and methods for routine use in large-scale cohorts

As work progresses in this field, it will become imperative that groups collaborate to define an optimal method for capturing biomarkers associated with food intake. Currently, these data are scattered across the literature and not easily presented for the nonexpert. There is an urgent need for an open-source database that captures biomarker data, the associated food, the study design used, and information on the validity of the biomarker. Recently, a simple classification method was suggested where biomarkers would be graded by the level of validation (Sumner et al., 2007). Initiatives such as the European Joint Programming Initiative, Healthy Diet for a Healthy Life, should facilitate the formation of such databases in the coming years.

Furthermore, there is a requirement for the scientific community to deposit and share metabolomics biomarker data in open-source databases. Examples of such databases are (1) MetaboLights (http://www.ebi.ac.uk/metabolights/) and (2) the Nutritional Phenotype database (van Ommen et al., 2010). The storage of data in such open-access databases could facilitate users in validating their findings in other studies, thus enabling faster validation of putative biomarkers. Due to the fast development of the technology, it is also necessary that researchers share samples stored from the many dietary intervention studies that form the basis for food biomarker developments. An example of a biobank specialised in this area is CUBE (http://cube.ku.dk/). So in addition to the biobanks associated with cohort studies, there is a need to expanding current biobank infrastructures to cover also small experimental biobanks initiated by the community.

9.8 Conclusion

Nontargeted metabolomics has the potential to revolutionise the field of dietary assessment, through the discovery of dozens of new intake/exposure biomarkers. These biomarkers once properly validated could be included in multitool strategies for dietary assessment, combining Internet questionnaires, digital camera images, and analysis of biomarker panels. Accuracy and precision of dietary assessment will be markedly increased, as required for modern nutritional epidemiology. However, several technical challenges have been identified that will have to be collectively tackled before the metabolomics approach reaches its full potential.

References

Afman, L., Muller, M., 2006. Nutrigenomics: from molecular nutrition to prevention of disease. J. Am. Diet. Assoc. 106, 569–576.

Altmaier, E., Kastenmuller, G., Romisch-Margl, W., Thorand, B., Weinberger, K.M., Illig, T., Adamski, J., Doring, A., Suhre, K., 2011. Questionnaire-based self-reported nutrition habits associate with serum metabolism as revealed by quantitative targeted metabolomics. Eur. J. Epidemiol. 26, 145–156.

Andersen, M.B.S., Reinbach, H.C., Rinnan, A., Barri, T., Mithril, C., Dragsted, L.O., 2013. Discovery of exposure markers in urine for Brassica-containing meals served with different protein sources by UPLC-qTOF-MS untargeted metabolomics. Metabolomics 9, 984–997.

Andersen, M.B., Kristensen, M., Manach, C., Pujos-Guillot, E., Poulsen, S.K., Larsen, T.M., Astrup, A., Dragsted, L., 2014a. Discovery and validation of urinary exposure markers for different plant foods by untargeted metabolomics. Anal. Bioanal. Chem. 406, 1829–1844.

Andersen, M.B., Rinnan, A., Manach, C., Poulsen, S.K., Pujos-Guillot, E., Larsen, T.M., Astrup, A., Dragsted, L.O., 2014b. Untargeted metabolomics as a screening tool for estimating compliance to a dietary pattern. J. Proteome Res. 13, 1405–1418.

Baldrick, F.R., Woodside, J.V., Elborn, J.S., Young, I.S., McKinley, M.C., 2011. Biomarkers of fruit and vegetable intake in human intervention studies: a systematic review. Crit. Rev. Food Sci. Nutr. 51, 795–815.

Beckmann, M., Lloyd, A.J., Haldar, S., Seal, C., Brandt, K., Draper, J., 2013. Hydroxylated phenylacetamides derived from bioactive benzoxazinoids are bioavailable in humans after habitual consumption of whole grain sourdough rye bread. Mol. Nutr. Food Res. 57, 1859–1873.

Bingham, S.A., Luben, R., Welch, A., Wareham, N., Khaw, K.T., Day, N., 2003. Are imprecise methods obscuring a relation between fat and breast cancer? Lancet 362, 212–214.

Bingham, S., Luben, R., Welch, A., Low, Y.L., Khaw, K.T., Wareham, N., Day, N., 2008. Associations between dietary methods and biomarkers, and between fruits and vegetables and risk of ischaemic heart disease, in the EPIC Norfolk Cohort Study. Int. J. Epidemiol. 37, 978–987.

Bondia-Pons, I., Barri, T., Hanhineva, K., Juntunen, K., Dragsted, L.O., Mykkanen, H., Poutanen, K., 2013. UPLC-QTOF/MS metabolic profiling unveils urinary changes in humans after a whole grain rye versus refined wheat bread intervention. Mol. Nutr. Food Res. 57, 412–422.

Champagne, C.M., Wroten, K.C., 2012. From food databases to dietary assessment: a beginning to an end approach for quality nutrition data. Nutr. Diet. 69, 187–194.

Corella, D., Peloso, G., Arnett, D.K., Demissie, S., Cupples, L.A., Tucker, K., Lai, C.Q., Parnell, L.D., Coltell, O., Lee, Y.C., Ordovas, J.M., 2009. APOA2, dietary fat, and body mass index replication of a gene-diet interaction in 3 independent populations. Arch. Intern. Med. 169, 1897–1906.

Cross, A.J., Major, J.M., Sinha, R., 2011. Urinary biomarkers of meat consumption. Cancer Epidemiol. Biomarkers Prev. 20, 1107–1111.

Daykin, C.A., van Duynhoven, J.P.M., Groenewegen, A., Dachtler, M., van Amelsvoort, J.M. M., Mulder, T.P.J., 2005. Nuclear magnetic resonance spectroscopic based studies of the metabolism of black tea polyphenols in humans. J. Agric. Food Chem. 53, 1428–1434.

Dragsted, L.O., 2010. Biomarkers of meat intake and the application of nutrigenomics. Meat Sci. 84, 301–307.

Edmands, W.M.B., Beckonert, O.P., Stella, C., Campbell, A., Lake, B.G., Lindon, J.C., Holmes, E., Gooderham, N.J., 2011. Identification of human urinary biomarkers of cruciferous vegetable consumption by metabonomic profiling. J. Proteome Res. 10, 4513–4521.

Fan, Y., Murphy, T.B., Byrne, J.C., Brennan, L., Fitzpatrick, J.M., Watson, R.W.G., 2011. Applying random forests to identify biomarker panels in serum 2D-DIGE data for the detection and staging of prostate cancer. J. Proteome Res. 10, 1361–1373.

Freedman, L.S., Potischman, N., Kipnis, V., Midthune, D., Schatzkin, A., Thompson, F.E., Troiano, R.P., Prentice, R., Patterson, R., Carroll, R., Subar, A.F., 2006. A comparison of two dietary instruments for evaluating the fat-breast cancer relationship. Int. J. Epidemiol. 35, 1011–1021.

Friel, P.N., Logan, B.K., Baer, J., 1995. An evaluation of the reliability of widmark calculations based on breath alcohol measurements. J. Forensic Sci. 40, 91–94.

Garcia, A.L., Mohan, R., Koebnick, C., Bub, A., Heuer, T., Strassner, C., Groeneveld, M.J., Katz, N., Elmadfa, I., Leitzmann, C., Hoffmann, I., 2010. Plasma beta-carotene is not a suitable biomarker of fruit and vegetable intake in German subjects with a long-term high consumption of fruits and vegetables. Ann. Nutr. Metab. 56, 23–30.

Gerlich, M., Neumann, S., 2013. MetFusion: integration of compound identification strategies. J. Mass Spectrom. 48, 291–298.

Gibney, M.J., Walsh, M.C., 2013. The future direction of personalised nutrition: my diet, my phenotype, my genes. Proc. Nutr. Soc. 72, 219–225.

Hartman, A.M., Brown, C.C., Palmgren, J., Pietinen, P., Verkasalo, M., Myer, D., Virtamo, J., 1990. Variability in nutrient and food intakes among older middle-aged men – implications for design of epidemiologic and validation studies using food recording. Am. J. Epidemiol. 132, 999–1012.

Heinzmann, S.S., Brown, I.J., Chan, Q., Bictash, M., Dumas, M.E., Kochhar, S., Stamler, J., Holmes, E., Elliott, P., Nicholson, J.K., 2010. Metabolic profiling strategy for discovery of nutritional biomarkers: proline betaine as a marker of citrus consumption. Am. J. Clin. Nutr. 92, 436–443.

Hercberg, S., 2012. Web-based studies: the future in nutritional epidemiology (and overarching epidemiology) for the benefit of public health? Prev. Med. 55, 544–545.

Hjerpsted, J.B., Ritz, C., Schou, S.S., Tholstrup, T., Dragsted, L.O., 2014. Effect of cheese and butter intake on metabolites in urine using a non-targeted metabolomics approach. Metabolomics 10, 1176–1185.

Hoiseth, G., Yttredal, B., Karinen, R., Gjerde, H., Morland, J., Christophersen, A., 2010. Ethyl glucuronide concentrations in oral fluid, blood, and urine after volunteers drank 0.5 and 1.0 g/kg doses of ethanol. J. Anal. Toxicol. 34, 319–324.

Jacobs, D.M., Fuhrmann, J.C., van Dorsten, F.A., Rein, D., Peters, S., van Velzen, E.J.J., Hollebrands, B., Draijer, R., van Duynhoven, J., Garczarek, U., 2012. Impact of short-term intake of red wine and grape polyphenol extract on the human metabolome. J. Agric. Food Chem. 60, 3078–3085.

Jenab, M., Slimani, N., Bictash, M., Ferrari, P., Bingham, S.A., 2009. Biomarkers in nutritional epidemiology: applications, needs and new horizons. Hum. Genet. 125, 507–525.

Johansson-Persson, A., Barri, T., Ulmius, M., Onning, G., Dragsted, L.O., 2013. LC-QTOF/MS metabolomic profiles in human plasma after a 5-week high dietary fiber intake. Anal. Bioanal. Chem. 405, 4799–4809.

Kall, M.A., Clausen, J., 1995. Dietary effect on mixed-function P450 1A2 activity assayed by estimation of caffeine metabolism in man. Hum. Exp. Toxicol. 14, 801–807.

Kamimori, G.H., Karyekar, C.S., Otterstetter, R., Cox, D.S., Balkin, T.J., Belenky, G.L., Eddington, N.D., 2002. The rate of absorption and relative bioavailability of caffeine administered in chewing gum versus capsules to normal healthy volunteers. Int. J. Pharm. 234, 159–167.

Kaput, J., 2008. Nutrigenomics research for personalized nutrition and medicine. Curr. Opin. Biotechnol. 19, 110–120.

Kind, T., Fiehn, O., 2007. Seven golden rules for heuristic filtering of molecular formulas obtained by accurate mass spectrometry. BMC Bioinformatics 8, 105.

Kipnis, V., Midthune, D., Buckman, D.W., Dodd, K.W., Guenther, P.M., Krebs-Smith, S.M., Subar, A.F., Tooze, J.A., Carroll, R.J., Freedman, L.S., 2009. Modeling data with excess zeros and measurement error: application to evaluating relationships between episodically consumed foods and health outcomes. Biometrics 65, 1003–1010.

Kirchmair, J., Williamson, M.J., Tyzack, J.D., Tan, L., Bond, P.J., Bender, A., Glen, R.C., 2012. Computational prediction of metabolism: sites, products, SAR, P450 enzyme dynamics, and mechanisms. J. Chem. Inf. Model. 52, 617–648.

Klebanoff, M.A., Levine, R.J., Dersimonian, R., Clemens, J.D., Wilkins, D.G., 1998. Serum caffeine and paraxanthine as markers for reported caffeine intake in pregnancy. Ann. Epidemiol. 8, 107–111.

Kristal, A.R., Peters, U., Potter, J.D., 2005. Is it time to abandon the food frequency questionnaire? Cancer Epidemiol. Biomarkers Prev. 14, 2826–2828.

Lampe, J.W., Navarro, S.L., Hullar, M.A.J., Shojaie, A., 2013. Inter-individual differences in response to dietary intervention: integrating omics platforms towards personalised dietary recommendations. Proc. Nutr. Soc. 72, 207–218.

Lang, R., Wahl, A., Stark, T., Hofmann, T., 2011. Urinary N-methylpyridinium and trigonelline as candidate dietary biomarkers of coffee consumption. Mol. Nutr. Food Res. 55, 1613–1623.

Lee, M.B., Storer, M.K., Blunt, J.W., Lever, M., 2006. Validation of ^{1}H NMR spectroscopy as an analytical tool for methylamine metabolites in urine. Clin. Chim. Acta 365, 264–269.

Lees, H.J., Swann, J.R., Wilson, I.D., Nicholson, J.K., Holmes, E., 2013. Hippurate: the natural history of a mammalian-microbial cometabolite. J. Proteome Res. 12, 1527–1546.

Lehtonen, H.M., Lindstedt, A., Jarvinen, R., Sinkkonen, J., Graca, G., Viitanen, M., Kallio, H., Gil, A.M., 2013. ^{1}H NMR-based metabolic fingerprinting of urine metabolites after consumption of lingonberries (*Vaccinium vitis-idaea*) with a high-fat meal. Food Chem. 138, 982–990.

Lenz, E.M., Bright, J., Wilson, I.D., Hughes, A., Morrisson, J., Lindberg, H., Lockton, A., 2004. Metabonomics, dietary influences and cultural differences: a H-1 NMR-based study of urine samples obtained from healthy British and Swedish subjects. J. Pharm. Biomed. Anal. 36, 841–849.

Levine, M., Conry-Cantilena, C., Wang, Y., Welch, R.W., Washko, P.W., Dhariwal, K.R., Park, J.B., Lazarev, A., Graumlich, J.F., King, J., Cantilena, L.R., 1996. Vitamin C pharmacokinetics in healthy volunteers: evidence for a recommended dietary allowance. Proc. Natl. Acad. Sci. U. S. A. 93, 3704–3709.

Li, L., Li, R.H., Zhou, J.J., Zuniga, A., Stanislaus, A.E., Wu, Y.M., Huan, T., Zheng, J.M., Shi, Y., Wishart, D.S., Lin, G.H., 2013. MyCompoundID: using an evidence-based metabolome library for metabolite identification. Anal. Chem. 85, 3401–3408.

Llorach, R., Urpi-Sarda, M., Jauregui, O., Monagas, M., Andres-Lacueva, C., 2009. An LC-MS-based metabolomics approach for exploring urinary metabolome modifications after cocoa consumption. J. Proteome Res. 8, 5060–5068.

Llorach, R., Garrido, I., Monagas, M., Urpi-Sarda, M., Tulipani, S., Bartolome, B., Andres-Lacueva, C., 2010. Metabolomics study of human urinary metabolome modifications after intake of almond (*Prunus dulcis* (Mill.) DA Webb) skin polyphenols. J. Proteome Res. 9, 5859–5867.

Llorach, R., Urpi-Sarda, M., Tulipani, S., Garcia-Aloy, M., Monagas, M., Andres-Lacueva, C., 2013. Metabolomic fingerprint in patients at high risk of cardiovascular disease by cocoa intervention. Mol. Nutr. Food Res. 57, 962–973.

Llorach, R., Medina, S., Garcia-Viguera, C., Zafrilla, P., Abellan, J., Jauregui, O., Tomas-Barberan, F.A., Gil-Izquierdo, A., Andres-Lacueva, C., 2014. Discovery of human urinary biomarkers of aronia-citrus juice intake by HPLC-q-TOF-based metabolomic approach. Electrophoresis 35 (11), 1599–1606.

Lloyd, A.J., Beckmann, M., Fave, G., Mathers, J.C., Draper, J., 2011a. Proline betaine and its biotransformation products in fasting urine samples are potential biomarkers of habitual citrus fruit consumption. Br. J. Nutr. 106, 812–824.

Lloyd, A.J., Fave, G., Beckmann, M., Lin, W.C., Tailliart, K., Xie, L., Mathers, J.C., Draper, J., 2011b. Use of mass spectrometry fingerprinting to identify urinary metabolites after consumption of specific foods. Am. J. Clin. Nutr. 94, 981–991.
Lloyd, A.J., Beckmann, M., Haldar, S., Seal, C., Brandt, K., Draper, J., 2013. Data-driven strategy for the discovery of potential urinary biomarkers of habitual dietary exposure. Am. J. Clin. Nutr. 97, 377–389.
Macdiarmid, J., Blundell, J., 1998. Assessing dietary intake: who, what and why of under-reporting. Nutr. Res. Rev. 11, 231–253.
Manach, C., Hubert, J., Llorach, R., Scalbert, A., 2009. The complex links between dietary phytochemicals and human health deciphered by metabolomics. Mol. Nutr. Food Res. 53, 1303–1315.
Marklund, M., Landberg, R., Andersson, A., Aman, P., Kamal-Eldin, A., 2013. Alkylresorcinol metabolites in urine correlate with the intake of whole grains and cereal fibre in free-living Swedish adults. Br. J. Nutr. 109, 129–136.
Marshall, J.R., Chen, Z., 1999. Diet and health risk: risk patterns and disease-specific associations. Am. J. Clin. Nutr. 69, 1351S–1356S.
May, D.H., Navarro, S.L., Ruczinski, I., Hogan, J., Ogata, Y., Schwarz, Y., Levy, L., Holzman, T., McIntosh, M.W., Lampe, J.W., 2013. Metabolomic profiling of urine: response to a randomised, controlled feeding study of select fruits and vegetables, and application to an observational study. Br. J. Nutr. 110, 1760–1770.
Menikarachchi, L., Hill, D., Hamdalla, M., Mandiou, I., Grant, D.F., 2013. In silico enzymatic synthesis of a 400 000 compound biochemical database for nontargeted metabolomics. J. Chem. Inf. Model. 53, 2483–2492.
Minihane, A.M., 2013. The genetic contribution to disease risk and variability in response to diet: where is the hidden heritability? Proc. Nutr. Soc. 72, 40–47.
O'Gorman, A., Morris, C., Ryan, M., O'Grada, C.M., Roche, H.M., Gibney, E.R., Gibney, M.J., Brennan, L., 2014. Habitual dietary intake impacts on the lipidomic profile. J. Chromatogr. B Analyt. Technol. Biomed. Life Sci. 966, 140–146. http://dx.doi.org/10.1016/j.jchromb.2014.01.032.
O'Sullivan, A., Gibney, M.J., Brennan, L., 2011. Dietary intake patterns are reflected in metabolomic profiles: potential role in dietary assessment studies. Am. J. Clin. Nutr. 93, 314–321.
Pere-Trepat, E., Ross, A.B., Martin, F.P., Rezzi, S., Kochhar, S., Hasselbalch, A.L., Kyvik, K. O., Sorensen, T.I.A., 2010. Chemometric strategies to assess metabonomic imprinting of food habits in epidemiological studies. Chemometr. Intell. Lab. 104, 95–100.
Pujos-Guillot, E., Hubert, J., Martin, J.F., Lyan, B., Quintana, M., Claude, S., Chabanas, B., Rothwell, J.A., Bennetau-Pelissero, C., Scalbert, A., Comte, B., Hercberg, S., Morand, C., Galan, P., Manach, C., 2013. Mass spectrometry-based metabolomics for the discovery of biomarkers of fruit and vegetable intake: citrus fruit as a case study. J. Proteome Res. 12, 1645–1659.
Rago, D., Mette, K., Gurdeniz, G., Marini, F., Poulsen, M., Dragsted, L.O., 2013. A LC-MS metabolomics approach to investigate the effect of raw apple intake in the rat plasma metabolome. Metabolomics 9, 1202–1215.
Rasmussen, L.G., Winning, H., Savorani, F., Toft, H., Larsen, T.M., Dragsted, L.O., Astrup, A., Engelsen, S.B., 2012. Assessment of the effect of high or low protein diet on the human urine metabolome as measured by NMR. Nutrients 4, 112–131.
Rothwell, J.A., Fillâtre, Y., Martin, J.F., Lyan, B., Pujos-Guillot, E., Fezeu, L., Hercberg, S., Comte, B., Galan, P., Touvier, M., Manach, C., 2014. New biomarkers of coffee consumption identified by the non-targeted metabolomic profiling of cohort study subjects. Plos One 9 (4), e93474.

Rozet, E., Marini, R.D., Ziemons, E., Boulanger, B., Hubert, P., 2011. Advances in validation, risk and uncertainty assessment of bioanalytical methods. J. Pharm. Biomed. Anal. 55, 848–858.

Scalbert, A., Brennan, L., Manach, C., Andres-Lacueva, C., Dragsted, L.O., Draper, J., Rappaport, S., van der Hooft, J.J., wishart,, D., 2014. The food metabolome: a window over dietary exposure. Am. J. Clin. Nutr. 99 (6), 1286–1308. http://dx.doi.org/10.3945/ajcn.113.076133.

Schatzkin, A., Kipnis, V., 2004. Could exposure assessment problems give us wrong answers to nutrition and cancer questions? J. Natl. Cancer Inst. 96, 1564–1565.

Silva, V., Barazzoni, R., Singer, P., 2014. Biomarkers of fish oil omega-3 polyunsaturated fatty acids intake in humans. Nutr. Clin. Pract. 29, 63–72.

Six, B.L., Schap, T.E., Zhu, F.M., Mariappan, A., Bosch, M., Delp, E.J., Ebert, D.S., Kerr, D.A., Boushey, C.J., 2010. Evidence-based development of a mobile telephone food record. J. Am. Diet. Assoc. 110, 74–79.

Spencer, J.P.E., Mohsen, M.M.A., Minihane, A.M., Mathers, J.C., 2008. Biomarkers of the intake of dietary polyphenols: strengths, limitations and application in nutrition research. Br. J. Nutr. 99, 12–22.

Stanstrup, J., Gerlich, M., Dragsted, L.O., Neumann, S., 2013. Metabolite profiling and beyond: approaches for the rapid processing and annotation of human blood serum mass spectrometry data. Anal. Bioanal. Chem. 405, 5037–5048.

Stanstrup, J., Schou, S.S., Holmer-Jensen, J., Hermansen, K., Dragsted, L.O., 2014. Whey protein delays gastric emptying and suppresses plasma fatty acids and their metabolites compared to casein, gluten and cod protein. J. Proteome Res. 13, 2396–2408.

Stella, C., Beckwith-Hall, B., Cloarec, O., Holmes, E., Lindon, J.C., Powell, J., van der Ouderaa, F., Bingham, S., Cross, A.J., Nicholson, J.K., 2006. Susceptibility of human metabolic phenotypes to dietary modulation. J. Proteome Res. 5, 2780–2788.

Stumbo, P.J., 2013. New technology in dietary assessment: a review of digital methods in improving food record accuracy. Proc. Nutr. Soc. 72, 70–76.

Subar, A.F., Kirkpatrick, S.I., Mittl, B., Zimmerman, T.P., Thompson, F.E., Bingley, C., Willis, G., Islam, N.G., Baranowski, T., McNutt, S., Potischman, N., 2012. The automated self-administered 24-hour dietary recall (ASA24): a resource for researchers, clinicians, and educators from the National Cancer Institute. J. Acad. Nutr. Diet. 112, 1134–1137.

Sumner, L.W., Amberg, A., Barrett, D., Beale, M.H., Beger, R., Daykin, C.A., Fan, T.W.M., Fiehn, O., Goodacre, R., Griffin, J.L., Hankemeier, T., Hardy, N., Harnly, J., Higashi, R., Kopka, J., Lane, A.N., Lindon, J.C., Marriott, P., Nicholls, A.W., Reily, M. D., Thaden, J.J., Viant, M.R., 2007. Proposed minimum reporting standards for chemical analysis. Metabolomics 3, 211–221.

Trujillo, E., Davis, C., Milner, J., 2006. Nutrigenomics, proteomics, metabolomics, and the practice of dietetics. J. Am. Diet. Assoc. 106, 403–413.

Tucker, K.L., Smith, C.E., Lai, C.Q., Ordovas, J.M., 2013. Quantifying diet for nutrigenomic studies. Annu. Rev. Nutr. 33, 349–371.

Tulipani, S., Llorach, R., Jauregui, O., Lopez-Uriarte, P., Garcia-Aloy, M., Bullo, M., Salas-Salvado, J., Andres-Lacueva, C., 2011. Metabolomics unveils urinary changes in subjects with metabolic syndrome following 12-week nut consumption. J. Proteome Res. 10, 5047–5058.

van Dorsten, F.A., Daykin, C.A., Mulder, T.P.J., van Duynhoven, J.P.M., 2006. Metabonomics approach to determine metabolic differences between green tea and black tea consumption. J. Agric. Food Chem. 54, 6929–6938.

van Dorsten, F.A., Grun, C.H., van Velzen, E.J.J., Jacobs, D.M., Draijer, R., van Duynhoven, J.P.M., 2010. The metabolic fate of red wine and grape juice polyphenols in humans assessed by metabolomics. Mol. Nutr. Food Res. 54, 897–908.

van Ommen, B., Bouwman, J., Dragsted, L.O., Drevon, C.A., Elliott, R., de Groot, P., Kaput, J., Mathers, J.C., Muller, M., Pepping, F., Saito, J., Scalbert, A., Radonjic, M., Rocca-Serra, P., Travis, A., Wopereis, S., Evelo, C.T., 2010. Challenges of molecular nutrition research 6: the nutritional phenotype database to store, share and evaluate nutritional systems biology studies. Genes Nutr. 5, 189–203.

van Velzen, E.J.J., Westerhuis, J.A., van Duynhoven, J.P.M., van Dorsten, F.A., Grun, C.H., Jacobs, D.M., Duchateau, G., Vis, D.J., Smilde, A.K., 2009. Phenotyping tea consumers by nutrikinetic analysis of polyphenolic end-metabolites. J. Proteome Res. 8, 3317–3330.

Vazquez-Fresno, R., Llorach, R., Alcaro, F., Rodriguez, M.A., Vinaixa, M., Chiva-Blanch, G., Estruch, R., Correig, X., Andres-Lacueva, C., 2012. ^{1}H-NMR-based metabolomic analysis of the effect of moderate wine consumption on subjects with cardiovascular risk factors. Electrophoresis 33, 2345–2354.

Vermeulen, M., van Rooijen, H.J.M., Vaes, W.H.J., 2003. Analysis of isothiocyanate mercapturic acids in urine: a biomarker for cruciferous vegetable intake. J. Agric. Food Chem. 51, 3554–3559.

Wang, Y.L., Tang, H.R., Nicholson, J.K., Hylands, P.J., Sampson, J., Holmes, E., 2005. A metabonomic strategy for the detection of the metabolic effects of chamomile (Matricaria recutita L.) ingestion. J. Agric. Food Chem. 53, 191–196.

Wang, Z., Tang, W.H., Buffa, J.A., Fu, X., Britt, E.B., Koeth, R.A., Levison, B.S., Fan, Y., Wu, Y., Hazen, S.L., 2014. Prognostic value of choline and betaine depends on intestinal microbiota-generated metabolite trimethylamine-N-oxide. Eur. Heart J. 35, 904–910.

Wishart, D.S., 2008. Metabolomics: applications to food science and nutrition research. Trends Food Sci. Technol. 19, 482–493.

Xia, J.G., Mandal, R., Sinelnikov, I.V., Broadhurst, D., Wishart, D.S., 2012. MetaboAnalyst 2.0 – a comprehensive server for metabolomic data analysis. Nucleic Acids Res. 40, W127–W133.

Zeisel, S.H., 2007. Nutrigenomics and metabolomics will change clinical nutrition and public health practice: insights from studies on dietary requirements for choline. Am. J. Clin. Nutr. 86, 542–548.

Zivkovic, A.M., Wiest, M.M., Nguyen, U., Nording, M.L., Watkins, S.M., German, J.B., 2009. Assessing individual metabolic responsiveness to a lipid challenge using a targeted metabolomic approach. Metabolomics 5, 209–218.

Metabolomics and nutritional challenge tests: what can we learn?

L. Brennan[1,2]
[1]University College Dublin, Dublin, Ireland; [2]Newcastle University, Newcastle upon Tyne, United Kingdom

10.1 Introduction

Traditionally, challenge tests such as oral glucose tolerance test (OGTT) and oral lipid tolerance test (OLTT) have been used to assess metabolic disorders such as type II diabetes. In recent years, the use of such meal challenges to identify subtle changes in nutrition studies has gained momentum (Berthiaume and Zinker, 2002; Lin et al., 2011; Zhao et al., 2009). The underlying concept behind applying these challenge tests in such a situation is that healthy humans have the ability to maintain homeostasis through a multitude of nutritionally regulated processes; thus, measurements at homeostasis will often not reveal differences between groups. Assessment of time-dependent changes in response to food provides information about the health of an individual and helps detect subtle changes following dietary interventions.

Glucose homeostasis is a complex physiological process involving the orchestration of multiple organ systems. During an overnight fasting, for instance, glucose levels are maintained through both glycogenolysis and gluconeogenesis, and the liver begins to generate ketone bodies. Ingestion of glucose following an overnight fasting triggers the rapid release of insulin from the pancreatic beta-cells. This in turn promotes glucose uptake in peripheral tissues and switches the body from catabolism to anabolism. Hence, the transition from fasting to feeding is accompanied by many changes in metabolite concentrations as the body makes adjustments to achieve glucose homeostasis. In order to obtain a systematic view of the physiological response to glucose ingestion, researchers have recently started to apply metabolomic analysis to samples collected during the time course of a challenge. This chapter will give a review of the current literature with respect to applying metabolomics to nutritional challenges in human studies.

10.2 Application of metabolomics to challenge tests

Applications of metabolomics to study the response to nutritional challenge tests in humans have grown in recent years and the key studies are summarised in Table 10.1. Shaham et al. (2008) was one of the first published papers to investigate

Metabolomics as a Tool in Nutrition Research. http://dx.doi.org/10.1016/B978-1-78242-084-2.00010-1

Table 10.1 Overview of key studies using metabolomics in conjunction with challenge tests

Reference	Challenge test	Target population	Duration	Methodology	Outcome
Ho et al. (2013)	OGTT	377 subjects: 189 (insulin normal), 188 (insulin-resistant) BMI: 30.1 $\pm$ 5.3 kg/m^2	2 h	LC–MS, plasma samples	91 metabolites significantly change with the OGTT
Pellis et al. (2012)	Standardised dairy shake containing contribution to energy as follows: 59% lipids 30% CHO 12% protein	Crossover double-blind study design Male BMI: 25.6–34.7 kg/m^2 (n = 36)	6 h	Plasma samples GC–MS	Alterations in 106 metabolites, 31 proteins, and 5 clinical chemistry parameters. The challenge test identified metabolic changes following the dietary intervention not observed in nonperturbed conditions
Krug et al. (2012)	Oral glucose and lipid tests, liquid test meals, physical exercise, and cold stress	Males (n = 15) BMI: 23.1 $\pm$ 1.8 kg/m^2	4 days	Plasma, urine, exhaled air, and breath condensate samples LC–MS ^{1}H-NMR	Physiological challenges increased interindividual variation even in phenotypically similar volunteers, revealing metabotypes not observable in baseline metabolite profiles
Zivkovic et al. (2009)	Dairy-based lipid challenge	Male (n = 2) Female (n = 1) BMI: 21 $\pm$ 0.25 kg/m^2 (SEM)	8 h	Plasma samples	Assessed metabolic response as a measure of metabolic phenotype

Zhao et al. (2009)	OGTT	Males and females ($n=16$)	2 h	Plasma samples UPLC–qTOF MS	Four major groups of metabolites were detected as the most discriminating OGTT biomarkers: free fatty acids (FFA), acylcarnitines, bile acids, and lysophosphatidylcholines
Shaham et al. (2008)	OGTT	*Healthy individuals*: Males ($n=17$) Females ($n=12$) BMI: 17.8–26.9 kg/m^2 *Prediabetics*: Males ($n=24$) Females ($n=26$) BMI: 18.8–41.2 kg/m^2	2 h	Plasma samples LC–MS MS	Identified novel changes to OGTT including bile acids, urea cycle intermediates, and purine degradation products, none of which were previously linked to glucose homeostasis

Values are means ± SD unless otherwise stated.

the metabolomic response to an OGTT. The analysis revealed that there were 18 plasma metabolites that changed significantly and reproducibly during an oral glucose challenge including bile acids, urea cycle intermediates, and purine degradation products, none of which were previously linked to glucose homeostasis. The metabolite dynamics also revealed insulin's known actions along four key axes – proteolysis, lipolysis, ketogenesis, and glycolysis – reflecting a switch from catabolism to anabolism. In prediabetes, a blunted response in all four axes was observed. Multivariate analysis revealed that declines in glycerol and leucine/isoleucine (markers of lipolysis and proteolysis, respectively) jointly provided the strongest predictor of insulin sensitivity. This study made a significant contribution to the literature and lay the groundwork for using metabolic profiling to define an individual's "insulin response profile".

Zhao et al. (2009) also investigated the changes of the plasma metabolome during an OGTT. Using a nontargeted metabolomic approach, the metabolic response to the challenge was investigated. Applying multivariate data analysis revealed four major groups of metabolites as the most discriminating OGTT biomarkers. These four groups included free fatty acids (FFA), acylcarnitines, bile acids, and lysophosphatidylcholines. Some of the interesting findings included a strong decrease of all saturated and monounsaturated FFA studied during the OGTT and a significant faster decline of palmitoleate (C16:1) and oleate (C18:1) FFA levels compared to their saturated counterparts. Moreover, the bile acids glycocholic acid, glycochenodeoxycholic acid, and glycodeoxycholic acid were highly discriminative showing a biphasic kinetic with a maximum of a 4.5- to 6-fold increase at 30 min after glucose ingestion. The application of metabolomics in combination with an OGTT in this study revealed detailed insights into the complex physiological regulation of the metabolism during an OGTT.

Applying metabolomics in conjunction with proteomics to an OGTT as part of a dietary intervention revealed subtle effects on human metabolic status induced by the intervention (Pellis et al., 2012). Assessment of the time course revealed that 106 metabolites, 31 proteins, and 5 clinical chemistry parameters changed over the course of the challenge test. The application of the approach to a dietary intervention study was performed to evaluate if profiling the challenge test could reveal additional metabolic changes compared to nonperturbed conditions. The intervention of interest consisted of a 5-week intervention with a supplement mix of anti-inflammatory compounds in a crossover design with 36 overweight subjects. Of the 231 quantified parameters, 31 had different responses over time between treated and control groups, revealing differences in amino acid metabolism, oxidative stress, inflammation, and endocrine metabolism. Overall, the results clearly demonstrated that the acute, short-term metabolic responses to the challenge test were different in subjects on the supplement mix compared to the controls. The challenge test approach provided additional metabolic changes related to the dietary intervention not observed in nonperturbed conditions. This study supports the concept that a metabolomics-based quantification of a challenge of metabolic homeostasis is more informative with respect to metabolic status and the subtle effects induced by dietary interventions compared to the quantification of the homeostatic situation.

In another study, a highly controlled 4-day challenge protocol was applied to 15 young healthy male volunteers (Krug et al., 2012). Using this approach, the dynamics of the human metabolome in response to environmental stimuli, by submitting 15 young healthy male volunteers to a highly controlled 4-day challenge protocol, including 36 h fasting, oral glucose and lipid tests, liquid test meals, physical exercise, and cold stress. Blood, urine, exhaled air, and breath condensate samples were analysed on up to 56 time points by MS- and NMR-based methods, yielding 275 metabolic traits with a focus on lipids and amino acids. The results revealed that physiological challenges increased interindividual variation even in phenotypically similar volunteers, revealing metabotypes not observable in baseline metabolite profiles again supporting the concept of the use of these challenges to yield biological information.

A metabolic profiling study of normal subjects ($n = 189$) and insulin-resistant subjects ($n = 188$) revealed that of the 110 metabolites profiled, 91 significantly increased or decreased following the challenge (Ho et al., 2013). The changes broadly agreed with the actions of insulin including changes to the following pathways: proteolysis, ketogenesis, TCA cycle, and glycolysis. More importantly, the analysis revealed changes to pathways that were unknown to be linked to glucose homeostasis. Specifically, alterations in the neurotransmitter serotonin and precursors and derivatives of B vitamins were observed following the glucose challenge. Furthermore, comparison of the subjects with and without insulin resistance revealed that the application of metabolomics in combination with an OGTT may be useful in unmasking phenotypes in the prediabetic state.

Strassburg and colleagues examined the response of oxylipins to high-fat challenges and demonstrated that the response depended on the fatty acid composition of the meal challenge (Strassburg et al., 2014). The oxylipins were measured using a targeted LC–MS-based method. Assessment of the changes allowed the authors to propose that saturated fat consumption creates a pro-atherogenic environment whereas consumption of $n-3$ PUFA promoted a harmful environment in terms of inflammatory mediators. This is an important demonstration of how we can employ metabolic profiling in conjunction with challenge tests to obtain new information in terms of health determinants.

10.3 Conclusion and future trends

The findings from the above-mentioned studies and those in Table 10.1 have revealed detailed insights into complex metabolic changes induced by challenge tests, such as OGTT and OLTT, and offer novel perspectives on the regulation of glucose and lipid metabolism. Furthermore, the application of the combination of metabolomics and challenge tests has revealed different responses between subjects with and without insulin resistance: the development of this strategy in the future should help in the identification of predisease phenotypes. The application of this approach to nutritional interventions has great potential in terms of identifying subtle changes. The response to the challenge tests following different treatment regimes (e.g. treated and control) revealed changes that were not observable in homeostatic condition. Further development of this approach has the potential to help identify subtle metabolic benefits of a range of foods.

In conclusion, the use of challenge tests in nutrition research is growing and still in its infancy. More examples of the potential use and benefits of combining challenge tests with metabolic profiling are needed. Furthermore, expanding the analysis to include transcriptomics and proteomics will be an important step in the future and the integration of these datasets to identify key metabolic pathways should be extremely fruitful. Overall, the use of challenge tests in combination with metabolomics may prove to demonstrate a better understanding of subclinical metabolic dysfunctions, and they could contribute to improved personalised nutrition management.

References

Berthiaume, N., Zinker, B.A., 2002. Metabolic responses in a model of insulin resistance: comparison between oral glucose and meal tolerance tests. Metabolism 51 (5), 595–598.

Ho, J.E., Larson, M.G., et al., 2013. Metabolite profiles during oral glucose challenge. Diabetes 62 (8), 2689–2698.

Krug, S., Kastenmüller, G., Stückler, F., Rist, M.J., Skurk, T., Sailer, M., Raffler, J., Römisch-Margl, W., Adamski, J., Prehn, C., Frank, T., Engel, K.H., Hofmann, T., Luy, B., Zimmermann, R., Moritz, F., Schmitt-Kopplin, P., Krumsiek, J., Kremer, W., Huber, F., Oeh, U., Theis, F.J., Szymczak, W., Hauner, H., Suhre, K., Daniel, H., 2012. The dynamic range of the human metabolome revealed by challenges. FASEB J. 26 (6), 2607–2619.

Lin, S., Yang, Z., Liu, H., Tang, L., Cai, Z., 2011. Beyond glucose: metabolic shifts in responses to the effects of the oral glucose tolerance test and the high-fructose diet in rats. Mol. Biosyst. 7 (5), 1537–1548.

Pellis, L., van Erk, M.J., van Ommen, B., Bakker, G.C., Hendriks, H.F., Cnubben, N.H., Kleemann, R., van Someren, E.P., Bobeldijk, I., Rubingh, C.M., Wopereis, S., 2012. Plasma metabolomics and proteomics profiling after a postprandial challenge reveal subtle diet effects on human metabolic status. Metabolomics 8 (2), 347–359.

Shaham, O., Wei, R., Wang, T.J., Ricciardi, C., Lewis, G.D., Vasan, R.S., Carr, S.A., Thadhani, R., Gerszten, R.E., Mootha, V.K., 2008. Metabolic profiling of the human response to a glucose challenge reveals distinct axes of insulin sensitivity. Mol. Syst. Biol. 4, 214.

Strassburg, K., Esser, D., Vreeken, R.J., Hankemeier, T., Müller, M., van Duynhoven, J., van Golde, J., van Dijk, S.J., Afman, L.A., Jacobs, D.M., 2014. Postprandial fatty acid specific changes in circulating oxylipins in lean and obese men after high-fat challenge tests. Mol. Nutr. Food Res. 58 (3), 591–600.

Zhao, X., Peter, A., Fritsche, J., Elcnerova, M., Fritsche, A., Häring, H.U., Schleicher, E.D., Xu, G., Lehmann, R., 2009. Changes of the plasma metabolome during an oral glucose tolerance test: is there more than glucose to look at? Am. J. Physiol. Endocrinol. Metab. 296 (2), E384–E393.

Zivkovic, A.M., Wiest, M.M., Nguyen, U., Nording, M.L., Watkins, S.M., German, J.B., 2009. Assessing individual metabolic responsiveness to a lipid challenge using a targeted metabolomic approach. Metabolomics 5 (2), 209–218.

Using metabolomics to describe food in detail

11

F. Capozzi, A. Trimigno
University of Bologna, Bologna, Italy

11.1 Introduction

Metabolomics is a relatively new "omic" science that aims to describe, in a snapshot, the complete set of metabolites constituting a defined biological system. This new omic approach has recently become widespread in many research areas, such as the study of human pathologies and diseases (see Chapter 8 for detailed discussion), drug discovery and toxicity assessment, human nutrition, and plant analysis. The broad application of metabolomics has been possible thanks to technological innovations that allow the high-throughput separation and identification of small molecules, even in complex biological matrices. These techniques include mass spectroscopy (MS) and high-resolution nuclear magnetic resonance (NMR) spectroscopy, together with separation methods such as capillary electrophoresis (CE) and chromatography (gas (GC), liquid (LC), ultra high-pressure liquid (UPLC), and high-performance liquid (HPLC)). Together with these scientific advances, the creation of databases containing spectral data and the corresponding signal assignments has driven the progress of metabolomics in various fields.

Along with genomics, transcriptomics, and proteomics, metabolomics provides the holistic definition of food according to the new foodomic approach. Foodomics has been defined as "the discipline that studies the food domain as a whole with the nutrition domain, applying the same advanced omics technologies to different samples, and integrates all results in order to have an overall vision allowing the improvement of health and well-being" (Capozzi and Bordoni, 2013).

Data obtained through the above-described techniques are then usually interpreted through statistical and multivariate data analyses in order to produce robust and comparable information because it is generally necessary to classify samples in separate categories (see Chapter 3 for detailed description).

Thanks to the possibility of identifying a great range of metabolites with the aforementioned analytical techniques and the potential of modern computers to handle a vast quantity of data for multivariate analysis, this kind of approach is now widely applied in every life science.

Food science has been increasingly linked to other fields such as medicine, veterinary science, agriculture, biology, and genetics. Metabolomics can help link those different fields by connecting food quality with health, while accounting for food quality changes related to human and environmental perturbations on the food metabolome (Figure 11.1). For this reason, a large portion of foodomics is centred on

Metabolomics as a Tool in Nutrition Research. http://dx.doi.org/10.1016/B978-1-78242-084-2.00011-3

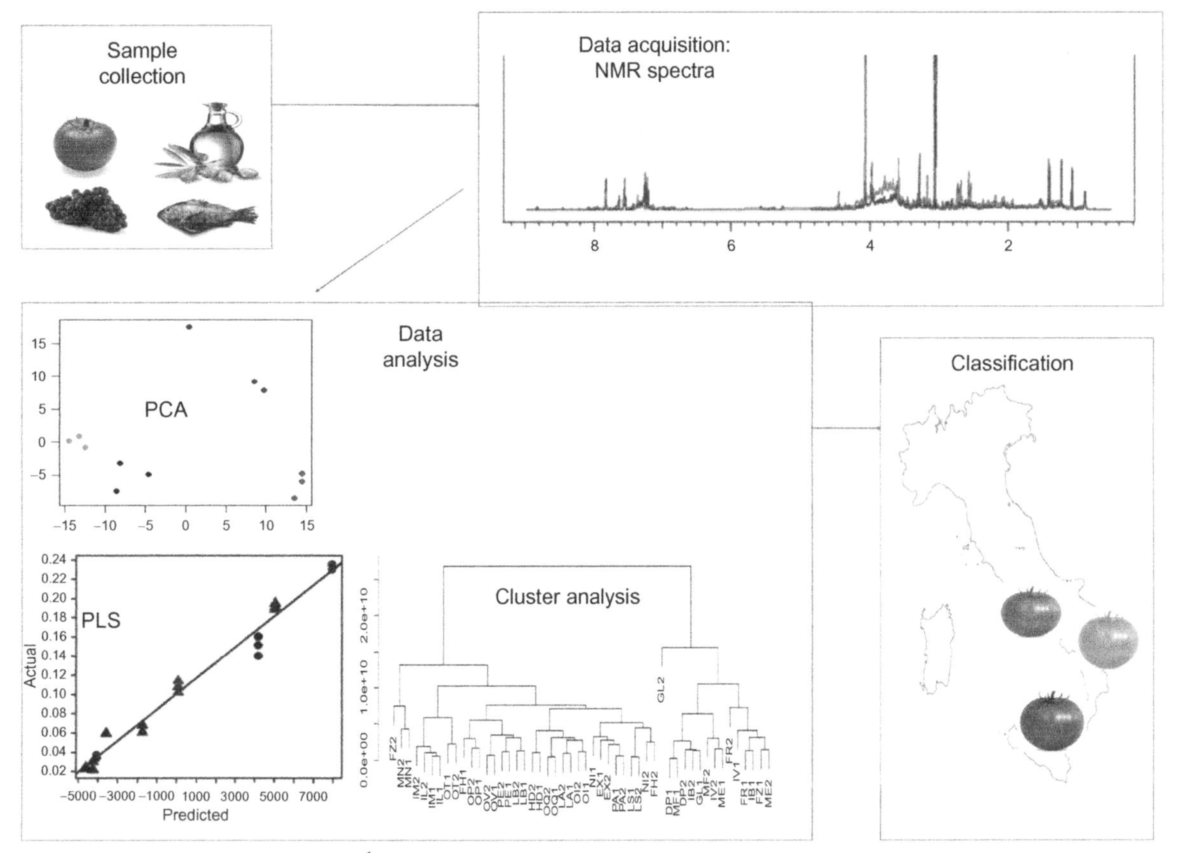

Figure 11.1 The metabolomics approach using ^{1}H NMR spectroscopy. After sample collection, NMR spectra are acquired and subjected to multivariate analysis. As in the illustrated case, spectra usually do not show much difference at first glance. Thus, statistical tools such as multivariate data analysis techniques (PCA, PLS, cluster analysis) are employed to emphasise possible differences. Using those methods, researchers can then classify the samples according to their different origins and characteristics.

metabolomics applied to the exploration of possible links between food quality and the nutritional value.

More and more studies are investigating the sources of variance in food quality, such as the effects of genetic modification of plants on their food quality and derivatives, or the origin of a determined food based on its metabolic profile. These studies are of increasing importance in our society because consumers are more concerned about food quality, which is often associated with its origin, as well as the impact of food transformation on the nutritional value of the product. Digestibility is another important attribute of food quality, and its assessment by metabolomics is of paramount importance for the development of foods tailored to fragile population categories such as infants and elderly people. Thus, being able to thoroughly prove food quality is a key tool for food producers and factories and for food consumers. This chapter highlights some of the key studies on this subject and future possibilities for the use of metabolomics in the evaluation of food quality.

11.2 Using metabolomics to assess the effects of genetic selection and modification

In recent years a lot of research has focused on the production of genetically modified (GM) or transgenic foods produced by DNA recombination in order to obtain favourable features. These new products are still seen as potentially harmful by consumers, however, and further analysis investigating the quality and possible unintended effects of GM foods is necessary, as is public education on the subject. Metabolomics is starting to be employed in this sense, thanks to its use of high-throughput techniques, and many studies have now been published.

GMs can have various unintended effects, they might or might not have an impact on food quality and safety, they might or might not be predictable. Therefore, research is needed to prove the nature of these possible effects. The substantial equivalence (SE) of GMs to their wild-type counterparts must be proven by assessing the variation of the overall composition of the modified genotype with respect to the original wild-type organism and by comparing such differences with those naturally occurring within the only wild-type category. This concept means that two plant variants (GM and not) are similar enough to be considered the same, and thus they can be treated in the same way regarding food safety concerns. Accordingly, no unintended or different phenotypic variances should be found in GMs crops, especially variations that negatively influence their nutritional profiles or can create harmful effects on consumers (Kok and Kuiper, 2003). Metabolomics can clearly help in this assessment, generating full metabolite profiles for GM products and comparing them to their original, unmodified counterparts.

A study from Fraser et al. (2007) examined normal and GM tomatoes with an overexpression of phytoene synthase1 through different approaches (protein activity, gene expression, physiological parameters, and metabolomics). This is one of the most thorough studies, employing many different techniques real-time polymerase chain reaction (PCR) for mutant gene expression, enzyme assays, HPLC (to identify carotenoids, isoprenoids, flavonoids, and phenylpropanoids), and GC-MS. Metabolic profiles were obtained through HPLC and time-of-flight mass spectrometry (TOF-MS), showing that transgenic tomatoes were different from the normal ones in various ways. The whole ripening process was different in the transgenic lines, and metabolomics was useful in assessing the specific changes occurring at the different ripening stages, linking gene expression and enzyme activity to the actual altered production of metabolites and uncovering the unexpected metabolic deviations caused by the different genetic profiles of those tomatoes. Having data from genomic and enzymatic assays, researchers could also link the results from those analyses to the metabolomics information to get a panoramic view of what is really happening in the food product after genetic insertion and modification.

Another study by Levandi et al. (2008) found differences between transgenic and conventional maize through CE–TOF-MS and subsequent spectral and statistical analysis (principal component analysis (PCA) and univariate statistical tests). As usual, the best extraction and analytical conditions were assessed at first, and after the optimisation, metabolites in the maize samples were identified thanks to the literature and metabolite databases. Peak areas were then compared between GM and wild-type samples to see which molecules were over- or underexpressed in the former type of maize. Twenty-seven metabolites were detected and identified in the samples, and just two among these were found to have enough statistical predictivity to differentiate the two types of crops. In effect, L-proline-betaine and, to a greater degree, L-carnitine were typical of GM maize; this was interpreted as a signal of alteration in fatty acid and glucose metabolism, because L-carnitine is employed in those pathways enhancing the transport of fatty acids in mitochondria for their subsequent oxidation and increasing glycogen storage, respectively. Further multivariate PCA confirmed these compounds as discriminating between the two classes. Thus, this kind of approach can clearly provide robust results, because different statistical analysis techniques, both supervised and unsupervised, are employed corroborating each other.

A later study on GM maize by Leon et al. (2009), employing Fourier transform ion cyclotron resonance mass spectrometry (FT-ICR-MS) and CE–TOF-MS followed by partial least squares–discriminant analysis (PLS-DA), confirmed L-carnitine as a discriminating marker between GM and conventional maize and highlighted at least nine other metabolites (mainly from the amino acid pathways) able to distinguish between the two types of maize. Initially, it was once again necessary to perform an optimisation of the analytical parameters. In this case, after peak identification, a supervised statistical method, PLS-DA, was employed to discriminate among samples, confirming the results of the previous studies, while exploiting different statistical techniques to increase the robustness of the results.

Other studies focused on GM wheat versus conventional wheat (Baker et al., 2006; Baudo et al., 2006) showed no clear difference between the two types of wheat, but these studies proved a higher differentiation due to environmental and farming conditions. The first example (Baker et al., 2006), employed NMR analysis combined with PCA and GC-MS coupled with analysis of variance (ANOVA) to study the metabolome. Conversely, the study from Baudo et al. (2006) mainly focused on transcriptomics analysis. The combination of different approaches (metabolomics and complementary traditional genomics and transcriptomics techniques) provided more information on how the genetic variation can cause effects on the phenotypic behaviour.

Another study by García-Villalba et al. (2008) focused on the comparative analysis of transgenic and conventional soybean through CE–ESI-TOF-MS. At first, the optimal conditions for extraction of metabolites from soybean samples were assessed, and then the best separation and CE-UV parameters were established. Afterward, metabolites were identified and quantified, using the best possible combination. Some differences among the samples were found GM soybean showed greater concentrations of some metabolites, including liquiritigenin, *p*-coumaroyl glucoside, naringenin 7-*O*-glucoside, and 6-methoxytaxifolin. On the other hand, conventional soybean seemed to contain larger amounts of proline, histidine, asparagine, gluconic acid, and trihydroxy-pentanoic acid. The main difference, though, was found to be 4-hydroxy-L-threonine, which was only identified in conventional soybean, and only this difference has been ascribed to the genetic modification. Again, the described metabolomic study allowed the identification of differences in the metabolic profiles of crops, exposing the biochemical modifications and identifying possible control mechanisms of the metabolic pathways. In this specific case, the amino acids and derivatives that showed different concentrations in GM maize and the corresponding wild-type counterpart shared a common precursor. Therefore, it was possible to verify that the 5-enolpyruvylshikimate-3-phosphate synthase, which differentiated the transgenic line, affected the synthesis of aromatic amino acids.

Picone et al. (2011a) studied the possible SE of GM grapes through a metabolomic approach employing NMR spectroscopy. The spectral matrix was subjected to multivariate statistical analysis (PCA) in order to project the overall variance of all wild-type and transgenic grapes on the orthogonal components of a metabolomics space. Subsequent ANOVA was applied to the first 20 principal component (PC) scores, and only the first two PCs appeared to be responsible for the discrimination between wild-type and GM grapes. Studying the respective PC loadings, it was clear that the whole metabolic profile was responsible for a clear differentiation between GM and conventional grapes, rather than a few metabolites. Among the spectral regions, however, the most affected were those referring to aromatic molecules (tryptophan and indole derivatives), with pathways expected to be affected by the genetic modification. Surprisingly, the region with organic acids also showed significant differences, thus pointing out that the ripening process could also be affected by genetic insertion. Interestingly, only one of the two studied cultivars showed a discriminant metabolic profile between GM and wild-type plants. In this case, it was demonstrated that the effect of the genetic modification was modulated by the host genotype. This metabolomics study proved to be an effective tool in investigating the SE, because the whole plant metabolic profile was analysed and quantified and not just some preselected molecules. NMR spectroscopy and multivariate data analysis (unsupervised in this case) can give robust results in this sense. An untargeted approach in metabolomics is fundamental as a preliminary analysis for the assessment of the pros and cons of new products.

The above-mentioned studies demonstrate how metabolomics reveals even the unexpected effects caused by a genetic alteration. Such effects are not always predictable by taking into account only the specific modified pathway, because cascade effects might occur, generated by feedback regulations. Thanks to the metabolomic approach, which allows analysis of the whole metabolic profile, it is possible to detect all variations, including those that may not be captured by target analysis.

11.3 Using metabolomics to assess the effects of organic versus conventional farming

Many studies attempted to assess differences in the metabolome of organic and conventional agricultural products (Woese et al., 1997). In recent years consumers have increasingly requested organic foods, mainly due to concerns about food quality and safety and the resulting perception that organic products are safer and healthier than their conventional counterparts. Nowadays, many unprocessed and processed organic food products are commercially available, and numerous studies have compared the actual composition and nutritional value of these food matrices. Organic foods are considered to be of higher quality than conventionally produced foods because consumers believe that they contain lower levels of pesticide and chemical fertilisers, as well as higher levels of nutrients and beneficial phytochemicals, together with better sensory characteristics (Williams and Hammitt, 2001; Harper and Makatouni, 2002; Makatouni, 2002). On the contrary, however, organic products may be more contaminated by microorganisms and their products, such as biogenic amines, as a result of the application of manure and the reduced utilisation of antibiotics and fungicides. Organic products are usually sold at higher prices in comparison to their conventional counterparts, and the increased prices generate the risk of fraud. Therefore, once again, proper analytical techniques are required to assess the true organic origin of these foods.

Usually, traditional analyses are carried out in order to compare organic and conventional food products, using techniques including target analyses of specific macro- (sugars, lipids, proteins) or micronutrients (minerals, vitamins, bioactive compounds, etc.). Other studies have focused on the analysis of stable isotopes of light elements (H, C, N, O, S) in order to verify, for example, the soil of cultivation and fertilisers used synthetic nitrogen fertilisers, banned in organic farming, tend to have lower $\delta^{15}N$ values, and manure, which is used in organically grown crops, has a higher content of this isotope. However, these techniques often result in unreliable data for the classification of farming procedures, unless they are combined with other multivariate approaches (Capuano et al., 2013).

Untargeted screening is therefore promising for the achievement of robust and unbiased results, and metabolomics is clearly one of the best applicable strategies for identifying and quantifying molecules for the comparison of different products. Considering that different farming procedures and practices might influence cellular processes and plant response, a metabolomics approach should be able to detect a change in the resulting plant metabolites (Wishart, 2008).

MS, coupled with other separation techniques, has been widely used in recent studies with the aim of discriminating between organically and conventionally grown food crops. An untargeted study carried out by Chen et al. (2010) proved discrimination of organic or conventional grapefruit samples (Citrus paradisi cv. Rio Red) analysed by MS, with two different separation techniques flow injection electrospray ionisation time-of-flight mass spectroscopy (FI-ESI-TOF-MS) and flow injection electrospray ionisation ion trap mass spectroscopy (FI-ESI-IT-MS). Data obtained from MS were then analysed by ANOVA and PCA. Year of harvest was the first source of variance among spectra, and farming mode was the second. This study was not capable of identifying the metabolites giving rise to those differences, but the metabolomics approach pointed out that a metabolic modification exists between the grapefruit cultivated with different protocols.

Zörb et al. (2006) successfully used GC-MS analysis to discriminate between dynamic, bio-organic and conventional wheat grains, looking at only 8 out of 52 different detected metabolites (amino acids, sugars, alcohols, phosphates, nucleotides, and organic acids). Wheat grain extracts were analysed by GC-MS. Tukey's test was then applied to the concentrations of 52 metabolites. Seven replicates were made, and the values were accepted only when the difference between those replicates was below 5%. Because only eight metabolites were found to have different concentrations in grains according to their cultivation practices, the authors concluded that the farming process does not have much impact on the nutritional value of the products, because sugar and sugar alcohols were not different in their content. In addition, the authors found no sign of limited photosynthesis in organic plants.

In 2010, Röhlig et al. investigated the influence of the farming system on the metabolome of maize kernels, showing that the main differences were due to cultivars and environmental factors, and the farming system caused only minor variation (organic vs. conventional). The molecular GC-MS profiles of organic and conventional maize were compared by ANOVA and PCA. Before PCA, data were scaled by the standard deviation of each variable in order to reduce the influence of abundant metabolites. PCA showed a clear separation in the metabolic profiles of the three analysed cultivars based on the first two components, which accounted for a total 39–59% of expressed variance. Within each cluster, organic products were slightly separated from conventional ones. Applied to the relative amount of each analyte, ANOVA revealed that 29% of 125 compounds so far considered in such univariate analyses were capable of discriminating between locations/cultivation systems. ANOVA found the main differences in the concentrations of myo-inositol, malic acid, and phosphate, which showed higher levels in the organic crops. Myo-inositol is an important metabolite in many biochemical pathways, intervening in stress response and osmoregulation. Its increased expression in organic kernels, though, has not yet been explained. On the other hand, phosphate is very important for plant growth and has been proved to change in various organically grown plants, depending on their farming procedures and protocols (i.e., organic fertilisation) (Steiner et al., 2007).

In a more recent study, Bonte et al. (2014) used GC-MS profiling to compare 11 wheat cultivars grown in controlled conventional and organic conditions, and they found significant differences in the concentration of specific metabolites in winter cultivars. Only a few metabolites were identified. As in the study by Röhlig and Engel (2010), myo-inositol, in particular, and malic acid were particularly high in grains from the organic crops, and some free amino acids (e.g. aspartate, asparagine, alanine) showed higher concentrations in the conventional farming system.

As stated, MS is usually employed in metabolomics studies. Ambient MS was recently found to be a very useful tool, capable of generating a specific fingerprint for low molecular weight metabolites (<1 kDa). This type of MS requires very little sample preparation and does not necessitate any kind of separation prior to spectral acquisition. Newly designed ambient MS techniques include desorption electrospray ionisation, atmospheric solids analysis probe, direct analysis in real time (DART). A pilot study tried comparing tomatoes and sweet bell peppers, either organically or conventionally grown, through the use of DART and TOF-MS analysis (Novotnà et al., 2012). This research demonstrated that DART might be applicable for a rapid assessment of plant samples and showed a reasonable differentiation of samples due to the type of farming system, though it assigned a greater impact on the metabolic fingerprint given by the production year. Models generated through PCA and subsequent linear discriminant analysis (LDA) on those data, however, were not completely reliable because a higher number of samples would be needed to generate a more robust classification (Novotnà et al., 2012).

Very few researchers have carried out studies on processed food produced by organic versus conventional farming. One of these studies concerned ketchup (Vallverdú-Queralt et al., 2011) and demonstrated, through LC coupled to MS in tandem mode (LC–ESI-QqQ) and statistical analysis (ANOVA), some differences in the composition of the organic and conventional products. The former showed significantly higher amounts of caffeoylquinic and dicaffeoylquinic acids, caffeic and caffeic acid hexosides, kaemp-ferol-3-*O*-rutinoside, ferulic-*O*-hexoside, naringenin-7-*O*-glucoside, naringenin, rutin, and quercetin. On the other hand, the latter products contained typical compounds (glutamylphenylalanine and *N*-malonyltryptophan) that were not found in the organic ones. The authors concluded that the metabolites found in organic ketchups are due to the secondary metabolism of plant, related to its self-defense mechanisms.

A further step in the application of metabolomics concerns a study from Laghi et al. (2014) employing NMR spectroscopy to assess the differences between red wines obtained from either organic or biodynamic grapes. PCA was applied to NMR spectra and showed a great variation due to the vinification protocol (biodynamic vs. organic). Tyrosine-related metabolites seemed to be the major source of distinction, exhibiting a higher concentration in organic wines. The second PC showed the effect of vineyard management causing a greater concentration of resveratrol and a lower amount of transcaffeic acid in organic grapes. Further cluster analysis also showed a marked difference between samples due to the vinification procedure and, to lesser extent, to vineyard management. In addition, ANOVA applied to the NMR spectra pointed out that the concentration of transcaffeic acid was higher in biodynamic wines, which also contained a lower concentration of glutamine. Melgarejo et al. (2010) described this inverse correlation, suggesting that some polyphenols might target biogenic amine-producing enzymes. This was further investigated by studying the spectral differences in wines from successive years, proving that switching from organic to biodynamic farming modifies the phenylpropanoid pathways, thus corroborating the hypothesis that the decrease of glutamine concentration is related to an antagonistic effect of polyphenol biosynthesis.

Thus, the metabolomic approach can be helpful in the investigation of the possible differences between organic and conventional food products. MS, coupled with newly advanced techniques, has been particularly exploited, but NMR spectroscopy was also found to be useful. Using this approach, it is possible to highlight the patterns of metabolites that discriminate between plants produced according to different cultivation protocols, and to give proof of possible distinctive characteristics in organically produced foods that could be investigated by nutritionists and food scientists looking for additional positive properties. Although univariate statistical analysis is not able to provide a clear set of diagnostic metabolites differentiating organic from conventional products, multivariate data analyses, such as PCA, provide combinations of compounds useful for classification, suggesting that patterns of metabolites, rather than single molecules, may be used as quality biomarkers.

11.4 Using metabolomics to identify the geographical origin of food products

Another important parameter for food quality is geographical origin, which becomes fundamental for some products. In effect, a particular geographical origin might be associated with added value for a product, in comparison with others, thus creating a need to protect foods of a certain origin. This added value associated with protected products has led to the increased production of fraudulent food products, sold as food with a protected origin. Thus, the food industry and governments must be able to assess the authenticity of these counterfeit products to confirm this attribute of food quality.

Metabolomics has been proposed as a new technique to aid in the certification of a product's geographical origin, as it could identify metabolic markers selected for the substantiation of the claim. Many recent studies have employed techniques based on MS coupled with statistical and multivariate data analysis in order to assess metabolic differences in food products related to their geographical origin. Most of this research relies on induced couple plasma combined with mass spectrometry (ICP-MS), in addition to multivariate data analysis, such as PCA, and canonical or LDA, in order to classify samples according to their origin. This approach has been applied to honey (Chudzinska and Baralkiewicz, 2010), olive oil (Benincasa et al., 2007), paprika (Brunner et al., 2010), tomatoes (Mallamace et al., 2014; Savorani et al., 2009), and tomato products (Lo Feudo et al., 2010).

Meat quality is very important both for health and for nutritional reasons, and metabolomics studies demonstrate how great variation can be seen in samples with different geographical origins. These differences can also be exploited for certification of origin, and many countries are now implementing metabolomic certification processes for security and for quality assessment.

Jung et al. (2010) investigated the effects of geographical origin on the metabolome of beef by applying ^{1}H NMR spectroscopy. PCA and orthogonal partial least squares – discriminant analysis (OPLS-DA) were employed to establish whether some metabolites were able to discriminate between beef from different geographical regions (Australia, Korea, New Zealand, and United States). At first, PCA was carried out in order to test, in an unsupervised manner, if there were differences among the different types of samples, and it did indeed show a separation among the four groups. Thus, the supervised OPLS-DA approach was used to maximise these differences, and the model was tested with validation procedures, producing accurate results. A few orthogonal components were sufficient to distinguish between beef origins, and many metabolites were important for that classification acetate, anserine, betaine, carnitine, carnosine, choline, creatine, creatinine, fumarate, glycerol, hypoxanthine, lactate, niacinamide, succinate, and all amino acids. Most of the metabolites were clearly higher in the New Zealand samples, especially amino acids, and Australian beef exhibited lower levels of those molecules. US samples were the highest in succinate concentration. It is clear that many conditions can alter beef composition, including breed, feed, rearing system, pre and postslaughter parameters, and environmental conditions. Breed can cause differences in both essential and nonessential amino acids, and the amino acids also increase due to postmortem ageing resulting from the hydrolysis of peptides and proteins. In addition, diet can affect the level of amino acids found in beef if fed silage, cattle will have meat that shows higher concentrations of many amino acids in comparison with the meat of concentrate-fed cattle. Further studies have analysed differences in fatty acid composition, metabolites that can again vary due to diet, environmental effects, and type of production system.

For vegetable products, metabolomics has been exploited as a tool for preventing fraud when geographical origin certification is a key element for the certification of food quality. Two case studies were carried out (Mallamace et al., 2014; Savorani et al., 2009) to establish differences among cherry tomatoes with respect to their origin (Pachino province in Sicily vs. other Italian locations). They both employed NMR techniques and multivariate statistical analysis to assess the metabolic profile of those products and to identify possible differences between cherry tomatoes of different geographical origins. The studies showed how the metabolomics approach could be useful for tracking food origin, because Pachino tomatoes were found to contain higher concentrations of metabolites such as fructose, glucose, glutamine, glutamate, aspartate, and gamma-aminobutyric acid (GABA) and lower levels of fatty acids, alanine, methanol, and acetylglutamic acid, in comparison to products cultivated in other, even neighbouring, areas.

Cajka et al. (2011) describe another example of applying metabolomics to the determination of geographical origin. These authors studied the possibility of recognising beer origin through metabolomics, employing DART–TOF-MS and statistical analysis (PCA, PLS-DA, LDA, and artificial neural networks with multilayer perceptrons (ANN-MLP)). After careful inspection, markers were chosen from among the DART–TOF-MS profiles, in order to select the ones that could perform better upon chemometric analysis. At first, the prediction ability of both positive and negative ions was tested through leave-one-out cross validation of a preliminary LDA model. PCA was then calculated in order to investigate possible clustering among samples, and it showed how beers from the Czech Republic were different from Belgian and Dutch beers. PLS-DA was then performed to assess the source of variance between one type of beer over the rest of the productions and between Trappist and nonTrappist beers, and models with high-recognition performances were obtained, though their predictive power was lower. LDA was used as an alternative supervised technique to find the metabolite patterns giving maximum separation among sample classes. In this case, a better model from PLS-DA was generated for the classification of one beer versus all the others, rather than that obtained by comparing Trappist and nonTrappist beers. Finally, ANN-MLP was tested as a further approach. The latter technique applies to situations in which there is a complex relationship between input classifiers and predicted variables. Even in this case, the model built by comparing one type over the other beers was better than the model obtained when testing if beers were Trappist or not. Moreover, models had better performance in the latter approach than in PLS-DA and LDA, although the results were similar. Taken together, these models can establish robust statistical differences between beer productions by finding the features of the metabolite fingerprint responsible for discrimination. Finally, the same study also compared another approach by analysing the same samples with solid-phase microextraction (SPME)–GC–TOF-MS instead of DART–TOF-MS. The different SPME–GC–TOF-MS trial proved to be more effective in the classification, while requiring more (although simple) preparation steps and thus more analytical time.

Although metabolomics proves that the geographic origin of a food product may be reflected in a unique molecular fingerprint, the actual source of differentiation is still questionable because multiple factors contribute to defining a "local production", including the restriction to use only autochthon genotypes, the practice of using traditional production protocols, and the existence of confined pedoclimatic conditions. For this reason, the definition of a geographic origin must rely on updated databases intended to monitor the changes in one or more of the multiple factors affecting the metabolite profile of the local production. In this way, robust models developed to predict the geographic origin of a product include correction functions based on the complete set of cofactors contributing to the definition of its molecular composition. Only then can robust models be adopted to assess fraudulent declarations of a certified origin, when the latter is an added value.

11.5 Using metabolomics to assess the effects of rearing conditions on the quality of meat, eggs, and fish

Many elements contribute to establishing the quality of food products of animal origin, such as the feeding, the use of antibiotics and medicines, and the choice of rearing conditions. Recently, metabolomics studies have attempted to connect the metabolic profiles of animal products to rearing protocols. Most studies have focused on the evaluation of differences in food products caused by the use of hormones or other chemicals (e.g. antibiotics) to improve cattle growth.

Regal et al. (2011) showed statistical differences between the LC high resolution mass spectra of sera sampled from control cattle and the spectra of sera from cattle treated with estradiol and progesterone. The authors performed their analysis using multivariate statistical analysis based on PCA, OPLS, and OPLS-DA. First, unsupervised PCA was performed in order to find possible sources of variations among samples. Then, OPLS and OPLS-DA were used to build more a robust model for samples classification. Eight molecular markers found by OPLS were finally selected for discrimination between treated and untreated animals and were therefore associated with perturbed metabolic pathways of hormones.

Another study by Graham et al. (2012) focused on bovine plasma samples in order to highlight the presence of illicit growth-promoting agents. These products are illegally used to improve feed efficiency, increasing animal weight gain. Growth-promoters cause alteration in blood and tissues composition, and many studies have attempted to detect those biological changes. Because metabolomics could be of great help, given its ability to produce a rapid and high-throughput screening of metabolic profile, this research employed two methods of NMR spectroscopy (classical 1-D and CPMG pulse sequence), followed by multivariate statistical analysis (OPLS-DA) to differentiate treated and nontreated cattle. The two NMR techniques were used in order to develop a high-throughput screening technique because they can show different classes of metabolites. NMR peaks were identified through libraries and literature data, and OPLS-DA was then performed on spectral data in order to visualise differences and clusters among samples. Treated animals showed altered metabolic profiles, especially in markers of metabolic balance and nitrogen flux, proving how growth-promoting agents can alter different biochemical processes such as protein metabolism, gluconeogenesis, and glycogen deposition.

The impact of different rearing conditions on the quality of bovine milk was investigated by Boudonck et al. (2009), through the use of GC-MS and LC-MS/MS metabolomics, followed by unsupervised data analysis (PCA). Ten different types of bovine milk were analysed. Samples varied in terms of brand, percentage of fat, expiration date, rearing method, and type of package. Metabolites exhibited in GC and LC mass spectra were identified by searching specific libraries using three criteria retention time, experimental precursor mass match to library standard, and MS/MS scores. Internal standards were used in both analytical methods in order to calibrate the experiment and control it. Data were then normalised by dividing the raw metabolite area by its median value in each run-day in order to correct for possible interday variation. After this prestatistical transformation, data were analysed first with the unsupervised PCA technique to explore possible separation and clustering, and then the expected and interesting classes were further tested with ANOVA. PCA showed that the first PC, accounting for the maximum variance, was related to difference in rearing practices (organic vs. conventional), and the second orthogonal PC was influenced by the fat percentage of the milk. One of the most interesting findings was the relation between farming (organic vs. conventional) and the consequent metabolic differences. A one-way ANOVA was performed on milk samples, and 25 metabolites in two types of milk were found to be significantly different in their concentrations, compared to the 11 different metabolites that would be expected in the case of random classification. Organic milk showed higher concentrations of tyrosine, isoleucine, mannose, glycerate, ribose, carnitine, hyppurate, and butyrylcarnitine when compared to conventional milk, and proline, trans-4-hydroxyproline, glucose-1-phosphate, ribose-5-phosphate, glycerol-3-phosphate, and glycerol-2-phosphate were found in lower concentrations. Hyppurate was one of the main markers for organic milk, and it has been positively linked to the following (i) fibre intake in diets (Holmes et al., 2008), (ii) consumption of products rich in polyphenols (Walsh et al., 2007), and (iii) exposure to determined environmental conditions (Holmes et al., 2008; Walsh et al., 2007). Thus, the observed discrimination is consistent with the different diets fed to animals in the two types of rearing because organically raised cattle is mainly fed forage (grass and clover), while conventional cows consume grain-based feed with cereals, maize, and protein supplements.

Two studies from van Ruth et al. (2011, 2013) demonstrated differences in the carotenoid profiles of organic, free-range, and barn eggs through HPLC and multivariate statistical analysis. A model was built with k-nearest-neighbour clustering analysis, allowing the correct prediction of organic (100% accuracy) and nonorganic (free-range and barn) samples (92% accuracy). Calibrated on Dutch eggs, the model was then tested with eggs from different countries, and it proved successful once again in discriminating samples by their production systems. The metabolomics approach thus proved to be useful, verifying the hypothesis that the different rearing conditions and, in particular, the access to different sources of feed for organic hens created differences in carotenoid profiles in eggs.

Other studies have focused on fish quality in relation to rearing practices. A study by Savorani et al. (2010) tried to assess the differences in the metabolic profiles of gilthead sea bream in relation to aquaculture methods through ^{1}H NMR metabolomics. NMR spectra were acquired on percloric acid extracts. After the normal processing steps (Fourier transform, baseline, and phase correction), spectra were normalised to total unit area in order to correct for possible vertical-scale errors due to dilution biases. After that, spectra were aligned using the iCoshift algorithm to allow the highest stability in the signal position among the different spectra. Finally, multivariate data analyses (PCA, PLS, extended canonical variates analysis (ECVA), and interval extendend canonical variates analysis (iECVA)) were performed on the spectral matrix. Only a few of the many signals present in the spectra could be assigned by using literature data; therefore, the nature of the other unknown signals was revealed by addition of pure standard compounds, and finally 38 additional peaks were assigned. Spectral analysis was useful for following the evolution of the main metabolite content during fish storage and for capturing the most important features to be recorded to describe declining fish quality. The main metabolites are amino acids and nucleotides. PCA was calculated by selecting only the aromatic region of the spectra the results pointed out that inosine and inosine

5′-monophosphate were mainly responsible for the differentiation due to storage time. However, specimens extracted after 16 days of storage under ice showed differences mostly caused by the farming system. Supervised ECVA confirmed that aquaculture practices give a higher variance of metabolite composition in stored fish rather than fresh fish. By using iECVA and omitting the effect of storage, the authors found that the compounds responsible for discrimination were glycine, histidine, alanine, and glycogen. Therefore, they showed that postmortem glycolysis is faster for fish farmed in pseudonatural environments, such as lagoons and off-shore cages, with respect to those reared in tanks, suggesting that the former aquaculture systems can induce higher levels of stress in animals or that a greater glucose metabolism rate is caused by higher exercise.

A later study by Picone et al. (2011b) was carried out on another fish species, *Spaurus aurata*, by applying a different chemometric approach. Picone and colleagues identified the same metabolites as those found in the previous study, with a paired *t*-test, by comparing the metabolic profile evolution during storage obviously, glycogen decreased significantly as a consequence of glycolysis, nucleotides were degraded into hypoxanthine as a consequence of postmortem processes, and trimethylamine *N*-oxide was converted into trimethylamine by microbial attack. Conversely, the amount of lactate did not change because it was already depleted at the start of the observation. PCA also captured some differences dependent on the farming system, with PC1 mainly collecting spectral changes in the hydroxylic region (amino acids, sugars, hydrophilic molecules) and PC2 being dominated by aliphatic signals.

The effects of storage temperature on the amino acid profile of Bogue fish was studied by Ciampa et al. (2012) using NMR metabolomics on spectra acquired at 600 MHz. In this case, the novelty of the approach concerned the normalisation algorithm based on the total nucleotide amount, which constituted a pool of interconverting metabolites. In this case, the normalisation to the total unitary area was impracticable because the solubilisation of compounds from protein hydrolysis during storage causes a clear increment of the total area in the spectra. The alternative normalisation step, based on internal standard addition, was also a poor choice because of the unknown dilution of extracts. For these reasons, the entire pool of metabolites originating from the adenosine triphosphate degradation pathway was used for normalisation. After this prestatistical step, the individual amino acid content was studied, pointing out different evolutions the concentration of taurine, not involved in any lysis, did not change much during storage; the amounts of alanine, phenylalanine, glycine, tryptophan, methionine, isoleucine, leucine, valine, glutamate, and tyrosine increased during storage, and a simultaneous decrease of histidine and serine was observed. These results confirmed similar changes in the amino acid content observed by other techniques. The advantage of using NMR spectroscopy is associated with its ability to quantify several classes of compound in one shot. By analysing the same spectra, the authors observed that, although the amount of amino acids changed at a constant rate during storage, some other molecules slowly changed up to day 4, then started varying faster due to bacterial development. To prove this trend, typical metabolites of bacterial development were quantified (e.g. lactate, acetate, glucose, succinate, and ethanol), and the hypothesis was then demonstrated. This study emphasises how a holistic view, obtained by applying the metabolomics principles to the whole molecular profile, can be helpful for understanding the processes going on during food storage, and this approach can be even more robust when a freshness index is built by accounting for all metabolites undergoing transformation. Basing their selection on a nontargeted approach, some unexpected alteration can be found, allowing for product quality assessment.

11.6 Using metabolomics to assess the effects of processing on food quality

Food quality is also affected by production technology and the processes that transform the raw material in food (fermentation, pasteurisation, cooking, etc.). Nowadays, more and more food products are subject to many transformation steps and processes, which might alter their nutritional, sensory, and biochemical properties. It is therefore necessary to assess any possible alteration caused by these procedures, in order to investigate the nature of transformed foods and to identify any possible differences caused by varying the manufacturing protocols or the presence/absence of treatments.

For example, milk is usually manipulated to lower its fat content, which can vary within a range of 3 percentage points. Only recently, though, studies have been carried out to assess the secondary changes occurring in the milk matrix regarding other nutrients. The aforementioned study from Boudonck et al. (2009) found further differences in milk due to the reduction of fat content. GC-MS and LC-MS/MS spectra from milk samples were subjected to a two-sample *t*-test in order to compare fat-free with whole milk and reduced-fat with fat-free milk. The authors found that 78 metabolites differed significantly in at least one of the four categories characterised by different fat percentages. Obviously, compared to reduced-fat or fat-free milk, whole milk contained higher amounts of the major free fatty acids (e.g. palmitate, oleate, stearate, and myristate), as well as more cholesterol, 1,2-dipalmitoylglycerol, and alpha-tocopherol. The nutritional value related to these nutrients is thus altered in the process of fat extraction, without any relation to milk brands. Other metabolites (amino acids, sugars, purines and pyrimidines, succinate, fumarate and casein peptides) also showed altered concentrations between groups, though these differences were related to brands.

Another field of application is the production of vegetable conserves. Capanoglu et al. (2008) studied the effect of processing in the industrial production of tomato paste. Samples taken from different processing steps and from different tomato batches were analysed by LC–QTOF-MS and untargeted metabolomics. The authors concluded that this approach shows higher throughput than a conventional technique based on the HPLC simply coupled to an online antioxidants detector. In effect, LC-MS provided a better insight into the actual alteration caused by the processing of tomato for paste production. Indeed, not only did the amount of carotenoids and vitamin C vary, but 40% of the 3177 mapped metabolites showed altered signals during the process. It seemed clear that two processing steps were accountable for the main differences the removal of seed and skin and the transition from fruit to breaker. The first causes a great reduction in the concentration of flavonoids and alkaloids because seeds and skin are richer in those compounds and they do not get completely extracted in the process. The other mentioned step showed an increase in flavonoids and alkaloids, maybe due to a wound response in the fruit tissues, though the total antioxidant activity decreases because of vitamin C loss during tomato breaking. Again, metabolomics proved to be a rapid and useful tool for investigating critical processes in the production of foods, and in the future, it might aid factories in assessing the best ways to reduce nutrient loss and alteration.

In this way, knowledge-driven industrial production systems could take advantage of metabolomics for the improvement of traditional food. Beleggia et al. (2011) investigated the effects of pasta making by following the process from semolina to the final product. Different techniques were employed GC-MS, LC-MS, and HPLC for carotenoid profiling, mineral profiling, and successive statistical analysis through ANOVA and PCA-FA (factor analysis). Results showed that metabolites varied because of the processing steps and processing conditions. PCA scores resulted in sample discrimination according to types of pasta (PC1) and processing phases (PC2). ANOVA confirmed these results. Investigation on the quantities of minerals and metabolites was then performed, and the differences among pasta samples prepared under varying processing conditions were identified. Phytosterols degrade because of oxidation, and this degradation is influenced by factors such as temperature and reaction time. Accordingly, the authors found that the drying step caused a reduction of these metabolites together with hydroxy fatty acids, tocopherols, and carotenoids, suggesting that an accurate temperature adjustment (lower drying temperature) might help maintain the levels of these molecules, leading to greater nutritional value in pasta. Variations were also observed in carotenoid degradation probably due to the kneading process, which favours lipoxygenase in its oxidation of polyunsaturated fatty acids and, as a consequence, of carotenoids. Different types of semolina showed different behaviours during this step, due to their characteristics and enzyme activities. Another change was observed in the content of total sugars, which showed an initial increase during the mixing step, due to optimal conditions for alpha-amylase, and a later decrease after the drying phase, probably due to a Maillard reaction and the inactivation of amylase. Again, the metabolomics approach clearly provides insight into many of the different biochemical changes occurring in food matrices during transformation steps, pointing out that the quality of the raw material is not the only parameter that influences the final product. Instead, optimal processing conditions are fundamental to the maintenance of high nutritional values in conventional and functional foods. Thus, it is clear how an analytical approach employing different techniques and ensuing multivariate and statistical data analysis is able to extract the relevant information from the many different operating conditions affecting the behaviour of food components and metabolites through processing procedures. This is necessary for the food industry in order to assess and then control the processing steps and conditions for the production of the best foods possible.

11.7 Using metabolomics to assess the effects of digestion on nutrient intake from particular foods

Assessing the quality of a food product is not enough to prove the real benefits of the food on human health. The food matrix undergoes the whole digestive process, and its beneficial components need to be released in the correct form in order to diffuse through the digestion fluid towards the gut membrane where they are absorbed and transferred to the blood stream, thus becoming bioavailable and ready to exert their bioactivity on the human body. In recent years, research has started focusing on the effects of digestion on the composition and structure of food products, and a very few studies have attempted to distinguish foods on the basis of their digestibility. This knowledge is fundamental for the understanding of the true nutritional and health properties of food products, however, and for their promotion.

Toydemir et al. (2013) investigated the effect of simulated gastrointestinal digestion on sour cherry fruit and nectar samples. They showed greater anthocyanin recovery after the digestion of nectar than that of fruit. This difference might be due to a greater stability of these metabolites in the nectar, possibly because of the matrix structure, the pH, the temperature, and other components present in the nectar. In effect, the nectar had more than 50% sucrose added, and it has been shown that this ingredient might preserve and stabilise anthocyanins (Hong and Wrolstad, 1990). This analysis employed spectrophotometric assays and HPLC in order to get a full phenolic profiling. Again, the use of compatible techniques is necessary to test the results obtained with each method.

Another study by Bordoni et al. (2011) compared *in vitro* digestion of Parmigiano Reggiano cheese, characterised by two different ageing times (15 and 30 months), by analysing the NMR spectra of digestates at different digestive steps. The authors found that the spectra of undigested aqueous extracts showed a greater presence of sharp signals (amino acids) in the 30-months-aged Parmigiano due to microbial fermentation during ageing. The main changes during the digestive steps were reportedly caused by an increase in broad signals from casein digestion. The study then focused on the analysis of particular spectral regions (amide and aromatic protons). The authors observed that higher amide areas were found in the 15-months-aged Parmigiano, associated with large-sized protein fragments, which were released during digestion of this cheese. On the other hand, the aromatic area showed the same trend in both types of samples, indicating that this kind of amino acid is most often released bound to small peptides. This research exploited a metabolomics approach, employing two different NMR techniques (1D-nuclear Overhauser effect spectroscopy and diffusion-ordered spectroscopy), while comparing different food products digested with the same protocol, thus highlighting the changes of their digestibility as a consequence of the food production protocol. In this way the authors were able to evaluate the actual digestibility of the foodstuff, and the multivariate data analysis could separate the digestion process into different components, each characterised by a different molecular profile observable during the sequential digestion phases (e.g. protein hydrolysis and peptide release in the oral, gastric, and duodenal tracts).

Three studies published in 2014 (Bordoni et al., 2014; Ferranti et al., 2014; Pan et al., 2014) shed light on meat digestion by *in vitro* simulation and metabolomics. Bordoni et al. (2014) focused on the evaluation of the protein bioaccessibility of Bresaola product (cured beef). Samples were digested and collected at five different check points in order to assess the protein hydrolysis pathway during the various digestive steps. Protein digestion was evaluated with a holistic approach, by employing a combination of Bradford assays, sodium dodecyl sulphate–polyacrylamide gel electrophoresis (SDS–PAGE), ^{1}H NMR and time domain nuclear magnetic resonance (TD-NMR). ^{1}H NMR spectra were normalised with reference to the L-carnitine signal, a metabolite that maintains an unaltered concentration during digestion. In this case other recurrent normalisation procedures could not be used, because the total spectral area changes during the digestive phases and the internal standard trimethylsilyl propanoic acid added for frequency calibration, disappears from solution during digestion due to their absorption on the matrix molecules. The obtained spectra were used to corroborate the results of the other techniques by following the appearance of small and medium-sized peptides not detectable by either the Bradford assay or the SDS–PAGE, with the latter techniques only identifying the disappearance of large proteins. TD-NMR gives further information on the modification of the matrix structure, indicating that, in the oral phase, mastication provokes the exit of 50% of the water from myofibrils and the entrance of 15% of digestion juices into the fibre bundles. Moreover, the same technique shows the unbundling of meat fibres during the gastric phase, favouring the action of pepsin.

Ferranti et al. (2014) also focused on Breasola digestibility in order to assess the possible release of bioactive peptides from the food matrix. In effect, during digestion, protein-rich matrices release small peptides with potential benefits for human health because some of them have been shown to have antihypertensive or antioxidant effects. This research employed *in vitro* digestion and sampling at five different check points along the digestion process. Samples were then analysed through SDS–PAGE, 2-dimensional electrophoresis (2-DE), subsequent protein spot hydrolysis, MALDI-TOF-MS analysis, and nano-HPLC–ESI-Q-TOF-MS/MS analysis of peptides. Through these various techniques, the profiles of peptide and protein mixtures have been established. 1D-SDS–PAGE and the coupled MS analysis showed that some proteins were already hydrolysed in the Bresaola samples before gastric digestion because, in the postmortem phase, proteins from the sarcoplasmic and myofibrillar tissues undergo hydrolysis by calpains and other endogenous proteases. The undigested compounds, studied by 2-DE and MALDI-TOF-MS, were found to be serum albumin, actin, tropomyosins, myosin light chains 1 and 3, and some of their fragments. During gastric and duodenal digestion, Bresaola proteins were subject to the attack of different proteases. The gastric phase showed the degradation of some sarcoplasmic proteins and the appearance of polypeptides, the latter undetectable by SDS–PAGE. reversed-phase high-performance liquid chromatography (RP-HPLC), and MALDI-TOF-MS were mainly employed to monitor the evolution of the peptide profiles during the digestive steps. RP-HPLC showed that myofibrillar proteins are demolished during duodenal digestion after being released during the gastric phase, whereas MALDI-TOF-MS spectra disclosed the size of the newly formed smaller peptides. Nano-HPLC–ESI-Q-TOF-MS/MS analysis showed the presence of bioactive ACE-inhibitors, peptides, or their precursors after digestion, though validation of their bioavailability in *in vivo* systems is still needed. This study showed how omics based on complementary analytical techniques can explain many underlying processes happening during food digestion.

Unlike the other two research groups, Pan et al. (2014) studied the digestion of ham to investigate its nutrients' bioaccessibility using SDS–PAGE, microscopy, and ^{1}H NMR spectroscopy. SDS–PAGE and NMR spectra showed the kinetics of protein degrading into smaller peptides. Unaffected by digestion, lactate was used as a normalisation reference for NMR spectra in order to quantify the nutrients in the different digestive steps and understand their fate. During the study, lipids and macromolecules appeared to increase greatly during gastric and duodenal digestion, though they stopped growing in quantity after 60 min of digestion. The NMR spectra of after-digestion samples also showed the presence of potential bioactive or positive compounds, such as carnosine or choline, and this can be used as an index of product digestibility or food quality associated with the accessibility of nutrients released upon digestion.

11.8 Conclusion

Metabolomics is now a widespread omic approach fruitfully exploited in many applied sciences. The key aspects of this new science, including the use of rapid and effective techniques, make it fundamental for many fields. Food science is not an exception, and it is now employing metabolomics in many avenues of research. Consumers' increasing demands for higher food quality and the substantiation of this quality have necessitated the development of new techniques for screening the metabolic and nutritional profiles of food products, and metabolomics can clearly serve as an explorative and classifying tool for this purpose.

Many studies now try to assess food quality by employing analytical techniques suitable for metabolomics, such as MS or NMR spectroscopy, and subsequent multivariate data analysis (Table 11.1). Today, this type of research methodology is the basis for a large portion of food research. Accordingly, this chapter highlights some of the many uses of metabolomics in food science, including the assessment of differences between GM and non-GM products and the identification of particular

Table 11.1 **Metabolomics studies applied to food science**

Type of study	Techniques	Statistical tools	Food analysed	Discriminant metabolites	Reference
Genetic modification	Real-time PCR, enzyme assays, HPLC, TOF-MS	–	Tomatoes	–	Fraser et al. (2007)
Genetic modification	CE–TOF-MS	PCA, Student's *t*-test	Maize	L-Proline-betaine, L-carnitine (typical of GM maize)	Levandi et al. (2008)
Genetic modification	FT-ICR-MS, CE–TOF-MS	PCA, PLS-DA	Maize	L-Carnitine	Leon et al. (2009)
Genetic modification	NMR, GC-MS	PCA, ANOVA	Wheat	–	Baker et al. (2006)
Genetic modification	Transcriptomic	–	Wheat	–	Baudo et al. (2006)
Genetic modification	CE–ESI-TOF-MS		Soybean	4-Hydroxy-L-threonine (only in conventional soybean)	García-Villalba et al. (2008)
Genetic modification	NMR	PCA, ANOVA, Student's *t*-test	Grapes	Tryptophan and indole derivatives (typical of GM grapes)	Picone et al. (2011a)
Organic vs. conventional	FI-ESI-TOF-MS, FI-ESI-IT-MS	ANOVA, PCA	Grapefruit	–	Chen et al. (2010)
Organic vs. conventional	GC-MS	Tukey's test	Wheat	–	Zörb et al. (2006)
Organic vs. conventional	GC-MS	ANOVA, PCA	Maize	Myoinositol, malic acid, and phosphate (in organic samples)	Röhlig and Engel (2010)
Organic vs. conventional	GC-MS	Student's *t*-test, PCA	Wheat	Myoinositol and malic acid (in organic crops)	Bonte et al. (2014)
Organic vs. conventional	DART, TOFMS	PCA, LDA	Sweet bell peppers	–	Novotnà et al. (2012)

Organic vs. conventional	LC–ESI-QqQ	ANOVA	Ketchup	Caffeoylquinic and dicaffeoylquinic acids, caffeic and caffeic acid hexosides, kaemp-ferol-3-*O*-rutinoside, ferulic-*O*-hexoside, naringenin-7-*O*-glucoside, naringenin, rutin and quercetin (in organic ketchup); glutamylphenylalanine and *N*-malonyltryptophan (in conventional ketchup)	Vallverdú-Queralt et al. (2011)
Organic vs. conventional	NMR	ANOVA, PCA	Red wines	Tyrosine, trans-caffeic acid, glutamine	Laghi et al. (2014)
Geographical origin	NMR	PCA, OPLS-DA	Beef	Different amino acids depending on the origin (Korea, Australia, United States, New Zealand)	Jung et al. (2010)
Geographical origin	NMR	PCA, LDA	Cherry tomatoes	–	Savorani et al. (2009)
Geographical origin	HR-MAS NMR	PCA, Student's *t*-test	Cherry tomatoes	Fructose and glucose, glutamine, glutamate, aspartate and GABA (higher in Pachino tomatoes), fatty acids, alanine, methanol and acetylglutamic acid (lower in Pachino tomatoes)	Mallamace et al. (2014)
Geographical origin	DART–TOFMS, SPME–GC–TOF-MS	PCA, PLS-DA, LDA, ANN-MLP	Beer	–	Cajka et al. (2011)
Rearing conditions	GC-MS, LC-MS/MS	PCA, ANOVA	Bovine milk	Hippuric acid (for organic milk)	Boudonck et al. (2009)
Rearing conditions	HPLC	k-Nearest-neighbour	Eggs	–	van Ruth et al. (2011)
Rearing conditions	HPLC	k-Nearest-neighbour	Eggs	–	van Ruth et al. (2013)

Continued

Table 11.1 Continued

Type of study	Techniques	Statistical tools	Food analysed	Discriminant metabolites	Reference
Rearing conditions	NMR	PCA, PLS, ECVA, iECVA	Gilthead sea bream	Molecules from the glucose metabolism (higher in farmed fish)	Savorani et al. (2010)
Rearing conditions	NMR	Paired *t*-test, PCA	Sparus aurata	Hydroxylic and aliphatic regions	Picone et al. (2011b)
Rearing conditions	NMR	–	Bogue fish	Amino acids	Ciampa et al. (2012)
Processing	LC-QTOF-MS, HPLC		Tomato paste	Flavonoids, alkaloids, vitamin C	Capanoglu et al. (2008)
Processing	GC-MS, LC-MS, HPLC	ANOVA, PCA-FA	Pasta	Minerals, phytosterols, fatty acids, carotenoids, tocopherols, sugars	Beleggia et al. (2011)
Digestion	Spectrophotometer, HPLC	–	Cherry fruit	–	Toydemir et al. (2013)
Digestion	NMR		Parmigiano Reggiano	Amino acids	Bordoni et al. (2011)
Digestion	SDS–PAGE, microscopy, NMR	PCA	Ham	–	Pan et al. (2014)
Digestion	Bradford assay, SDS–PAGE, NMR, TD-NMR	–	Bresaola	–	Bordoni et al. (2014)
Digestion	SDS–PAGE, 2-DE, MALDI-TOF-MS, nano-HPLC–ESI-Q-TOF-MS/MS	–	Bresaola	–	Ferranti et al. (2014)

metabolites typical of food from a certified geographical origin. Metabolomics will increasingly aid food science research, and it needs to develop new high-technology methods and protocols in order to completely and automatically assess food quality.

References

Baker, J.M., Hawkins, N.D., Ward, J.L., Lovegrove, A., Napier, J.A., Shewry, P.R., Beale, M.H., 2006. A metabolomic study of substantial equivalence of field-grown genetically modified wheat. Plant Biotechnol. J. 4, 381–392.

Baudo, M.M., Lyons, R., Powers, S., Pastori, G.M., Edwards, K.J., Holdsworth, M.J., Shewry, P.R., 2006. Transgenesis has less impact on the transcriptome of wheat grain than conventional breeding. Plant Biotechnol. J. 4, 369–380.

Beleggia, R., Platani, C., Papa, R., Di Chio, A., Barros, E., Mashaba, C., Wirth, J., Fammartino, A., Sautter, C., Conner, S., Rauscher, J., Stewart, D., Cattivelli, L., 2011. Metabolomics and food processing from semolina to pasta. J. Agric. Food Chem. 59, 9366–9377.

Benincasa, C., Lewis, J., Perri, E., Sindona, G., Tagarelli, A., 2007. Determination of trace element in Italian virgin olive oils and their characterization according to geographical origin by statistical analysis. Anal. Chim. Acta 585, 366–370.

Bonte, A., Neuweger, H., Goesmann, A., Thonar, C., Mäder, P., Langenkämper, G., Niehaus, K., 2014. Metabolite profiling on wheat grain to enable a distinction of samples from organic and conventional farming systems. J. Sci. Food Agric. 94, 2605–2612. http://dx.doi.org/10.1002/jsfa.6566.

Bordoni, A., Picone, G., Babini, E., Vignali, M., Danesi, F., Valli, V., Di Nunzio, M., Laghi, L., Capozzi, F., 2011. NMR comparison of in vitro digestion of Parmigiano Reggiano cheese aged 15 and 30 months. Magn. Reson. Chem. 49, S61–S70.

Bordoni, A., Laghi, L., Babini, E., Di Nunzio, M., Picone, G., Ciampa, A., Valli, V., Danesi, F., Capozzi, F., 2014. The foodomics approach for the evaluation of protein bio-accessibility in processed meat upon in vitro digestion. Electrophoresis 35 (11), 1607–1614. http://dx.doi.org/10.1002/elps.201300579.

Boudonck, K.J., Mitchell, M.W., Wulff, J., Ryals, J.A., 2009. Characterization of the biochemical variability of bovine milk using metabolomics. Metabolomics 5, 375–386.

Brunner, M., Katona, R., Stefánka, Z., Prohaska, T., 2010. Determination of the geographical origin of processed spice using multielement and isotopic pattern on the example of Szegedi paprika. Eur. Food Res. Technol. 231, 623–634.

Cajka, T., Riddellova, K., Tomaniova, M., Hajslova, J., 2011. Ambient mass spectrometry employing a DART ion source for metabolomic fingerprinting/profiling a powerful tool for beer origin recognition. Metabolomics 7, 500–508.

Capanoglu, E., Beekwilder, J., Boyacioglu, D., De Vos, R.C., Hall, R.D., 2008. Changes in antioxidant and metabolite profiles during production of tomato paste. J. Agric. Food Chem. 56, 964–973.

Capozzi, F., Bordoni, A., 2013. Foodomics: a new comprehensive approach to food and nutrition. Genes Nutr. 8, 1–4.

Capuano, E., Boerrigter-Eenling, R., van der Veer, G., van Ruth, S.M., 2013. Analytical authentication of organic products: an overview of markers. J. Sci. Food Agric. 93, 12–28.

Chen, P., Harnly, J.M., Lester, G.M., 2010. Flow injection mass spectral fingerprints demonstrate chemical differences in Rio Red grapefruit with respect to year, harvest time, and conventional versus organic farming. J. Agric. Food Chem. 58, 4545–4553.

Chudzinska, M., Baralkiewicz, D., 2010. Estimation of honey authenticity by multielements characteristics using inductively coupled plasma-mass spectrometry (ICP-MS) combined with chemometrics. Food Chem. Toxicol. 48, 284–290.

Ciampa, A., Picone, G., Laghi, L., Nikzad, H., Capozzi, F., 2012. Changes in the amino acid composition of Bogue (Boops boops) fish during storage at different temperatures by 1H-NMR spectroscopy. Nutrients 4, 542–553.

Ferranti, P., Nitride, C., Nicolai, M.A., Mamone, G., Picariello, G., Bordoni, A., Valli, V., Di Nunzio, M., Babini, E., Marcolini, E., Capozzi, F., 2014. In vitro digestion of Bresaola proteins and release of potential bioactive peptides. Food Res. Int. 63, 157–169. http://dx.doi.org/10.1016/j.foodres.2014.02.008.

Fraser, P.D., Enfissi, E.M., Halket, J.M., Truesdale, M.R., Yu, D., Gerrish, C., Bramley, P.M., 2007. Manipulation of phytoene levels in tomato fruit effects on isoprenoids, plastids, and intermediary metabolism. Plant Cell 19, 3194–3211.

García-Villalba, R., León, C., Dinelli, G., Segura-Carretero, A., Fernández-Gutiérrez, A., Garcia-Cañas, V., Cifuentes, A., 2008. Comparative metabolomic study of transgenic versus conventional soybean using capillary electrophoresis–time-of-flight mass spectrometry. J. Chromatogr. A 1195, 164–173.

Graham, S.F., Ruiz-Aracama, A., Lommen, A., Cannizzo, F.T., Biolatti, B., Elliott, C.T., Mooney, M.H., 2012. Use of NMR metabolomic plasma profiling methodologies to identify illicit growth-promoting administrations. Anal. Bioanal. Chem. 403, 573–582.

Harper, G.C., Makatouni, A., 2002. Consumer perception of organic food production and farm animal welfare. Br. Food J. 104, 287–299.

Holmes, E., Loo, R.L., Stamler, J., Bictash, M., Yap, I.K.S., Chan, Q., Ebbels, T., De Iorio, M., Brown, I.J., Veselkov, K.A., Daviglus, M.L., Kesteloot, H., Ueshima, H., Zhao, L., Nicholson, J.K., Elliott, P., 2008. Human metabolic phenotype diversity and its association with diet and blood pressure. Nature 453, 396–400.

Hong, V., Wrolstad, R.E., 1990. Characterization of anthocyanin-containing colorants and fruit juices by HPLC/photodiode array detection. J. Agric. Food Chem. 38, 698–708.

Jung, Y., Lee, J., Kwon, J., Lee, K.S., Ryu, D.H., Hwang, G.S., 2010. Discrimination of the geographical origin of beef by 1H NMR-based metabolomics. J. Agric. Food Chem. 58, 10458–10466.

Kok, E.J., Kuiper, H.A., 2003. Comparative safety assessment for biotech crops. Trends Biotechnol. 21, 439–444.

Laghi, L., Versari, A., Marcolini, E., Parpinello, G.P., 2014. Metabonomic investigation by 1H-NMR to discriminate between red wines from organic and biodynamic grapes. Food Nutr. Sci. 5, 52.

Leon, C., Rodriguez-Meizoso, I., Lucio, M., Garcia-Cañas, V., Ibañez, E., Schmitt-Kopplin, P., Cifuentes, A., 2009. Metabolomics of transgenic maize combining Fourier transform-ion cyclotron resonance-mass spectrometry, capillary electrophoresis-mass spectrometry and pressurized liquid extraction. J. Chromatogr. A 1216, 7314–7323.

Levandi, T., Leon, C., Kaljurand, M., Garcia-Cañas, V., Cifuentes, A., 2008. Capillary electrophoresis time-of-flight mass spectrometry for comparative metabolomics of transgenic versus conventional maize. Anal. Chem. 80, 6329–6335.

Lo Feudo, G., Naccarato, A., Sindona, G., Tagarelli, A., 2010. Investigating the origin of tomatoes and triple concentrated tomato pastes through multielement determination by inductively coupled plasma mass spectrometry and statistical analysis. J. Agr. Food Chem. 58, 3801–3807.

Makatouni, A., 2002. What motivates consumers to buy organic food in the UK? Results from a qualitative study. Br. Food J. 104, 345–352.

Mallamace, D., Corsaro, C., Salvo, A., Cicero, N., Macaluso, A., Giangrosso, G., Ferrantelli, V., Dugo, G., 2014. A multivariate statistical analysis coming from the NMR metabolic profile of cherry tomatoes (The Sicilian Pachino case). Physica A 401, 112–117. http://dx.doi.org/10.1016/j.physa.2013.12.054.

Melgarejo, E., Urdiales, J.L., Sánchez-Jiménez, F., Medina, M.Á., 2010. Targeting polyamines and biogenic amines by green tea epigallocatechin-3-gallate. Amino Acids 38, 519–523.

Novotnà, H., Kmiecik, O., Gazka, M., Krtková, M., Hurajová, A., Schulzová, V., Hallmann, E., Rembia³kowska, E., Hajšlová, J., 2012. Metabolomic fingerprinting employing DART-TOFMS for authentication of tomatoes and peppers from organic and conventional farming. Food Addit. Contam. Part A Chem. Anal. Control Expo. Risk Assess. 29, 1335–1346.

Pan, X., Smith, F., Cliff, M.T., Capozzi, F., Mills, E.C., 2014. The application of nutrimetabolomics to investigating the bioaccessibility of nutrients in ham using a batch in vitro digestion model. Food Nutr. Sci. 5, 17.

Picone, G., Mezzetti, B., Babini, E., Capocasa, F., Placucci, G., Capozzi, F., 2011a. Unsupervised principal component analysis of NMR metabolic profiles for the assessment of substantial equivalence of transgenic grapes (Vitis vinifera). J. Agric. Food Chem. 59, 9271–9279.

Picone, G., Balling Engelsen, S., Savorani, F., Testi, S., Badiani, A., Capozzi, F., 2011b. Metabolomics as a powerful tool for molecular quality assessment of the fish Sparus aurata. Nutrients 3, 212–227.

Regal, P., Anizan, S., Antignac, J.P., Le Bizec, B., Cepeda, A., Fente, C., 2011. Metabolomic approach based on liquid chromatography coupled to high resolution mass spectrometry to screen for the illegal use of estradiol and progesterone in cattle. Anal. Chim. Acta 700, 16–25.

Röhlig, R.M., Engel, K.-H., 2010. Influence of the input system (conventional versus organic farming) on metabolite profiles of maize (Zea mays) kernels. J. Agric. Food Chem. 58, 3022–3030.

Savorani, F., Capozzi, F., Engelsen, S.B., Dell'Abate, M.T., Sequi, P., 2009. Pomodoro di Pachino: an authentication study using 1H-NMR and chemometrics-protecting its P.G.I. European certification. In: Guðjónsdóttir, M., Belton, P.S., Webb, G.A. (Eds.), Magnetic Resonance in Food Science: Challenges in a Changing World. The Royal Society of Chemistry, London, 319, pp. 158–166.

Savorani, F., Picone, G., Badiani, A., Fagioli, P., Capozzi, F., Engelsen, S.B., 2010. Metabolic profiling and aquaculture differentiation of gilthead sea bream by ^{1}H NMR metabonomics. Food Chem. 120, 907–914.

Steiner, C., Teixeira, W.G., Lehmann, J., Nehls, T., de Macêdo, J.L.V., Blum, W.E., Zech, W., 2007. Long term effects of manure, charcoal and mineral fertilization on crop production and fertility on a highly weathered Central Amazonian upland soil. Plant and Soil 291, 275–290.

Toydemir, G., Capanoglu, E., Kamiloglu, S., Boyacioglu, D., de Vos, R.C., Hall, R.D., Beekwilder, J., 2013. Changes in sour cherry (*Prunus cerasus* L.) antioxidants during nectar processing and *in vitro* gastrointestinal digestion. J. Funct. Foods 5, 1402–1413.

Vallverdú-Queralt, A., Medina-Remón, A., Casals-Ribes, I., Amat, M., Lamuela-Raventós R.M., 2011. A metabolomic approach differentiates between conventional and organic ketchups. J. Agric. Food Chem. 59, 11703–11710.

van Ruth, S.M., Alewijn, M., Rogers, K., Newton-Smith, E., Tena, N., Bollen, M., Koot, A., 2011. Authentication of organic and conventional eggs by carotenoid profiling. Food Chem. 126, 1299–1305.

van Ruth, S.M., Koot, A.H., Brouwer, S.E., Boivin, N., Carcea, M., Zerva, C.N., Haugen, J.-E., Höhl, A., Köroglu, D., Mafra, I., Rom, S., 2013. Eggspectation: organic egg authentication method challenged with produce from ten different countries. Qual Assur. Saf. Crop 5, 7–14.

Walsh, M.C., Brennan, L., Pujos-Guillot, E., Sébédio, J.-L., Scalbert, A., Fagan, A., Higgins, D.H., Gibney, M.J., 2007. Influence of acute phytochemical intake on human urinary metabolomic profiles. Am. J. Clin. Nutr. 86, 1687–1693.

Williams, P.R., Hammitt, J.K., 2001. Perceived risks of conventional and organic produce: pesticides, pathogens, and natural toxins. Risk Anal. 21, 319–330.

Wishart, D.S., 2008. Metabolomics applications to food science and nutrition research. Trends Food Sci. Technol. 19, 482–493.

Woese, K., Lange, D., Boess, C., Bögl, K.W., 1997. A comparison of organically and conventionally grown foods – results of a review of the relevant literature. J. Sci. Food Agric. 74, 281–293.

Zörb, C., Langenkämper, G., Betsche, T., Niehaus, K., Barsch, A., 2006. Metabolite profiling of wheat grains (*Triticum aestivum* L.) from organic and conventional agriculture. J. Agric. Food Chem. 54, 8301–8306.

Appendix: abbreviations

2-DE	2-dimensional electrophoresis
ANN-MLP	artificial neural network with multilayer perceptrons
ANOVA	analysis of variance
ASAP	atmospheric solids analysis probe
CA	cluster analysis
CE	capillary electrophoresis
DART	direct analysis in real time
DESI	desorption electrospray ionisation
ECVA	extended canonical variates analysis
EPSPS	5-enolpyruvylshikimate-3-phosphate synthase
ESI	electrospray ionisation
FI	flow injection
FT-ICR	Fourier transform-ion cyclotron resonance
GABA	gamma 4-aminobutyric acid
GC	gas chromatography
GM	genetically modified
HPLC	high-performance liquid chromatography
ICP	induced couple plasma
iECVA	interval extendend canonical variates analysis
IT	ion trap
LC	liquid chromatography
LC–ESI-QqQ	liquid chromatography coupled to MS in tandem mode
LDA	linear discriminant analysis
MALDI	matrix-assisted laser desorption/ionisation
MS	mass spectrometry
MS/MS	tandem mass spectrometry
NMR	nuclear magnetic resonance

OPLS-DA	orthogonal partial least squares – discriminant analysis
PC	principal component
PCA	principal component analysis
PCA-FA	principal component analysis – factor analysis
(Real time) PCR	polymerase chain reaction
PLS	partial least squares
PLS-DA	partial least squares – discriminant analysis
QTOF	quadrupole time-of-flight
RP-HPLC	reversed-phase high-performance liquid chromatography
RSD	relative standard deviation
SDS–PAGE	sodium dodecyl sulphate–polyacrylamide gel electrophoresis
SE	substantial equivalence
SPME	solid-phase microextraction
T_0	time point 0
T_{16}	time point 16
TD-NMR	time domain nuclear magnetic resonance
TOF	time-of-flight
TOF-MS	time-of-flight mass spectrometry
UV	ultraviolet

Future perspectives for metabolomics in nutrition research: a nutritionist's view

12

M. Ferrara
Institut National de la Recherche Agronomique (INRA), Clermont-Ferrand, France

12.1 Introduction

In order to better understand how numerous food components interact with the complex biochemical networks of living organisms, nutrition science needs to rely on more holistic approaches, rather than simply analysing a handful of nutrients or metabolic pathways. Given that metabolites provide a direct readout of functional activity, metabolomics fills a critical gap in the domain of systems biology, complementing genomics and proteomics (Patti et al., 2012; Sassone-Corsi, 2013). Thus, global metabolite analysis, or the metabolome, describes a biological system at a level that surpasses genetic information while revealing the impact of environmental components, including diet (Chen et al., 2014; Pellis et al., 2012; Rezzi et al., 2007) and gut microflora activity (McHardy et al., 2013; Ursell et al., 2014; Xie et al., 2013). The metabolome therefore reflects more closely the ultimate phenotypes (Fiehn, 2002; Keurentjes, 2009; Matsuda et al., 2012), and metabolomics is set to be a key tool for nutrition research (Brennan, 2013) because it offers a snapshot of the molecular composition of food (Hu and Xu, 2013; Ibanez et al., 2012) and the individual's metabolic status (Roberts et al., 2014; Xu et al., 2013).

The previous chapters describe how metabolomics approaches have developed in diverse fields of nutrition, and these approaches clearly show that the characterisation of all metabolites may provide an overview of metabolism, consequently serving as a biomarker for an organism's biological state. Despite the high potential of metabolomics approaches, the applications of metabolomics in nutrition are still in their infancy. The two major pitfalls of the field are identified by all of this book's authors: metabolite identification and the biological interpretation of the voluminous data produced by these approaches. Given these challenges, advancements in the field of human nutrition depend on the biological relevance of metabolomic analyses. These analyses involve the identification and quantification of metabolites observed in various pathophysiological and nutritional states, as well as the observation of changes in metabolite concentration and their effects. The approaches must also embrace the dynamic nature of metabolism and its compartmentalisation in a large number of living organisms.

Metabolomics as a Tool in Nutrition Research. http://dx.doi.org/10.1016/B978-1-78242-084-2.00012-5

12.2 Metabolites identification and biological relevance

The fast and accurate identification of molecules largely depends on the analytical performance of devices and the standardisation of current practises in data mining. Thus, in recent years, a major step was realised when biologists increased their use of high-resolution appliances, while optimising the annotation process for organic compounds (Courant et al., 2012; Da Silva et al., 2013; Kiefer et al., 2008; Liu et al., 2014). The constant improvement of measuring instruments is a basic element in advancing the detection and identification of metabolites; however, this improvement depends on the manufacturers, and it is outside the competence of biologists and platforms associated with their activities. In addition to these future conceptual and technological advances, the combination of existing technologies and the sharing of standardised databases could significantly improve the identification of metabolites.

The combined use of isotopic labelling and metabolomics seems to be a promising strategy for accurate metabolite quantification not only for *in vitro* systems but also for complex matrices such as biofluids and tissues. de Jong and Beecher (2012) have described a novel isotopic-labelling method that uses the creation of distinct biochemical signatures to eliminate current bottlenecks and to enable accurate metabolic profiling. This isotopic ratio outlier analysis (IROA) method is a non-targeted analysis that utilises a specific isotopic balance to create definable metabolite patterns. This makes the mass-spectral signals complex but increases the information that can be extracted from these signals. The power of stable isotope- and mass spectrometry-based metabolomics is also demonstrated in the field of xenobiotic metabolism (Li et al., 2013). These are two examples of how the combination of isotope labelling and MS technology can be of crucial importance to metabolomics applied to higher organisms.

Stable isotope labelling is an established approach for investigating the dynamics of metabolic pathways, and its combination with metabolomics promises to provide a comprehensive understanding of metabolic networks in biological systems (Klein and Heinzle, 2012). The needed tools are available, given the general application of high-resolution MS-based metabolomics and recent bioinformatics advances for automated isotopomer detection (Creek et al., 2012), and there are already some examples of metabolic profiling in whole animal and human models (Fan et al., 2012). Thus, this type of development should eventually enable enriched descriptions of metabolic networks with a temporal element, which is often essential for explaining the variations observed in biofluid metabolite concentrations in response to diet.

12.3 *In vivo* metabolomics

In the mammalian body, global metabolism involves multiple organs and tissues. Indeed, metabolites are present in different compositions and concentrations within tissues and even cell compartments. The use of common sample preparations for metabolomics analysis does not enable access to spatial information. A more holistic view requires a multi-organ system approach aimed at screening metabolites in various tissues. Astarita and Piomelli (2011) give an example of such an approach by studying the dysregulations of docosahexaenoic acid metabolism in Alzheimer's disease. Recently developed *in situ* metabolomics approaches (Caprioli, 2014; Gessel et al., 2014; Jungmann and Heeren, 2012; Miura et al., 2012) can provide detailed spatial distributions of metabolites that go beyond the simple measurement of metabolite level. In addition to nuclear magnetic resonance imaging (MRI), mass spectrometry imaging (MSI) can now produce images of a large number of compounds in tissue sections with a spatial resolution better than 150 μm (Lanekoff et al., 2013), providing a spatial distribution of metabolites *in situ* (Hart et al., 2011; Lietz et al., 2013). Such an approach was used to visualise the metabolic changes in response to disease progression in a rat brain during infarct formation after ischemia–reperfusion (Irie et al., 2014). In food science, MSI is also a powerful method for characterising nutrients and contaminants with a high chemical and spatial sensitivity (Handberg et al., 2014). Compared to the fields of protein and peptide MSI, metabolite MSI is still in its infancy, but it is rapidly growing. Analysis of these small molecules has been difficult due to the large amount of chemical interference in the low-mass region, but recent advances in the resolution power of different devices, as well as ion transmission optics, have increased the confidence levels and sensitivities of these types of experiments. Continued improvement in sample preparation techniques, instruments, and software will enable MSI of metabolites to become a routine approach.

12.4 Conclusion

In recent years, metabolomics has progressed from improvements in the sensitivity and precision of measuring devices, through the development of new technologies, to the synergistic use of different approaches combined with advances in signal analysis (Zeng et al., 2014) and data mining (Booth et al., 2013). All of these developments offer metabolomics the potential to couple the characterisation and quantification of metabolites with a spatiotemporal dimension, giving it greater relevance for the biological interpretation of data.

Nutrition science has clearly just begun to explore the potential of metabolomics, but this field offers a range of approaches that might better explain the responses of cells, tissues, and organs to different foods, which are also more finely characterised by the same technologies. By identifying food composition, as well as the individual's health and nutrition status, metabolomics could likely enable diagnosis, prognosis, and prediction of individual responses to diet. Through its various facets, metabolomics also promises to identify individual variations in dietary requirements, classifying individuals into specific groups. In addition, the development of integrated analytical platforms will provide the possibility to uncover the precise functional connectivity between nutrition and metabolism at the system level, in order to move towards the definition of nutrient requirements across the lifespan, while targeting nutrition to achieve optimal health and wellness.

References

Astarita, G., Piomelli, D., 2011. Towards a whole-body systems [multi-organ] lipidomics in Alzheimer's disease. Prostaglandins Leukot. Essent. Fat. Acids 85, 197–203.

Booth, S.C., Weljie, A.M., Turner, R.J., 2013. Computational tools for the secondary analysis of metabolomics experiments. Comput. Struct. Biotechnol. J. 4, e201301003.

Brennan, L., 2013. Metabolomics in nutrition research: current status and perspectives. Biochem. Soc. Trans. 41, 670–673.

Caprioli, R.M., 2014. Imaging mass spectrometry: molecular microscopy for enabling a new age of discovery. Proteomics 14, 807–809.

Chen, M., Zhou, K., Chen, X., Qiao, S., Hu, Y., Xu, B., Xu, B., Han, X., Tang, R., Mao, Z., Dong, C., Wu, D., Wang, Y., Wang, S., Zhou, Z., Xia, Y., Wang, X., 2014. Metabolomic analysis reveals metabolic changes caused by bisphenol A in rats. Toxicol. Sci. 138, 256–267.

Courant, F., Royer, A.L., Chereau, S., Morvan, M.L., Monteau, F., Antignac, J.P., Le Bizec, B., 2012. Implementation of a semi-automated strategy for the annotation of metabolomic fingerprints generated by liquid chromatography-high resolution mass spectrometry from biological samples. Analyst 137, 4958–4967.

Creek, D.J., Chokkathukalam, A., Jankevics, A., Burgess, K.E., Breitling, R., Barrett, M.P., 2012. Stable isotope-assisted metabolomics for network-wide metabolic pathway elucidation. Anal. Chem. 84, 8442–8447.

Da Silva, L., Godejohann, M., Martin, F.P., Collino, S., Burkle, A., Moreno-Villanueva, M., Bernhardt, J., Toussaint, O., Grubeck-Loebenstein, B., Gonos, E.S., Sikora, E., Grune, T., Breusing, N., Franceschi, C., Hervonen, A., Spraul, M., Moco, S., 2013. High-resolution quantitative metabolome analysis of urine by automated flow injection NMR. Anal. Chem. 85, 5801–5809.

de Jong, F.A., Beecher, C., 2012. Addressing the current bottlenecks of metabolomics: Isotopic Ratio Outlier Analysis, an isotopic-labeling technique for accurate biochemical profiling. Bioanalysis 4, 2303–2314.

Fan, T.W., Lorkiewicz, P.K., Sellers, K., Moseley, H.N., Higashi, R.M., Lane, A.N., 2012. Stable isotope-resolved metabolomics and applications for drug development. Pharmacol. Ther. 133, 366–391.

Fiehn, O., 2002. Metabolomics—the link between genotypes and phenotypes. Plant Mol. Biol. 48, 155–171.

Gessel, M.M., Norris, J.L., Caprioli, R.M., 2014. MALDI imaging mass spectrometry: spatial molecular analysis to enable a new age of discovery. J. Proteome 107C, 71–82. http://dx.doi.org/10.1016/j.jprot.2014.03.021.

Handberg, E., Chingin, K., Wang, N., Dai, X., Chen, H., 2014. Mass spectrometry imaging for visualizing organic analytes in food. Mass Spectrom. Rev. http://dx.doi.org/10.1002/mas.21424.

Hart, P.J., Francese, S., Claude, E., Woodroofe, M.N., Clench, M.R., 2011. MALDI-MS imaging of lipids in ex vivo human skin. Anal. Bioanal. Chem. 401, 115–125.

Hu, C., Xu, G., 2013. Mass-spectrometry-based metabolomics analysis for foodomics. TrAC Trends Anal. Chem. 52, 36–46.

Ibanez, C., Valdes, A., Garcia-Canas, V., Simo, C., Celebier, M., Rocamora-Reverte, L., Gomez-Martinez, A., Herrero, M., Castro-Puyana, M., Segura-Carretero, A., Ibanez, E., Ferragut, J.A., Cifuentes, A., 2012. Global Foodomics strategy to investigate the health benefits of dietary constituents. J. Chromatogr. 1248, 139–153.

Irie, M., Fujimura, Y., Yamato, M., Miura, D., Wariishi, H., 2014. Integrated MALDI-MS imaging and LC-MS techniques for visualizing spatiotemporal metabolomic dynamics in a rat stroke model. Metabolomics 10, 473–483.

Jungmann, J.H., Heeren, R.M., 2012. Emerging technologies in mass spectrometry imaging. J. Proteome 75, 5077–5092.

Keurentjes, J.J., 2009. Genetical metabolomics: closing in on phenotypes. Curr. Opin. Plant Biol. 12, 223–230.

Kiefer, P., Portais, J.C., Vorholt, J.A., 2008. Quantitative metabolome analysis using liquid chromatography-high-resolution mass spectrometry. Anal. Biochem. 382, 94–100.

Klein, S., Heinzle, E., 2012. Isotope labeling experiments in metabolomics and fluxomics. Wiley Interdiscip. Rev. Syst. Biol. Med. 4, 261–272.

Lanekoff, I., Burnum-Johnson, K., Thomas, M., Short, J., Carson, J.P., Cha, J., Dey, S.K., Yang, P., Prieto Conaway, M.C., Laskin, J., 2013. High-speed tandem mass spectrometric in situ imaging by nanospray desorption electrospray ionization mass spectrometry. Anal. Chem. 85, 9596–9603.

Li, F., Pang, X., Krausz, K.W., Jiang, C., Chen, C., Cook, J.A., Krishna, M.C., Mitchell, J.B., Gonzalez, F.J., Patterson, A.D., 2013. Stable isotope- and mass spectrometry-based metabolomics as tools in drug metabolism: a study expanding tempol pharmacology. J. Proteome Res. 12, 1369–1376.

Lietz, C.B., Gemperline, E., Li, L., 2013. Qualitative and quantitative mass spectrometry imaging of drugs and metabolites. Adv. Drug Deliv. Rev. 65, 1074–1085. http://dx.doi.org/10.1016/j.addr.2013.04.009.

Liu, X., Ser, Z., Locasale, J.W., 2014. Development and quantitative evaluation of a high-resolution metabolomics technology. Anal. Chem. 86, 2175–2184.

Matsuda, F., Okazaki, Y., Oikawa, A., Kusano, M., Nakabayashi, R., Kikuchi, J., Yonemaru, J., Ebana, K., Yano, M., Saito, K., 2012. Dissection of genotype-phenotype associations in rice grains using metabolome quantitative trait loci analysis. Plant J. 70, 624–636.

McHardy, I.H., Goudarzi, M., Tong, M., Ruegger, P.M., Schwager, E., Weger, J.R., Graeber, T.G., Sonnenburg, J.L., Horvath, S., Huttenhower, C., McGovern, D.P., Fornace Jr., A.J., Borneman, J., Braun, J., 2013. Integrative analysis of the microbiome and metabolome of the human intestinal mucosal surface reveals exquisite inter-relationships. Microbiome 1, 17.

Miura, D., Fujimura, Y., Wariishi, H., 2012. In situ metabolomic mass spectrometry imaging: recent advances and difficulties. J. Proteome 75, 5052–5060.

Patti, G.J., Yanes, O., Siuzdak, G., 2012. Innovation: Metabolomics: the apogee of the omics trilogy. Nat. Rev. Mol. Cell Biol. 13, 263–269.

Pellis, L., van Erk, M.J., van Ommen, B., Bakker, G.C., Hendriks, H.F., Cnubben, N.H., Kleemann, R., van Someren, E.P., Bobeldijk, I., Rubingh, C.M., Wopereis, S., 2012. Plasma metabolomics and proteomics profiling after a postprandial challenge reveal subtle diet effects on human metabolic status. Metabolomics 8, 347–359.

Rezzi, S., Ramadan, Z., Martin, F.-P.J., Fay, L.B., van Bladeren, P., Lindon, J.C., Nicholson J.K., Kochhar, S., 2007. Human metabolic phenotypes link directly to specific dietary preferences in healthy individuals. J. Proteome Res. 6, 4469–4477.

Roberts, L.D., Koulman, A., Griffin, J.L., 2014. Towards metabolic biomarkers of insulin resistance and type 2 diabetes: progress from the metabolome. Lancet Diabetes Endocrinol. 2, 65–75.

Sassone-Corsi, P., 2013. Physiology when metabolism and epigenetics converge. Science 339, 148–150.

Ursell, L.K., Haiser, H.J., Van Treuren, W., Garg, N., Reddivari, L., Vanamala, J., Dorrestein, P.C., Turnbaugh, P.J., Knight, R., 2014. The intestinal metabolome: an intersection between microbiota and host. Gastroenterology 146, 1470–1476.

Xie, G., Zhang, S., Zheng, X., Jia, W., 2013. Metabolomics approaches for characterizing metabolic interactions between host and its commensal microbes. Electrophoresis 34, 2787–2798.

Xu, F., Tavintharan, S., Sum, C.F., Woon, K., Lim, S.C., Ong, C.N., 2013. Metabolic signature shift in type 2 diabetes mellitus revealed by mass spectrometry-based metabolomics. J. Clin. Endocrinol. Metab. 98, E1060–E1065.

Zeng, Z., Liu, X., Dai, W., Yin, P., Zhou, L., Huang, Q., Lin, X., Xu, G., 2014. Ion fusion of high-resolution LC-MS-based metabolomics data to discover more reliable biomarkers. Anal. Chem. 86, 3793–3800.

Index

Note: Page numbers followed by *f* indicate figures and *t* indicate tables.

A

Acylcarnitines
  anti-inflammatory M2 macrophage phenotype, 148–149
  HepaRG cells, 148
  HF diet, 148
  inborn errors of metabolism, 146
  insulin resistance, 146, 147*t*, 148
  lauroyl carnitine, 148–149
  lipotoxic phenotype and reactive oxygen species production, 148
  liver histological status, 146–148
  mitochondrial β-oxidation dysfunction, 146–148
  NASH and steatotic patients, 146–148
  obesity, 148
  proinflammatory status, 148–149
ADD. *See* Average Danish diet (ADD)
Antioxidants, 18
Artificial neural networks with multilayer perceptrons (ANN-MLP), 212–213
Average Danish diet (ADD), 23–24

B

BioCyc database, 88–89, 95, 97
Biomarker mapping
  HumanCyc, 97, 100*f*
  human genome-scale metabolic network, 105–106, 105*f*
  KEGG Global Map, 97, 98*f*
  KEGG glycine, serine, and threonine metabolism pathway, 97, 99*f*
Biomarkers. *See also* Dietary biomarker discovery
  cohort study and identification (*see* Cohort study)
  definition, 170
  dietary intake and nutritional exposures, 170
  hepatic CYP1A2 metabolism, 170–171
  host factors, 170–171
  isolating *in situ* biomarkers, 159–160
  long-chain omega-3 fatty acids, 171–172
  nutrition and chronic metabolic diseases (*see* Nutrition and chronic metabolic diseases)
  objective phenotypic assessments, 170
  plasma trimethylamine oxide, 170–171
  predict measurement errors, 170–171
  short-term nutritional biomarkers, 170–171
  validation, 185–186
Bipartite graph, 102, 103*f*, 104
Body mass index (BMI), 18
Branched-chain amino acids (BCAAs), 147*t*, 149–151, 156

C

Cancer and Nutrition (EPIC)-Potsdam study, 155–156
Canonical correlation analysis (CCA), 41
Capillary electrophoresis (CE), 203
Cardiovascular Risk in Young Finns study, 158
CCA. *See* Canonical correlation analysis (CCA)
Challenge tests. *See* Oral glucose tolerance test (OGTT)
Chemometrics methods
  data integration (*see* Data integration methods)
  definition, 37
  Gene Set Enrichment Analysis, 51
  hierarchical clustering methods, 38
  information-rich omic technology, 37
  knowledge-based methods, 51
  multivariate calibration methods, 39–40
  protein–protein interaction, 51
  proteomic data and metabolic profile data, 51

Chemometrics methods *(Continued)*
supervised pattern recognition methods, 38–39
topological properties, 51–52
unsupervised pattern recognition methods, 38
Cohort study
Cancer and Nutrition (EPIC)-Potsdam study, 155–156
Cardiovascular Risk in Young Finns study, 158
experimental study protocol, 154–155, 154*f*
Framingham Heart study, 154–155, 158
Framingham Offspring study, 154–156
high-throughput metabolite profiling, 158
KORA study, 156–158
Malmö Diet Cancer Cardiovascular Cohort study, 154–155, 158
metabolites with T2DM, 156–158, 157*f*
MURDOCK CV study, 158
San Antonio Family Heart study, 155–156
T2DM and IFG, 156–158
triacylglycerols (TAGs) profiling, 155–156
TwinsUK and Health Ageing study, 156–158

D

DASH. *See* Dietary Approaches to Stop Hypertension (DASH)
Data integration methods
calibration transfer methods, 43–44
CCA, 41, 47–48
conceptual integration, 40
correlation-based approaches, 46–47
CPCA, 41, 42
model-based integration, 40
multiple factor analysis, 42
nonlinear kernel-based classification method, 43
OnPLS method, 42–43
OPLS modelling strategy, 42
PARAFAC, 44–45
statistical integration, 40, 41, 48–51
Tucker decomposition, 45–46
Denaturing gradient gel electrophoresis (DGGE), 122–123
DGGE. *See* Denaturing gradient gel electrophoresis (DGGE)
Dietary Approaches to Stop Hypertension (DASH), 18
Dietary assessment
chemical standards, 189
FooDB and PhytoHUB, 186–189
HMDB database, 186–189
marker identification, 174*t*, 186–189, 187*f*
MetaboLights, 190
METLIN and LIPID MAPS, 186–189
nutritional phenotype database, 190
raw data, 189
standard operational procedures, 189
24 h recalls method, 168–169
Dietary biomarker discovery, 172–173, 174*t*, 184
Dietary pattern effect, 23–25
Direct analysis in real time (DART), 210
Dysbiosis, 116–117, 118*t*

E

5-Enolpyruvylshikimate-3-phosphate synthase, 207
Enzymatic Commission (EC), 92
Extendend canonical variates analysis (ECVA), 215–216

F

Flow injection electrospray ionization ion trap mass spectroscopy (FI-ESI-IT-MS), 209
Flow injection electrospray ionization time-of-flight mass spectroscopy (FI-ESI-TOF-MS), 209
Fluorescent in situ hybridization (FISH), 122–123
Food frequency questionnaires (FFQs), 168–169
Foodomics, 77, 203
Food quality
digestibility, 205, 220–221
eggs, 215
fish, 216–217
geographical origin, 211–213
in vitro digestion, 219–220
in vitro simulation and metabolomics, 220
metabolomics approach, 203–205, 204*f*

nutrients' bioaccessibility, 221
OPLS, 214
OPLS-DA, 214
organic milk, 214–215
organic *vs.* conventional farming, 208–211
PCA, 214–215
process, 217–219
Fourier transform ion cyclotron resonance mass spectrometry (FT-ICR-MS), 206
Framingham Heart study, 154–155, 158
Framingham Offspring study, 154–156
FTO and *MC4R* genes, 138

G

Gas chromatography/electrospray ionization time-of-flight mass spectrometry (GC–EI-TOF-MS), 42
Gas-liquid chromatography coupled with mass spectrometry (GC-MS), 4
Gene Set Enrichment Analysis, 51
Genetic modification (GM), 205–207
Genome Analyzer system, 117–122
Genome Sequencer FLX+ System, 117–122
Genome-wide association studies (GWAS), 24–25, 167–168
Genome-wide association studies with metabolic traits (mGWAS), 138
Gut microbiota
compositional/functional diversity, 116–117
diversity, 116–117, 124–125
dysbiosis, 116–117, 118*t*
extragenome organ, 115–116
host–microbe interaction (*see* Host–microbe interaction study)
metagenomics (*see* Metagenomics)
microbiome–metabolome interactions, 127–128
microbiota composition, 116–117
personalised nutrition, 128–130
symbiotic signalling interactions, 124–125

H

High performance liquid chromatography coupled with mass spectrometry (LC-MS), 4
High-performance liquid chromatography (HPLC), 203
High-resolution nuclear magnetic resonance (NMR) spectroscopy, 203
Host–microbe interaction study
bile acid metabolism, 126–127
diverse microbial niches and inhabitants, 124–125
functional metagenome, 125
GC-MS and LC-MS based metabolomics approach, 125
vs. human host, 124–125
IBD, 127
impact, 125–126
SCFA, 125
symbiotic signalling interactions, 124–125
UPLC-MS profiling approach, 126
urinary and faecal metabolites, 125
HumanCyc, 97, 100*f*
Human metabolic networks
adipocyte model, 91
biochemical reconstruction, 87–88
Brenda, 91
cell/tissue-specific networks, 89, 91, 92*f*
Entrez Gene databases, 88–89
exchange formats, 93, 94*f*
genome-based reconstruction method, 86–87
genome-scale networks, 89, 90*t*
in vivo/*in vitro* biomarker metabolites, 85
limitations, 92–93
manual *vs.* automatic network analysis, 106–108, 107*f*
metabolic stories, 108
metabolism modelling (*see* Human metabolism modelling)
metabolite identifiers, 95–96, 96*t*
metabolite mapping, 97
metabolomics dataset, 94–95, 96*t*
multi-omics analysis, 108
off-target drug effects, 85–86
organism-specific BioCyc databases, 88
reaction paths, 105–106, 105*f*
UniProt, 91
Human metabolism modelling
FBA methods, 101–102
graph modelling, 102–104, 103*f*
highly informative methods, 101
HumanCyc, 97, 100*f*
KEGG global map, 97, 98*f*

Human metabolism modelling *(Continued)*
KEGG glycine, serine, and threonine metabolism pathway, 97, 99*f*
limitation, 101
objective function, 101–102
steady-state assumption, 101

I

Impaired fasting glucose (IFG), 156–158
Induced couple plasma combined with mass spectrometry (ICP-MS), 211
International Study of Macronutrients and Micronutrients and Blood Pressure (INTERMAP), 24
Interval extended canonical variates analysis (iECVA), 215–216
In vivo metabolomics, 232–233
Isotopic ratio outlier analysis (IROA) method, 232

K

KORA study, 156–158

L

LIPID Metabolites and Pathways Strategy (LIPID MAPS), 12
Lipidomics
ageing and maturation, 73
AMDMS-SL, 72
biochemical mechanisms, 66
bioinformatics, 72
compliance, progress, and dietary guidance, 73
control food quality, 77
diets/challenge tests, 73–75
environmental changes/lifestyle modifications, 73
hypothesis-driven targeted analysis, 68
hypothesis-generating, non-targeted analysis, 68
individual nutritional status, 73
LIMSA, 72
LipidInspector, 72
LIPID MAPS consortium, 71
LipidProfiler, 72
LipidQA/LipidBlast, 71–72
LipidXplorer, 72
liquid chromatographic separation, 68, 69–71, 70*f*
metabolic syndrome, 75–77
sample preparation, 66–67
shotgun lipidomics, 68–69
side effects and unexpected metabolic responses, 73
VANTED and Pathway Editor, 72–73
Lipids
fatty acid building blocks, 65–66
fatty acyls, 63
glycerolipids, 63–64, 64*f*
linoleic acid and α-linolenic acid, 65–66
nutrition and health, 65–66
polyketides, 63
prenol lipids, 63
saccharolipids, 63
sphingolipid, 64–65, 65*f*
sterols, 65
Low-density lipoproteins (LDL), 65
Lysophospholipids, 147*t*, 151–152

M

MALDI-TOF-MS spectra, 220–221
Malmö Diet Cancer Cardiovascular Cohort study, 154–155, 158
Mass spectrometry imaging (MSI), 17, 232–233
Mass spectroscopy (MS), 203
Metabolic dysfunction. *See* Biomarkers
Metabolic profiling
applications, 20–21
breast-feeding, 18–19
environmental factor, 18
epidemiological studies, 25
functional foods, 23
genetic determinants, 18
gut microbiota, 18
high-resolution spectroscopic techniques, 17
instrumental methods, 26–27
interventional studies, 25
mapping dietary patterns, 23–25
meat and fish, 22
Mediterranean and DASH diets, 18
metabonomics/metabolomics, 20
metagenomics/microbiomics, 20
milk products, 22–23
natural products, 21–22

nutrigenomics, 19–20
nutriproteomics, 20
obesity, 17–18
postgenomic technology, 17
prevalence, 17–18
sample analysis, 27–29, 27*f*, 29*f*
scope of, 19
wheat and fibre, 22
Metabolites identification and biological relevance, 232
Metabolome-wide association study (MWAS), 24–25, 50
Metabotype
advantages and disadvantages, 138
baseline metabolic profile, 139–140, 141
choline depletion study, 139–140
diet and gut microflora, 138, 139*f*
dietary preferences, 140
distinctive patterns, 140
k clusters, 138
lower serum 25(OH)D and higher levels of adipokines, 138–139
nutrityping/phytoprofiling, 141–142
partial least squares-discriminant analysis, 139–140
PCA, 138
personalised dietary advice, 140, 140*f*
sources, 142
targeted and nontargeted LC-MS approaches, 139–140
uncorrelated shrunken centroid, 139–140
Metagenomics
bacterial phyla, 122–123, 122*f*
compositional and functional characteristics, 117–122
cultivation-based techniques, 117–122
DGGE and FISH, 122–123
Genome Analyzer system, 117–122
Genome Sequencer FLX+ System, 117–122
gut microbiota-host co-metabolism, 123
^{1}H-nuclear magnetic resonance (NMR) spectroscopy, 123
mass spectrometry (MS), 123
metabolic nature, 123–124
metabolic profiling approach, 123
microbial community structure, 123
microbiome, 123
oxidative and conjugative nature, 123–124
Sanger sequencing approach, 117–122
16S rRNA gene sequencing, 122–123, 122*f*
Multi-dimensional mass spectrometry-based shotgun lipidomics (MDMS-SL), 68–69
Multiple factor analysis (MFA), 42
Multivariate analysis of variance (MANOVA), 72
Multiway/multimodal analysis methods
PARAFAC, 44–45
tucker decomposition, 45–46
MURDOCK CV study, 158

N

Nano-HPLC–ESI-Q-TOF-MS/MS analysis, 220–221
New Nordic Diet (NND), 23–24
Nonlinear kernel-based classification method, 43
Nuclear magnetic resonance imaging (MRI), 232–233
Nuclear magnetic resonance (NMR) spectroscopy, 4, 17, 221
Nutritional epidemiology
biomarkers, 170–172
dietary assessment (*see* Dietary assessment)
dietary patterns and metabolomic profiles, 184–185
diet records, 168–169
FFQ, 168–169
food composition, 169
food metabolome, 172
GWAS, 167–168
mobile phone applications, 169–170
sources, 167–168
24 h recalls method, 168–169
Nutritional metabolomics
analytical platform, 6–7, 7*f*
biological interpretations, 10–11
data sets and statistical analyses, 7–8
definition, 4
dietary polyphenols, 3
experimental design, 5–6
genotype-phenotype gap, 3–4, 4*f*
high-throughput technology, 3–4, 4*f*
identify-bioactive molecules, 3
linoleic and linolenic acids, 3
metabolite identification pipeline, 8–10
metabolomic analysis, 4–5, 5*f*

Nutritional metabolomics *(Continued)*
omic technology, 4
optimization, 3
standardization procedures, 11–12
Nutritional transition, 145
Nutrition and chronic metabolic diseases
acylcarnitines, 146–149
2-aminoethanesulphonic acid, 152
BCAA, 147*t*, 149–151
bile acids, 153
diet-induced hepatic IR, 153
lysophospholipids, 147*t*, 151–152
normal diet/HF diet, 152
taurine, 152

O

Oral glucose tolerance test (OGTT)
applications, 197–200, 198*t*
dietary intervention, 200
glucose homeostasis, 197
human metabolomic response, 201
plasma metabolome changes, 200
Oral lipid tolerance test (OLTT). *See* Oral glucose tolerance test (OGTT)
Organic *vs.* conventional farming
DART and TOF-MS analysis, 210
FI-ESI-IT-MS, 209
FI-ESI-TOF-MS, 209
GC-MS analysis, 209
macro/micronutrients, 208
myo-inositol, 209
PCA, 210–211
stable isotopes, 208
Tukey's test, 209
untargeted screening, 208
Orthogonal partial least squares (OPLS), 42, 214
Orthogonal partial least squares–discriminant analysis (OPLS-DA), 212, 214

P

Partial least squares (PLS) regression, 72
Partial least squares–discriminant analysis (PLS-DA), 206, 212–213
PCA. *See* Principal component analysis (PCA)
Peroxisome proliferator-activated receptor gamma coactivator 1α (PGC-1α), 148
Personalised nutrition. *See* Metabotype
Principal component analysis (PCA), 8, 72, 138, 206–207, 209, 212–213, 214–215

R

Reversed-phase high-performance liquid chromatography (RP-HPLC), 220–221

S

San Antonio Family Heart study, 155–156
Self-modelling curve resolution (SMCR), 40
Single-ion monitoring (SIM), 70–71
Sodium dodecyl sulphate–polyacrylamide gel electrophoresis (SDS–PAGE), 221
Statistical data integration
metabolic phenotypes/metabotypes, 50
mQTL approach, 50
MWAS, 50
quantitative trait locus mapping, 50
sample types, 48–49
Subnetwork extraction algorithm
manual *vs.* automatic network analysis, 106–108, 107*f*
metabolic stories, 108
multi-omics analysis, 108
reaction paths, 105–106, 105*f*
Systems biology markup language (SBML), 93, 94*f*

T

Time-of-flight (ToF) mass analyser, 159
Triacylglycerols (TAGs) profiling, 155–156
Trimethylamine *N*-oxide (TMAO), 173
TriVersa NanoMate device, 67
TwinsUK and Health Ageing study, 156–158
Type 2 diabetes mellitus (T2DM), 156–158

U

Ultra high-pressure liquid chromatography (UPLC), 203
UniProt, 91

V

Very low-density lipoproteins (VLDL), 65

Lightning Source UK Ltd.
Milton Keynes UK
UKOW06n2346050615

252967UK00001B/5/P

9 781782 420842